Healthy Garden Healthy You

BY MILO SHAMMAS
Dr. Earth

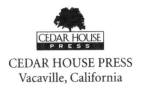

CEDAR HOUSE PRESS
Vacaville, California

Cedar House Press
P.O. Box 6804
Vacaville, California 95696
707-448-4678

Milo Shammas

Library of Congress Cataloging-in-Publication Data
Healthy Garden, Health You
Includes index.
Library of Congress Control Number: 2010929239
ISBN 978-1-4507-1729-851995

Printed in the United States of America
Walsworth Publishing Company
Marceline, Missouri 64658

Designed by Colortek
Book Jacket: Tom Zipp • Book Layout: Jody Goetz & Megan Webb
Set in Minion

Disclaimer of Liability
This book offers information and recommendations on the general relationships among food, human and animal health, and disease prevention. Some information is based on the author's personal and professional experiences. Additional information on the composition and contents of foods and the results of research on the health effects of various foods in one's diet come from sources the author and publisher believe to be reputable and accurate. However, each person has his or her unique biochemical makeup and health history. Whether the reader should use any fact, recommendation or inference in this book as a guide to his or her own health or the health of any other person is strictly a matter of personal choice and responsibility. Results may vary from one person to another. THIS BOOK IS NOT A SUBSTITUTE FOR QUALIFIED MEDICAL DIAGNOSIS AND TREATMENT. The author and publisher take no responsibility and cannot be held liable for the consequences to the reader of acting or failing to act on anything written here.

Healthy Garden
Healthy You

Contents

ooooo

· PART 1 ·
SOIL HEALTH

ooooo

• PART 2 •
PLANT HEALTH

ooooo

• PART 3 •
ANIMAL HEALTH

ooooo

• PART 4 •
HUMAN HEALTH

ooooo

• PART 5 •
GARDENING BASICS

ooooo

• PART 6 •
100 PLANTS YOU CAN GROW & EAT
FOR HEALTH AND WELL-BEING

ooooo

Dedication

{ *I dedicate this book to all the Shammas family, including the unborn generations that will contribute kindness, respect and dignity to humanity.* }

Acknowledgements

My father, Lou Nicholas Shammas has always believed in me and trusted my intuition. He was very strict with me when I was a child, always forcing me to study harder and achieve better grades. He drove into my mind that with a good education I could achieve anything. Later, he trusted my intuition to start the Dr. Earth Company at a young age when I knew nothing about manufacturing. He completely funded my dream, and, because of him, I live a very good life today. I met my wife Patricia because of my father's trust in me, and I lead a revolution in the organic movement because of him. He has had the greatest impact on my life, and I love him dearly.

My mother, Jeannette Shammas, introduced me to the garden. This book is possible because of her. She always gave me guidance when I needed it. When I was a child, we had a very special relationship. Unlike most mother-son relationships, we were good friends and still are. I love and respect everything she has done for our family and for me. My mother is the glue that keeps the family together. If everybody had a father and mother like mine, the world would be a better place.

My wife, Patricia Ann Williams-Shammas, is my best friend. She knows me and how difficult I am to live with. I especially appreciate her patience over the thousands of hours I spent writing a book that deprived us of our time together. She knows and accepts that I am a man with a purpose: to educate people on the healthy lifestyle. My purpose makes me happy, and that is the meaning of life.

Thank you, too, to my elder sister and brother, Rouba and Nicholas. They were great guidance counselors for me as a kid growing up. I am the youngest child, and whenever I needed direction my sister and brother were quick to offer it unselfishly. My brother is a meticulous architect. He always taught me to be the best at whatever I do. He used to say even a simple act like taking out the garbage had to be done to the best of my ability. "Adopt this philosophy and greatness awaits you." Those words he said to me when I was 10 years old have continued to help guide my life.

My lifelong friends have seen me morph into who I am today and supported my far-reaching ideas. I respect them all and list their names in alphabetical order to avoid offending any of them. (Also, I want to make sure at our next get together they do not tie my shoelaces together when I am not looking.) I thank Gerry Arteaga, Lorin Brady, Bobby Chambers, Steven Dunn, Shannon Fenady, Danny King, Peter Lupo and Jay Moh.

Three people influenced my business career and gave me unselfish guidance when I was a young businessman. Each helped to shape my life today. They are brilliant and deserve recognition: Tom Adikes, Dennis Kuga and Larry Simpson.

Tyler Kemper and Dennis Briskin worked diligently to help make this book accurate and thorough yet easy to read. Tyler Kemper is a brilliant young research scientist who spent hundreds of hours helping compile the details for Part 6 on how eating plants promotes human health, as well as other technical details that appear within my book. As an editor, Dennis added true word mastery, a keen eye for detail and devotion to high standards of clarity and economy of language.

Finally, to all my readers and everyone who cares for their family, gardens and the bio-diversity of our environment: Thank you! Have a purpose in your life, and you will be happy.

Forward

It is a real privilege and honor to write the forward to Healthy Garden, Healthy You. Milo Shammas, founder of Dr. Earth, writes in an easy-to-understand manner based on his years of gardening experience. Milo's vision for a healthy garden and environment helping to maximize human health is similar to mine. Dr. Earth's line of probiotic, organic fertilizers caught my attention some years ago. Whereas probiotic bacteria help keep the human gastrointestinal tract functioning in an optimum fashion, so do probiotic bacteria aid the plant kingdom in a similar fashion.

When reading Healthy Garden, Healthy You, it becomes obvious that the founder of Dr. Earth loves animals, the environment and people. This book will help the reader achieve a real interest in healthy gardening and healthy living. The synergy between human health, the environment and gardening (think stress reduction and physical activity) has been well documented in hundreds of scientific studies. If you do not have a yard, then buy some houseplants and enjoy their beauty and the fresh, clean air which they will help provide to your home.

Milo's vision is to see homegrown foods as a possible answer to some of the ills that plague our planet. Remember, you are only as healthy as the environment in which you live and work.

I have authored a number of books on health and beneficial lifestyle choices. Healthy Garden, Healthy You is a must read for every gardener and person who makes a decision to follow a lifestyle conducive to maximizing human, environmental and planetary health.

Steven G. Pratt MD, FACS, ABIHM
Scripps Memorial Hospital, La Jolla, California
author of *SuperFoods Rx, SuperFoods HealthStyle, The SuperFoods Rx Diet, SuperHealth*

Introduction

∞∞∞

HUMAN HEALTH STARTS IN THE SOIL

{
He who owns land possesses the greatest potential to live the longest life, for he has the ability to grow his own food and determine the ultimate control of his health, thus, his destiny.
-Milo
}

What is vital for life? Your health. The future of your health is imminent. To live a long life full of joy and vitality, your lifestyle choices today determine the state of your health tomorrow. This is true, whether we think about those choices or let ignorance and apathy make them for us.

The great news is you control your own destiny, because you control every decision in your life. Healthy eating and living are personal life choices. In your own backyard you can find the potential to create a future of good health for yourself, your family and the entire planet. This is the start of your journey to a better life.

To create an environment that nurtures you and provides you with enjoyment and health, you need a detailed plan similar to a road map. My mission is to help you plan and take this wondrous journey.

Being healthy is simple if you understand how to garden in your own backyard. Growing your own healthy food right outside your door will make you look at your home in a new, wonderful way. With so much excitement running through your veins, your enthusiasm may push you to act too soon. Before you grab a piece of paper, scribble many ideas, run down to your local plant nursery, and buy as many seeds, plants, soils and fertilizers as you can load up, let me guide you from my 20 years of experience and leadership in gardening. I want to teach you what I know that is true and effective.

Let's Get Dirty First!

Some people think of soil as nothing more than an anchor that holds plants in the ground, a dark, dusty place that critters crawl in that makes our hands dirty. Soil is not just "dirt" but the basis of all life. Healthy soil is alive with billions of microbes that feed all living things on our planet. Your body needs it to be healthy. It provides you with the sustenance you need to generate the energy for everything you do. Everyone who is alive today and everyone who ever lived, needed the benefits of soil to survive and prosper.

Soil health is the fundamental basis for the health of all plants, animals and people. This book shows you the link between soil and human health. The connection is simple: Healthy soil creates a healthy garden, which produces healthy plants to provide nutrients for us, for the animals we love and care for as pets, as well as the plants we consume as food.

Why should you grow a vegetable garden? Food is so cheap and easily accessible if you live in a modernized country. Much of what we can buy is more convenient to prepare than cooking garden produce from scratch. I can run down to a fast food drive-through and grab a value meal (for about $5) that is 2,500 calories of deep fried, grease-laden, processed food. You can get your fill of genetically modified, processed meat and potatoes for far less than one-tenth of a penny per calorie.

Maybe you do not care if that hamburger came from a cow fed with genetically modified grains and was shipped 2,500 miles to get to you. Maybe you believe it makes no difference if your fries are processed and grown with genetically modified potatoes. Your 32-ounce soda was full of simple sugars that went down smoothly with those salty fries.

Is a bargain meal a bargain if you pay for it with your health?

Why you should garden: It's good for your health. Besides giving you the best nutrients you can get, gardening is healthy work. You have to cultivate the soil, amend it, plant seeds or cuttings, fertilize, water, weed and mulch. Finally, you must harvest and preserve your crop for future use. Is eating healthy from your own garden worth all that effort? Yes!

If you read this book with an open mind and the attitude of caring about your health, the health of others and the well-being of our only home—the good earth itself—it will open your eyes to the importance of creating your healthy backyard garden. You will learn why eating food you nurture and harvest yourself is one of the most rewarding things you can do.

This book is also unique in taking the approach of starting from the ground up, explaining how human health begins in the soil, then providing clear examples of what to grow, how to grow it, and the nutritional benefits to you and your family, your friends and your community.

I know thousands of gardeners and have interviewed hundreds of them over the past 20 years. I have also met with many medical doctors, soil scientists, plant biologists, nutritionists and master gardeners. All this involvement and research has more than convinced me that a healthy garden will give you joy and bounty.

I live the organic lifestyle, and it all starts in my backyard. Even the smallest thing you do will make a huge difference toward living a long and healthy life and raising a healthy family. A garden can help you to achieve these goals.

Americans are on a new journey, seeking natural and organic solutions to their health problems. People from all backgrounds are on a personal quest to be healthy while making the right environmental decisions in the process.

I hope this book will inspire you and benefit you in the same way.

PART 1

SOIL HEALTH

Chapter 1

ooooo

YOU ARE WHAT YOU EAT. THE GIFT OF HEALTH

{
Forget not that the earth delights to feel your bare feet and the winds long to play with your hair.
-Kahlil Gibran
}

Every fiber that makes up the human body was once a biological or elemental part of the soil, air and water. We have heard the saying from the Bible, "Earth to earth, ashes to ashes, dust to dust." We come from the earth. We live off the earth. We return to the earth. The food we eat is inextricably linked to soil particles that existed millions of years ago. What you eat today is part of a food chain that was here before our species walked the earth.

Eating can be such an arbitrary act, simply a way to fill your stomach. Or you can eat consciously, with awareness, and insist that everything you allow into your body must be healthy and pure. When you intentionally choose healthy food, eating becomes more than a practical action to sustain your physical body. It becomes a lifestyle, a way of being in the world, an expression of your desire and choice to live longer and healthier. The only one way you can have ultimate control of that decision is to nurture the soil and then grow your own food in that soil. This is the basis of healthy living.

The large corporations that control most of our food supply and our farmland are set up to produce large quantities of food while making huge commercial profits. Sadly for the health of our nation, the quality of that food has been left far behind. And the quality of the food we eat, its ability to nourish us and sustain our health, rests simply on the quality of our soil.

The health and balance of our ecosystem also depends on the vitality of our soil. (Notice that word vitality. My dictionary defines it as "of or manifesting life." It comes from the Latin word vita, which means "life.") "Vital soil" has life in it and gives life to everything that grows in it.

Humans and animals depend on the health of the soil. Along with the other ancient elements (air, water and fire), earth-soil is the main thing supplying our plants with the sustenance they need to properly develop into naturally thriving, insect-resistant, nutrient-packed produce. When we eat a piece of a living plant that came out of living soil, our body draws out the life from it (nutrients) we need to stay alive. Looking at this life process in reverse, we stay alive by extracting the life from living plants that depend on "lively" soil.

As part of the movement to gain more life and health from our food, many people over the past 15 to 20 years have tried to buy or grow organic food. Organic has finally become mainstream. We see the number of organic goods multiply in stores, ranging from foods and clothing to household items and cosmetics. It's cool to be organic!

Many high-profile celebrities and activists support this movement. They have fostered a more positive image through their association with green goods. For many large companies, the term organic is part of successful marketing strategies. Malcomb Cork, president of Commerce Corporation, has said, "We are witnessing a national movement. Green goods are on Main Street, and they are here to stay." Tom Medhurst, President of L&L Nursery Supply, told me recently, "Just 10 years ago, you really had to convince many nurseries that organic products are the future. Today, we have to make sure we are constantly in stock."

Commercial agriculture supplies our grocery stores with all the produce we can imagine, organic or not. Some is grown locally, some on the other side of the nation, or even imported from other continents. The National Sustainable Agriculture Coalition says that much of our produce travels 1,500 to 2,500 miles to arrive at our tables. Aggressive marketing and efficient transportation networks enable us to eat fruits and vegetables from all over the world all year round. (If you're willing to pay the price, you can eat summer fruit from the Southern Hemisphere in the dead of winter in the frozen North.)

If you want to eat organic food, do you need to care about certification? A careful consumer may ask, "What gives a farming operation the ability to say they're organic? How does that change the treatment of their food? Does it matter if it is organic as long as it is healthy and does not contain chemical residues?"

What makes gardening for personal use organic is somewhat ambiguous for those of us growing our own produce. In essence, there are no policies or rules for home gardeners. We have no manual to follow. Our instinctive compass must guide us. If what we grow seems healthy and good enough for our bodies, we are generally free to grow it. Home growers have freedom of action but need to understand what they are doing and the probable consequences. Many prospective organic gardeners agree on the need to avoid synthetic pesticides, fertilizers, herbicides and genetically modified organisms. Beyond those popular conventions, we find a variety of gardening strategies. Some people take it to the extreme, believing that to be organic, a plant must not receive any type of nutritive treatment other than what is naturally found at hand. Others, slightly more involved, treat the soil and feed the foliage only certified organic materials.

For your growing and mine, this is not needed. If you use your neighbor's leaf litter as compost and are positive they don't apply any chemicals to their soil or plants, you don't need to worry about the quality of the leaf litter. Certification is more important to commercial growers who must prove they are growing by accepted public standards or a set of rules in order to truthfully label their produce organic. For the home gardener, certified is a useless term.

However, if you do not understand the techniques of organic practices, you cannot claim to know the effect your plants have on people, pets, children, health or the surrounding environment. Before you assert, "Organic is good," you should understand how and why. Otherwise, you may easily fall into the trap of believing, and paying to consume, someone's deceitful marketing scheme.

Organic gardening, growing and farming are all highly beneficial. The benefits, however, depend on the organic methods you use. Many who practice organic growing techniques want to conserve the beautiful biological diversity on our planet, while giving people and animals the resources they need to enjoy a comfortable, healthy life. However, some organic practices (discussed later) are not necessarily beneficial to people, animals or the environment. Saying "Natural is good" is too simple, as are claims that synthetic pesticide or weed control is good. We must understand the effects of our treatments before using them, so that we can properly apply them to gain the benefits while avoiding their adverse effects.

Whether planning quaint home gardening projects or large plantations, we must focus our energy on nurturing the soil, which serves as the basis for healthy sustainable growth. Look deeply into your particular situation to understand how and why the practices you choose meet your needs while protecting yourself and your soil.

I grow as much of my own food as I can. The rest I buy from my local farmers market and a good local produce market that stocks organic produce. Only when I buy produce from a market that the word certified matters to me. I know what I do in my backyard is healthy and pure. This is why it is so important to grow your own just as humans first did long ago.

Chapter 2

THE HISTORY OF FARMING & TODAY'S SOIL QUALITY

{
...the hills and groves were God's first temples, and the more they are cut down and hewn into cathedrals and churches, the farther off and dimmer seems the Lord himself.
- John Muir
}

To understand where we are, we need to know where we were and how we got here. The development of agriculture stands as one of the most important advances of early civilization. Without this innovation, who knows if we would still be alive on earth?

Let's look at a brief history of how people learned to grow their own food in places they deemed fitting. Following that, we will look at modern concerns and examine successful and well-respected methods to help maximize our health potential and that of our ecosystem.

Archeologists believe the earliest forms of agriculture date from around 10,000 B.C. Evidence of early agriculture was found in an area of the Near East known as Mesopotamia, a crescent-shaped region encompassing what is now Lebanon and Israel, curving up and around Iraq and Jordan, ending in southern Iran. (The name Mesopotamia, Greek in origin, means "the land between the rivers." The Tigris and Euphrates rivers that split this region also contain mountains and flatlands.) About 12,000 years ago, nomadic groups of hunter-gatherers settled in this area because of the abundant wild barley and wheat they found growing there. Although it is more arid now, ancient Mesopotamia had an unlimited water supply. These favorable conditions enabled many plants to thrive.

As people learned to plant, cultivate and harvest food, their thought processes, interactions, even their biology, changed. No longer needing to wander over large areas to find food, humans settled down to produce their food themselves, soon developing villages with a surplus of crops growing nearby. Now they could use their time, and physical and mental energy, on other activities and needs. As they farmed and developed not only a surplus of food but specialized labor, they also learned to trade, first among themselves and eventually with other developing societies. Human populations multiplied exponentially and brought many new challenges. These changes required new ways of thinking.

Early farmers must have relished their life of plentiful food, work and new commodities to trade. Yet, just as humans sometimes still resist change, those accustomed to hunting and gathering may have been disturbed to see land cleared for cultivation. Those first farmers could not have imagined how agriculture would spread widely thanks to irrigation and new technologies.

As farming spread and people adopted agriculture worldwide, they faced unforeseen consequences. Problems such as lack of sanitation, the spread of disease and pollution required regulation and more structured, uniform practices. Early farmers also created laws to govern human activity so that people could live close together in large numbers.

Soon, human tribes and settlements began to alter the balance of nature. They weeded out undesirable plants that robbed nutrients from the soil and threatened the harvests. They separated domesticated animals and crops. Early irrigation methods diverted waterways. They also learned to clear trees from the land for space and additional sunlight. As agriculture spread, it became the major source of food for most people. Now well fed, people multiplied, which further increased the demand for food.

Until well into the 20th Century, wherever capitalism allowed individuals to own private property, such as the U.S., most food came from small farms run by individual families. Once Industrialization and labor saving machinery became common, family farms could not compete with large corporate farms run as big businesses in search of big profits. Production large enough to meet demand became the goal and the new standard. Because agro-businesses could deliver larger crops, faster and at lower prices, over a short time more than four million privately owned farms were lost due to competitive pressures. Since World War II, the percentage of the U.S. population living and working on farms has shrunk dramatically. In 1960, for example, one American farmer fed 25 people. Fifty years later, one farmer feeds 129 people. *(Source: National Cattlemen's Beef Association.)*

Part of the profit picture had to do with replacing farm workers, who manually tended and harvested the crops, with machinery. New technologies were developed to increase yields, including using chemical fertilizers, herbicides, pesticides, and recently, genetically modified seeds and crops. The health and vital quality of commercially produced crops has suffered. As each decade passes, such crops contain decreasing concentrations of essential vitamins, minerals and micronutrients. Moreover, as soils became depleted, the plants need extra help in the form of fertilizers. What was once a largely natural process of growing food has become more and more unnatural.

One lesson we gain from the history of farming from ancient times to the present: Organic methods are the best. They are simple and pure and leave the soil rich and capable of supporting crops year after year. All farmers practiced organic methods until about 60 years ago, when food production became dominated by large-scale corporate farms run as "food factories." Now, slowly but progressively, we are returning to what mankind began doing about 12,000 years ago. Growing our own food in our own backyards takes us back in time and gives us ultimate control over our food, our health and our quality of life.

Chapter 3

ooooo

GET TO KNOW YOUR SOIL

{

We should take care not to make the intellect our god; it has, of course, powerful muscles, but no personality.

-Albert Einstein

}

If you pause to contemplate your garden or the plant life around you, you may wonder:

- What makes plants so large?
- What makes them healthy?
- What causes plants of a species to develop differently from each other?
- What keeps causing plants to wilt right away?
- How do you get a "green thumb"?
- How do you give plants the best chance at healthy development?
- What determines the health of plants?

While the science to answer these questions can be quite complex, it is easy to understand in general terms. In their natural environment, plants rely on environmental conditions, their genetics and a healthy soil foundation to spread their roots. Location (mountains, valleys, river banks) weather and air quality shape environmental conditions. Each plant needs a proper balance (specific to its species) of sunlight, hydration and nutrients such as carbon dioxide and nitrogen from the air or soil. Exposure to wind, rain and other living organisms also help determine a plant's life course. Any factor out of proper balance in "the equation of life" (too much, too little or at the wrong time) can lead to a plant's demise. Genetics also help determine whether a plant can survive, especially those that mature in extreme environments with high competition for nutrients.

Home gardeners who want maximum plant growth potential cannot control environmental factors nor plant genetics. Especially for organic growers, controlling the genetics of each seed is not an option. By using greenhouse growing to shelter plants from unsuitable environments, we have created pseudo environments. Because so many factors affect plant development, we cannot completely control our results. For these and other reasons, our strongest power to influence the health of plants is to control the health of the soil. If you want your plants to grow tall and be nutrient rich and resistant to pests, you must have healthy, balanced soil.

The interaction between plants and soils, sometimes over an entire life course, has received a lot of research attention during the past century. Among the important findings: When we control the health of the soil, we influence plant health in many ways. Scientists also agree that the best, most fertile soils have great consistency and structure for root extension, water retention and an abundance of organisms living in symbiosis with plants.

With regard to your own garden, consider your soil as a given that you learn to deal with. Since you cannot completely dig it out and replace it, you must get to know its nature and characteristics, and modify it as best you can to cultivate it successfully. Among the important soil qualities are:
- Texture
- Composition (heavy clay or light sand, for example)
- pH (the acid-alkaline spectrum)

With this information, you can intelligently choose the most suitable plant material for your environment. These factors also determine the best ways to modify your soil (adding amendments and nutrients) to gain the full potential for a healthy garden.

Living organisms are the bridge that connects nutrients stored in the soil to plant growth. Organisms ranging from bacteria, fungi to earthworms and insects perform a wide variety of tasks that create a regulated balance of nutrients. Soil organisms vary in size from microscopic up to small mammals like moles, groundhogs and mice. On the microscopic level, healthy topsoil contains billions of living organisms growing, reproducing and dying in each gram of soil. These species are crucially important to all life on earth, for they recycle nearly 100 percent of organic waste. They are able to provide nutrients in a form usable by plants through their digestive enzymes, changing complex molecules into a simpler form and making them bioavailable for plant root absorption. These invisible helpers serve as vehicles to transport stores of nutrients in the soil to plants, then to animals and ultimately to us.

Soil organisms play many different roles in the soil ecosystem. All living things must die and eventually decompose. Because animals and humans eat plant materials grown in the soil, organic waste must be broken down and recycled back into the soil to nourish future generations of plants. This waste may consist of animal or plant materials or both. Decomposers break down this organic matter to feed our plants, which feed our animals, both the ones we call our pets and the ones we eat for our health. They complete the cycle of living and prevent the build up of wastes. (Imagine not having the decomposers. Nothing would break down. Animals and plants that died millions of years ago would rest under mountains of waste. If dinosaurs were still on the side of the road, nutrients would never make their way back into the soil. We would run out of plant nutrients and all life would stop.)

This is why "living soil" is so crucial. The decomposers, (under attack by commercial farming practices) create a healthy balance of nutrients available in the soil to perpetuate life as we know it.

Briefly, here are some major contributors to the soil and its life.

Bacteria make up an enormous portion of living matter in the soil, weighing more than a ton per acre. In each gram of fertile soil, we can find about one million different species of bacteria just on the surface. Bacteria also exist far below the surface, more than a mile down. But they are most active around the root depth of plants, known as the rhizosphere. These hard workers are decomposers and recyclers. Some are responsible for decomposing naturally occurring organic matter such as dead cells released by roots or other organic plant and animal remains. Through their metabolism, they release carbon dioxide and other crucial nutrients supporting plant and animal life.

Other types of bacteria provide plants the essential nutrients they need to survive by transforming inorganic matter into forms plants can use. These organisms need carbon dioxide to function. Bacteria also provide plants essential nitrogen through a process called "nitrogen fixation." The Rhizobia bacteria, for example, are symbiotic with the legume family of plants, which includes more than 18,000 different species. They convert atmospheric nitrogen (which makes up 79 percent of our air) from its gaseous form to a water-soluble form that plants can take up through their roots. Nitrogen then becomes available to plants. Through both types of functions, bacteria are essential to plant nutrition.

Actinomycetes are decomposers and recyclers. They break down organic matter and convert gaseous nitrogen from the atmosphere into soluble particles for plants to feed on. The nitrogen fixers have little filaments that invade or grow into root hairs and form small aggregates there. Actinomycetes are most popular as a source of antibiotics. Even at microscopic levels, we find a system of checks and balances. They help keep bacterial populations from growing out of control and throwing off the delicate balance of nutrient cycling to benefit plants. Around the time scientists observed the relationship between actinomycetes and plant health, they also discovered antibiotics like penicillin to fight bacterial diseases..

Fungi decompose fallen leaves on forest floors and in our back yards and digest dead plant and animal remains. Fungi come in many different species with a plethora of functions. Some fungi work to degrade organic matter in sequence, from tough fibrous matter down to soft simple matter that produces nutrients in the soil usable by existing plants and animals. Other species form mutual relationships with plants and protect them by consuming nematodes or other bugs before they eat plant roots.

The fungus that is perhaps the most directly beneficial to plant life is known as mycorrhizae, which forms a symbiotic relationship with roots. Two types exist, endo-mycorrhizae and ecto-mycorrhizae. The endo- version embeds some of its arms within plant roots. The ecto- version attaches to the outside of the roots. In both cases, the fungi extend their arms (hyphae/filaments) out into the soil to increase the reach of the roots wider and deeper. These mycorrhizae webs allow entire populations of plants to share nutrients. *(See Chapter 6 for more detail on mycorrhizae.)*

Algae contribute much organic matter to the soil. In some species, such as blue green algae, they fix nitrogen from air, helping prevent the depletion of the critical nutrient for plant growth. The organic matter composed of algae helps improve soil structure by assisting soil particles stick loosely together, which in turn enhances water retention and decreases erosion. They are also food for other bugs living in the soil. In some cases, they form alliances with fungi, giving them sustenance that strengthens their ability to absorb even trace nutrients from the soil for plants to consume. Common lichen are an example of this alliance.

Nematodes, pot worms and earthworms decompose organic matter into humus and secrete a sticky substance that helps the soil form nice cake-like aggregates. These creatures exist in the highest numbers on or near grassland, prairies and pastures. They feed on plant debris as well as some bacteria or actinomycetes that share the same topsoil. Some nematodes will feast on insects within the soil. As a result, some gardeners use nematodes as a natural form of pest control. In turn, some bigger bugs and even mycorrhizal fungi feast on nematodes.

Earthworms are larger than the other two types. They travel through the soil by burrowing, eating minerals and organic matter as they go. As they do, they minutely perforate and loosen the soil, producing a similar effect as machine tillers. Throughout digestion, the matter consumed is mixed and many unusable minerals are transformed for plants to consume later. In addition, the remains of an earthworm, commonly referred to as "castings," are much higher in nitrogen, phosphorus, potassium, calcium, trace minerals and beneficial bacteria than the surrounding soil. By these processes, earthworms create more nutrient-rich, fertile soils with a pH close to neutral. Having many earthworms in your yard is a good sign that you have good soil.

Mites and spring tails decompose many types of organic substances in the soil. They are known as arthropods, which have characteristic exoskeletons and jointed legs. They are the most abundant soil dwellers. Of the arthropods, mites and springtails are the most vital source in the creation of humus, breaking down everything from nematodes and pot worms to fungus and leaf litter. Their main job is to break down leaf litter and other relatively large remains into smaller pieces so microbes can continue the nutrient cycling.

These are only a few of the billions of organisms in or around our gardens that have been evolving for millions of years. Growing methods that clear the soil of these organisms undermine the goal of producing healthy food through healthy soil. Agricultural practices that disrupt the bio-diversity of organisms responsible for sustaining growth of all types of plants throughout the world seem like a recipe for disaster.

The soil is a living, breathing, unique and dynamic force. Soil management practices of giant agribusiness are inefficient and inferior. Their focus is directed to large-scale, single-crop growth and "miracle" results by applying broad-spectrum chemical fertilizers. Many modern practices ignore the need for complex and highly diversified soil enrichment. Instead, they use the continuous applications of three water-soluble fertilizers: nitrogen, phosphorous and potassium (N-P-K). This practice compromises the biological health of soils, leading to poor plant health and ultimately poor human health.

The amount of nitrogen fixed for plants by rhizobia bacteria, actinomycetes and green algae is double the amount of applied nitrogen in commercial fertilizers. Starting in our backyard, we can begin to change this trend by supporting the organisms that provide our plants with the sustenance they need to give us the nutrients and vitamins we need for our health.

Chapter 4

ooooo

MAXIMUM SOIL HEALTH

{
We know more about the movement of celestial bodies than about the soil underfoot.

-Leonardo da Vinci
}

You may think of soil as little more than an anchor to hold plants in place. That's like thinking the ocean is nothing more than a liquid to float ships on. The soil itself is like an ocean filled with life and needing regular feeding.

As an organic gardener concerned with being healthy and living on a healthy planet, you must understand the difference between feeding the soil and feeding plants. Organic fertilizers and synthetic fertilizers work in fundamentally different ways. Organic fertilizers feed the living microorganisms in the soil. Synthetic fertilizers feed plant roots directly. You might ask, what is the difference as long as my plants grow? The difference is a short-term result that looks good for a while (synthetic chemicals), as opposed to the lasting benefits of improved soil health, plant health, and in the case of edibles, even your own health (from organics).

When you feed the soil with organic fertilizers, you build nutrient reserves. Plant roots can regularly tap into these reserves. This approach builds soil structure and makes it more porous, encouraging roots to expand into the rhizosphere. Using organic fertilizers also suppresses disease, creates biological diversity, supports a neutral pH, forms humus and adds minerals and micronutrients to a living soil.

Chemical fertilizers feed plants directly while ignoring the soil. Plants can grow this way, because the growth factors in chemical fertilizers are in a form that plants can absorb immediately. While this sounds attractive, it adds nothing beneficial to the soil. In fact, repeated use of chemicals over time can actually deplete the soil.

Organic fertilizers and amendments feed the soil that feeds your plants, slow and steady as Mother Nature intended. Because organic fertilizers and amendments are pure, natural ingredients, beneficial microbes in the soil digest them as a food source. Then the microbes convert the organics into a simpler form that plant roots can absorb as needed.

By contrast, chemical fertilizers leach through the soil, contaminate the water table and waste nutrients. The notion that plants will look good and be healthy if we add the right mix of chemical salts of nitrogen, phosphorus and potassium to the soil, is yesterday's view.

Do not be misled by the giant agribusiness scientific community that touts "miracle" results by using advanced blue liquid potions. The corporate agricultural industry has a large financial interest in selling water-soluble blue potions that have high dollar profit margins. Because of this, I have become quite pessimistic about governmental agencies and universities that receive research funding from giant agribusinesses ever focusing on the vital concept of nurturing the soil.

Expanded awareness leading to changes in widespread practices will have to come from people like us who care about our family's health and what we put into our bodies. It is up to us in the organic community, including amateur gardeners, to lead the way in discovering (or rediscovering) methods to nurture and protect the soil.

Everyone wants good looking, healthy plants, but many prefer, organic, sustainable ways to reach those goals. Organic gardeners provide plants with the nutrients they need for maximum health potential through the addition of organic fertilizers, soils, kelp meal and fish bone meal. They use non-toxic insect controls. Marketers have claimed chemistry creates a better life. However, our greatest opportunity for a better life, through better soil health, is to leave chemistry behind and move toward biology instead.

The soil is alive. Instead of just adding a particular chemical needed by plants, our soil treatment should support and nurture a diverse web of soil life, as complex and well organized as an ocean ecosystem. By doing so, we nurture our own web of life on earth.

Chapter 5

SOIL MICROBES (PROBIOTICS)

{

The capacity to blunder slightly is the real marvel of DNA.
Without this special attribute, we would still be anaerobic bacteria
and there would be no music.

-Lewis Thomas

}

Soil is alive! In the beginning there was life, and life was in the soil. Understanding the life in the soil is as important for a gardener as digging in the soil. In addition to parent rocks and minerals, complex webs of microorganisms interact to perpetuate life for each other as well as plants and any subsequent consumers in the food chain. The great digesters of the earth, invisible to the naked eye, constantly break down organic material into a more usable form that plant roots can identify, absorb and incorporate for new growth. Below our feet lie the wonders of a variety of living organisms hard at work converting complex organic compounds such as tannins, lignins, proteins, carbohydrates, cellulose and pectin into simpler, more usable forms plants can absorb for growth. Nutrient compounds must be broken down. All organic materials must be digested through microbial digestive enzymes for nutrients to be available to the plant roots. Without microbes, organic nutrients would simply sit in the soil and add nothing to plants.

Soil microbes also help physically change the soil structure. They bind soil particles to better facilitate water and air infiltration. Different microbes perform different tasks. Besides producing enzymes that simplify the molecular structure of complex organic compounds, microbes release "humic glues" that bind organic soil particles to mineral soil particles and help to stabilize it all. They create semi-stable soil aggregates, in lay terms, the soil every gardener dreams of: easy to work with, dark in color, teeming with a wide variety of biological life and giving off that wonderful, distinctive earthy smell.

Probiotics

The microbes are on the pathogen patrol to clean up our soils. They produce antibiotics to suppress fungal pathogens. Fungus can be a good friend or a troublesome enemy. Beneficial mycorrhizal fungi are one of our best friends for the health and success of our plants. They are able to succeed in the garden under all kinds of growing conditions. Conversely, some of our worst enemies in the garden are harmful pathogenic fungi such as pythium and rhizoctonia (damping-off), thielaniopsis (black root rot) and root rot and wilt organisms such as fusarium and phytophthora. Healthy plants can fall victim to the devastating effects of pathogenic fungi that can quickly destroy an entire garden. Conventional approaches to fungus control rely on fungicide drenches and soil fumigants. Yet, for millions of years we have had natural control of harmful fungus through a process called "general suppression." Probiotics suppress disease by releasing antibiotic compounds such as phenols and penicillin. They also proliferate bacterial and fungal microflora that suppress pathogens through antagonism, competition, predation and induced resistance.

General suppression naturally controls pathogens without the human interference of harsh chemicals. Healthy soil is full of beneficial bacteria and mycorrhizal fungi. Pathogenic fungus flourish in damp, wet conditions where they do not have to compete with other organisms. Pathogens rarely take over a healthy soil, which has a balanced mix of organic components. These hold many beneficial microbes to suppress fungal pathogens naturally without harming plants, people or pets.

Healthy soils properly inoculated with probiotics can fight off pathogens that harm plants. Productive soil promotes plants survival so that pathogens will not multiply in great numbers. Beneficial microbes fill up the available spaces in the soil so that pathogens cannot become established. Think of a parking lot at the supermarket. If every parking space is occupied, there is no space to park another car. Similarly, if all the available space in the soil is full of beneficial microbes, there is no room for destructive pathogens. When you create an environment rich in beneficial microbes, fungal diseases do not have a chance to become established. Probiotics naturally kill and control fungal pathogens, keeping your soil and plants healthy throughout the year.

Healthy soil should contain no less than 10 million bacteria per gram. As plants grow, they require more nutrients, as do microbes in the soil. As the weather warms, both plants and microbes respond at a similar rate. This self-regulating cycle is an established natural process. As microbes become more active in warm weather in the soil, they digest organic materials and convert them for plants to absorb. As the weather cools, both plants and microbes require less nutrition. Since fewer nutrients are being released in the soil, the soil builds food reserves in cooler weather.

The particular contents and physical characteristics of soil depend on its native rock source, shape of the land, climate, native vegetation, environmental history and how long the native rocks were subjected to weathering. Around the globe, infinite combinations of these features produce different ecological systems. Where you live affects how well your garden will grow. Even in a favorable growing area, local activities may affect your gardening experience. For example, if you bought a house in a beautiful new development where soil has been disturbed or layers removed during construction you probably have poor soil. Often such soil is lifeless and consists of heavy, compacted mineral soils that are intended to support the weight of a house. (You can't build a stable, 50-ton building on soft, well aerated soil.) If you live in the middle of a city, similar to where I grew up in Los Angeles, you will need to invest time in building the soil with organic amendments to restore good physical properties and biological diversity.

To know how to develop healthy plants while preserving the diversity and balance of an ecosystem, we must first understand the soil system. While we still have much to learn about the deep interactions between the soil and plants, research has come far enough to understand the basic components and functions of the living communities beneath our feet. Despite the wide variation in the complexity of each soil system, from an arid desert to the Amazon jungle, most have one major thing in common. On top of broken down rocks, they all contain living and dead organic matter.

Microbes are essential to the health of all productive soils. Increasing biological activity and building up existing bacterial populations in the soil make your plants and garden resistant to diseases, frost and insects while adding maximum growth and health potential. Your soil is alive; don't treat it like dirt! Learn to work with and nurture the natural bio-diversity of your soil.

Chapter 6

∞∞∞

MYCORRHIZAE: THE GOOD FUNGUS

{
Life preys upon life. This is biology's most fundamental fact.
-Martin H. Fischer
}

It would take an entire book to do justice to mycorrhizal fungi. This chapter explains what they are and why they are important.

The word "mycorrhizae" derives from the Greek words mykes meaning fungus and rhiza meaning root.

Imagine a giant underground network, a transportation system, complex by nature yet simple in concept. In the network, all established plants grow in harmony together, sharing nutrients with each other, the plant on the east side of your house sharing nutrients with Bob's tree across the street. How can this be? Mycorrhizae make it possible. The largest biomass on earth is a network of mycorrhizal hyphae in a mature established forest. It is invisible to the human eye and much smaller than any obvious root system. These threads of life share the nutrients with each other. The tall evergreen tree provides nutrients to the small fern growing at its base through mycorrhizae. The giant flowering tree on the west side of your yard provides nutrients to your tomato plants on the east side of the garden through mycorrhizae. The essence of mycorrhizae's role is to create an extensive network of microscopic filaments that facilitates nutrient transfer among plants. Mycorrhizae help absorb nutrients, assist in drought tolerance and create ideal garden soil structure, soil that drains, breaths and retains optimum moisture. The near perfect "coffee-grounds" soil texture we often find in fastidiously maintained organic gardens comes from long-term mycorrhizal soil activity.

Using a biologically active soil or fertilizer to introduce mycorrhizae to your garden makes a huge difference in the health and performance of all the plants.

This is why healthy soils are teeming with mycorrhizae. On the evolutionary scale, they are as important to the health of all plants as plants are important to us.

The Bridge for Life

Mycorrhizae were the bridge for plants millions of years ago when they first made the transition from water to land, scientists believe. The earth was a harsh environment with little nutrients available to plants. The earth was salty, the sun was hot and soils were void of biological activity, creating a rocky, harsh environment for plants. Dr. Mike Amaranthus, a friend and colleague, is a leading world expert on mycorrhizae. He says, "It is believed mycorrhizae are one of the primary reasons plants were able to survive the drastic transition from the nutrient-rich oceans to this harsh, nutrient-poor soil environment."

If hearty mycorrhizae gathered nutrients from the soil for plants during this harsh transitional period, imagine what they can do for your backyard plants today. Here is how mycorrhizae contribute and why they are needed.

Mycorrhizae are beneficial soil fungi that form a symbiotic relationship with your backyard plants and about 90 percent of all plants on earth. They penetrate growing plant root tissues, surround the root mass and extend far into the surrounding soil, encompassing a much greater volume of soil than that occupied by the plant's own root system. The fungi's long thread-like mycelia capture moisture and nutrients from the soil, particularly nitrogen and phosphorous. The fungi consume these nutrients, but, more importantly, they generously share them with the roots of the host plant. In return, the host plant provides the fungi with photosynthesized nutrients such as the simple sugars (sucrose, fructose and glucose) to keep them energized and viable.

Mycorrhizae are also important soil-binding agents, which adds to friable soil texture. Countless long filaments called hyphae tend to accumulate in the soil over a period, persisting for months or even years. Hyphae filaments tend to hold together larger soil particles, particularly the sand-sized fraction. The filaments tend to have sticky surfaces from sugars processed and exuded by the mycorrhizae. Also, the tips of developing root hairs secrete a similarly sticky, plant-produced substance. Together, these sticky materials enable the hyphae to strongly adhere to soil particles, physically binding and enmeshing them together to form better soil for growing. This condition increases in the root zone, encouraging further root growth, which in turn attracts more mycorrhizae, leading to a more stabilizing aggregation of soil particles. The cycle repeats and supports the creation of desirable soil for gardeners.

Chapter 7

∞∞∞

SOIL MINERALS: FOOD FOR STRONG PLANTS, ANIMALS & PEOPLE

{

Suburbia is where the developer bulldozes out the trees, then names the streets after them.

-Bill Vaughn

}

Minerals make up about 90 percent of garden soil. Unless we dig up an entire garden and import new soil, (and we don't want to do that), mineral soil particles are important for holding onto many plant nutrients. Creating a desirable soil structure enables plant roots to absorb these nutrients. With proper attention to the soil, you can build a viable, productive, nutrient-rich environment for growth.

Geologic forces move slowly to build perfect soil like that found in a tropical forest. It takes tens of thousands of years for rocks to wear down into small particles of sand, silt and clay small enough to be valuable to garden soil. Large rocks cannot hold onto plant nutrients. If you were blessed to inherit grandma's fastidiously maintained garden, you may know she spent a lifetime working to cultivate and maintain a good soil structure. That is what it took her to make it perfect, adding compost, removing large chunks of rocks, weeding, constantly turning the soil and adding amendments three times a year. Dedication to the garden requires dedication to the soil.

Getting down to the rocks and minerals of the soil, the texture can range from sand, silt, clay to peat. Each of these forms may vary in texture, structure, aggregation and water retention ability. Also, to be productive a soil must allow air to reach the roots and also retain water without becoming waterlogged. Taken together, these characteristics are known as a soil's tilth. Great tilth equals a high fertility potential.

The variety of rock structures and environments around the world create thousands of varieties of soil. The ground-down particles of rock form the underlying basis of the soil, sand, silt, clay or, the ideal, loam. All of these contain organic elements from the decomposed remains of plants and animals.

On the farmland of a country like the United States, which has been cultivated for hundreds of years, the soil includes the underlying geological strata plus the products of years of farming. This, too, leaves us with highly variable soils. Clays, sands and loams all give color and texture to the patchwork of fields once typical of the countryside.

Rich, dark soils are particularly good at supporting crops such as vegetables and grasses. The dead organic remains from previous crops retain moisture, feed biological life and ensure good soil structure. Other edible crops prefer lighter, more freely draining soils with higher levels of mineral nutrients. The good news is you can always improve the structure of your soil by amending it with the appropriate materials to achieve the desired structure for the plants you are growing.

In our gardens, soils are even more varied than those under the plow on farms. Most soils can support a colorful range of healthy plants. Even those from the most remote or exotic parts of the world seem to find an agreeable climate somewhere in our gardens. However, in order to grow a wide range of healthy plants, you need to know what your soil is composed of, and if necessary, how to improve it.

Chapter 8

ooooo

SOIL STRUCTURE

{
We cannot always build the future for our youth, but we can build our youth for the future.

-Franklin Delano Roosevelt
}

To the naked eye, soils look pretty much the same except sandy desert soils or tropical rain forest soils. Yet a gardener needs to know the soil's unseen composition. Correct analysis of the soil, and correcting any defects you find, is fundamental to your success in growing, whether you have a fruit and vegetable garden or plants of any other type. The kind and quality of your soil determines which plants you can grow.

Soil consists of mineral particles, organic matter, air and water of different kinds and in a variety of proportions. The nature of your soil depends on the nature of the underlying rock. If you live in a river valley, particles there have been ground down to form silt or clay. In other areas that have only a thin covering of soil, the land may well be rocky or sandy. These underlying conditions also determine how acid or alkaline the soil is. The acid/alkaline balance (also called "pH") is another important factor in determining what you can grow in your soil. *(See Chapter 9 for more on pH.)*

You can improve your soil structure with a little work. We know that roughly 90 percent of soil consists of non-living solid mineral material. Of that 90 percent, half is air space known as pores. Organic matter makes up the other 10 percent of substance in soil. Some of the living matter will move freely, grow and expand, such as organisms and roots. However, the majority of the visible biomass will be plant roots. Even though living matter makes up 10 percent of soil mass, it is responsible for far more than 10 percent of plant health. Nature can cope well with poor soil conditions, ensuring that only suitable plants will survive to propagate themselves. But the gardener wants a far wider scope. To grow a larger range of plants than nature will allow in your locale, you must improve the soil in various ways.

As an aside, hunter-gatherers lived off what they found and had to adapt to it. What we might call "agricultural man" or "gardening man" takes what he finds and adapts it to fit his needs and desires. Both the organic gardener and the corporate farmer take steps to modify what they find in the ground. Two key differences between them are how far they go to modify or interfere with the natural processes in their environment and the consequences they are willing to accept.

You will find a spectrum of different textures in natural soil. Depending on the type of soil you have, adding compost and/or organic fertilizer may not be enough to get a beautiful tilth. You may need to add other substances such as grit to get the desired texture. Experiment to find the best way to achieve a super fertile soil.

Plants will not thrive unless they have enough oxygen for their roots. Heavy clay soil has such small particles that very little air penetrates it. With clay soils the gardener must create a more porous texture in the soil, normally by adding lots of organic matter and possibly some grit. Another way to improve heavy clay soil is to add gypsum. If the soil is waterlogged and fails to drain well, you may also consider some form of artificial drainage.

Light sandy soil, by contrast, drains too freely and retains very little moisture. In periods of drought, plants in sandy soil will suffer and possibly die. Again, the answer is to add plenty of bulky organic matter to help bind the soil particles together and hold onto precious water.

To learn what your soil consists of, take a lump in your hand and crumble it between your fingers. If the soil is very sandy, you will hear the sound of grains rubbing together and feel them between your fingers. A less sandy soil, often found in areas surrounding a riverbed, is silt, which has a soapy feel. Clay is very heavy and sticky, with a glaze on its surface that causes it almost to shine. You will find one of these basic soil types in your garden.

To succeed at gardening you must create a loamy soil, a rich mixture of soil that feels light and friable to the touch and has a pleasant earthy smell. Loamy soil encourages earthworm activity and is well aerated. Because it is neither too dense nor too crumbly, this soil type holds moisture to the right degree with plenty of oxygen for microbes, mycorrhizae and, most importantly, healthy plants.

Clay has the finest particles of minerals and the least amount of air in its structure. Unless you work a lot of grit and organic matter into it, it will be hard to grow a good range of plants.

Silt lies somewhere between sand and clay in particle size. Provided it contains lots of organic matter, silt makes good garden soil. Silt has a silky feel and is often found in river valleys.

Sand has the coarsest mineral particles and, although it is well aerated, water runs through it very easily. Sand needs lots of organic matter added to bind the particles and improve its moisture retaining properties.

Pores are spaces between soil particles where water and air can flow. In the best conditions, about half the volume of soil consists of pores. The water and air will fill these gaps and attach to the particles. Pore space is crucial to good tilth. Without them, any type of fertilizer will not be able to get into the soil to feed the plants or even the microbes. Also, pores enable moisture to make its way up from beneath the roots through capillary action.

Loam is what all gardeners aim for. This soil structure has a good combination of organic matter with the basic mineral particles, whether sand, silt or clay. The structure is achieved by generous and regular applications of composted material, which helps create valuable pore space for roots to travel through and accumulate the necessary nutrients for their growth.

How well a soil holds together can be influenced by the action of microbes that digest organic materials in the soil. Their action helps stabilize the soil by physically binding soil particles together. Microbes also release a by-product called glomalin that acts like a glue to help bind mineral particles and organic materials together. This greatly contributes to building better soil structure by creating semi-stable soil aggregates.

Plant health largely depends on the amount of water and oxygen that can enter the soil. Tightly compacted soils do not let plants breathe and allow minimal amounts of water to penetrate deep into the root zone, inhibiting root growth. To get a friable soil with good tilth, two things that will always help are amending it with organic matter and cultivating the soil as often as possible.

Chapter 9

ooooo

UNDERSTANDING SOIL pH

$\Bigg\{$ *It's surprising how much memory is built around things unnoticed at the time.*

-*Barbara Kingsolver* $\Bigg\}$

I have given more than one thousand public talks on soil health. Without exception, when I get to the pH part, faces go blank. pH is an abstract discussion that requires real depth of thought. Yet, pH is very important to know and get right so your plants will benefit from everything else you do in your garden.

The basic requirements for a successful garden are often highly visible, such as sunlight, water and organic amendments. Unfortunately, you cannot see pH, also an essential consideration but hidden deep in the soil. Proper pH promotes plant growth by making it easier for roots to absorb essential nutrients. If this often-neglected consideration of soil fertility is ignored, the results are highly visible in poor plant growth. Many times gardeners diagnose a plant as being chlorotic (nitrogen, iron, or magnesium deficiencies) and add more nutrients to the soil without checking soil pH first. Adding nutrients has limited benefit if soil pH is not right.

Soil pH Basics
The fundamental concept of soil pH is simple. Acidity and alkalinity are measured as pH (parts Hydrogen). Acidity means an increase in hydrogen ions. Alkalinity means an increase of hydroxyl ions. The differences affect how molecules or potential plant nutrients interact in the soil.

The pH measure is expressed as a number from 0 to 14 on a logarithmic scale. Logarithmic here means each whole number on the scale is an exponent that expresses a size ratio. Thus, 3 on the scale means 10^3 (ten to the third power or 10 x 10 x10, which equals 1,000). The number 4 on the scale means 10^4 (ten to the fourth power or 1,000 x 10, which equals 10,000). Log scales are convenient to use when dealing with numbers covering a wide range, such as the number of hydrogen ions in a liquid or solid.

A pH of 7.0, like pure water, is neutral because the concentrations of hydrogen and hydroxyl ions are equal. As the pH number goes lower than 7, the hydrogen ions increase, and the soil becomes more acidic. As the pH number goes higher than 7, the concentration of hydroxyl ions increases, and the soil becomes more alkaline. Most garden plants grow best in a slightly acidic soil with a pH level 6.5, which is the best for most of our edible varieties (unless a nursery professional advises you otherwise for a specific plant type). Some plants like acidic soils. Other plants prefer alkaline soils. In either case, knowing the pH helps you get the best results.

Acid soils, common on the East Coast where rain leaches out calcium and the underlying rock is largely magnesium, typically range from pH 4 to 6. Alkaline soils in the dry Southwestern states come from calcium-rich rock and range from pH 7 to 9.

pH Affects Nutrient Uptake

You can give your plants a nutrient feast, but roots may not be able to absorb it well if the soil pH is not appropriate. Phosphorous is a good example. Phosphorous is a close second to nitrogen in its importance to plants. Phosphorous is essential for DNA, membrane development and energy production. Phosphorous also participates in photosynthesis and sugar formation. However, most of the phosphorous in soil particles is tied up in insoluble forms that are not available to roots. Phosphorous must be in solution in the form of orthophosphate for the plant to absorb it. At very low pH levels, the phosphorous is tightly bound to iron and aluminum in the soil. At high pH levels, phosphorous is locked inside insoluble forms of calcium and magnesium.

When a pH window is between 6 and 7, the mineral grip on phosphorous loosens and more orthophosphate dissolves. Also, the pH of orthophosphate in solution determines its electrical charge, which is between 6.0 and 7.0.

Buy a pH meter at your local nursery and test your soil in a few random spots around your yard and then calculate the average pH. The pH number should be between 6.0 and 7.2, with the ideal 6.5 to 6.7. This affects uptake. Around pH 6.0, orthophosphate has one negative charge, the form most favored for root absorption. Above pH 7.5, most of the orthophosphate has two negative charges and is absorbed more slowly.

Because of pH and its major influence, adding phosphorous to a garden can be tricky. Just because you put on three pounds does not mean three pounds will be available. Adding a fertilizer such as super phosphate temporarily makes more orthophosphate available, but most of the added phosphorous gradually turns into insoluble forms.

The good news is the role of pH is less dramatic with other plant nutrients. Nitrogen, usually taken up by roots as nitrate nitrogen (NO_3^-), is very soluble in the soil solution. Soil pH does not influence the uptake of nitrogen by roots. The same is true of potassium, which clings tightly to soil particles in layers of crystalline sandwiches and does not leach out rapidly like nitrate.

Plants require minute amounts of other minerals, including calcium, magnesium, sulfur, iron and zinc. Although the ideal pH for these elements varies, a pH of 6.5 is usually adequate to make sufficient amounts available. In alkaline soils, you often see poor growth and yellow leaves, because plants cannot absorb enough iron and other nutrients when they become insoluble.

The first step toward proper pH is from agricultural experiment stations or private labs. If your soil is too alkaline, you can increase the acid level by mixing in materials such as peat moss or soil sulfur. Clay soils demand more of these amendments.

You can counter the low pH of acid soils by mixing in crushed limestone or wood ash. The amount needed depends on the pH change and the soil texture. Know what pH you have in your garden. You can get a clearer understanding of your plants' growing requirements when you know your soil's pH. Knowledge equals success! Measure your garden's pH values. Kits available at your local nursery will give you a good approximation of your soil pH value. Results that are more exact come.

The great thing about gardening organically is you usually will not have to concern yourself with pH as a major problem. Organic materials tend to bring soils to a slightly acid range after they have gone through decomposition and contributed to the humus reserve in the soil. Alkaline soils can be lowered and acidic soils can be elevated to a more neutral level by using organic components. Also, microbes help stabilize the soil and create a pH environment that is more productive for plants and microbes equally.

Chapter 10

HUMUS, THE LIVING DEAD

{

Science, like life, feeds on its own decay. New facts burst old rules; then newly divined conceptions bind old and new together into a reconciling law.

-William James

}

Humus comes from the death and decay of organic materials that have fallen from leaf litter or other raw organic matter that get incorporated into the soil. You could say plants grow their own soil. Also, the contributions of beneficial soil microbes and fungus make soil more productive.

When plants die, it may appear they have fallen to the ground to rot away as waste. Mother Nature never wastes anything. The beauty of plant design is it only looks this way. A plethora of different varieties of microbes and fungi eat dead plants. As they do, the microbes and fungi release nutrients back into the soil for future plant generations.

In addition to returning to the soil all the elements that plants once borrowed from it, microbes contain the nutrient energy plants captured from the sun as they grew and thrived. The microbes and fungi pass on their accumulated nutrients to the soil as they actively decompose the plant remains. These remains are in turn decomposed by other microorganisms and consumed over and over, life to death, death feeds life, life to death and so on…consumed several times by many different organisms. This cycle creates stable humus and helps form rich, healthy soil.

Gardeners have known for centuries that to grow vegetables when they have nutrient poor, rocky soil they must crush the rocks to tiny particles, the smaller the better, and mix them with decaying organic materials. The organic matter added to plant materials, animal waste and the bodies of dead animals enriches a soil's physical and chemical properties. Remember "ashes to ashes, earth to earth." Everything that goes back in to the soil helps to build it by providing the essential nutrients right where plants need them, at the root zone.

Humus is usually dark brown, spongy and gooey. Some types of humus contain highly soluble molecules that readily break down further, known as active humus, the kind gardeners value most for feeding soil microbes. Others resist breaking down, because their larger, insoluble molecules bind tightly to clay molecules. Stable humus is crucial to fertile soil's physical qualities. A nice balance between both types is best and helps maintain exceptional soil health and tilth. For this reason, you should add both raw organic matter and composted organic matter to your garden. This keeps the biology going strong and adds the physical properties to create beautiful, healthy soil.

Many plant fibers and animal tissues are what we call recalcitrant, meaning they resist decomposition. The tough fibers of dead plants like leaf veins and other woody materials are connected together to form long chains of complex organic molecules that do not easily break down.

Because organisms vary in how easily they break down, we need a highly diversified soil food web. All organisms in garden soil serve different functions. One might be great at digesting cellulose, another at carbohydrates, fats or lignins. Many macro-organisms such as worms and small insects prepare recalcitrant organic materials by passing them through their digestive processes, which prepares them for other microscopic digesters to fully break them down into a simpler molecular structure. When nutrients break down into simpler forms, plant roots can absorb them to grow. This is the essence creating humus.

Organic matter gets consumed a number of times. As microbes and fungus continue to break down the remains of various organisms into simpler compounds more available to plants, they also add stable organic matter to the soil. This organic matter is vital as the primary source of nutrients for plants in the form of carbon, hydrogen, oxygen, nitrogen, phosphorus, potassium and trace elements or micronutrients. *(See Chapter 15 for more on essential micronutrients.)* Humus also acts as an important reserve between the fresh organic matter from which it comes and the simpler forms of carbon dioxide, water, and minerals that returns to the soil, sometimes several years later.

Humus formation varies with air temperature. When the temperature rises above 80°F, organic matter decays faster than it is generated. Conversely, when temperatures drop below 40° F, biological activity in the soil slows down, building humus reserves for plants to draw on later.

Eventually, this digested organic matter transforms into tiny particles of dark humus. Humus is delicious for plants, loaded with nutrients and full of structural integrity. Plants love humus and you will love what it does for your garden.

Among the environmental benefits of humus in your backyard garden (and in large farming operations that use organic practices): It holds carbon dioxide, sequestered in the humus soil particles, until microbes digest them and liberate the carbon dioxide gas back into the atmosphere. Carbon dioxide is also held in the soil while complex chains of organic compounds wait for microbes to digest them in preparation for plant root absorption.

Carbon dioxide plays a role in the troubling phenomenon of global warming, a reality of our time. Organic gardening works organic materials back into the soil until microorganisms use it as an energy source. The energy then passes to actively growing plants in different compounds for their use. Animals and humans consume these plants, further sequestering carbon dioxide that otherwise would release into the atmosphere. In this way, even your little backyard makes a difference on a global level.

Chapter 11

ⲟⲟⲟⲟⲟ

COMPOSTING, COMPOST TEA AND MULCH

{ *Every parting is a form of death, as every reunion is a type of heaven.*

-Tryon Edwards }

Composting

The most common form of composting is basic and simple. Gather up as many leaves as you can one morning. Rake them into a pile. After dinner that night, collect all your vegetable kitchen scraps, throw them on top of the pile and wait. Do it again daily with the kitchen scraps. Keep adding weekly with the yard litter.

This approach works well if you have a ranch-like setting and do not mind the odor of a decomposing pile on your property. It also works if you have an area that is out of sight, or if you don't care what your guests think of how your house smells when they come to visit. I didn't mind for a long time, even in the middle of Los Angeles with my barbeque going every weekend and a pile rotting away right next to it. Most people can create a compost pile, especially if you have a large yard that generates a lot of leaves, pruned branches and other bulky stuff. However, a giant heap is not enough. When it comes to handling messy kitchen waste, new and experienced compost enthusiasts need an enclosed composting bin to make the process carefree and convenient.

I have composted in open piles for almost 20 years. Often my dog digs into it and destroys it, or possums, raccoons and skunks get into it for worms and other kitchen scraps. When Los Angeles began a composting program in the early 1990's, I was finally able to set clear boundaries by getting a free, enclosed compost bin. This was a major improvement over my open pile, because it gave the compost form and structure and didn't look too bad. Besides solving critter problems, this method hides the shiny left over salads with chopped tomatoes covered with olive oil along with a yellow splash of banana peels. It all disappears from view.

Enclosed compost bins provide visual relief, and you can put them just about anywhere. To make a home composting system work, you need to make each stage of the process quick and easy. You need a container for collecting fruit and veggie trimmings in the kitchen along with a weatherproof enclosed composter, which can range from a covered pit to a modified garbage can to a state-of-the-art tumbler. If your composter is located more than 15 feet from your back door, you may need a transfer station container (sort of a drop off point) for kitchen overflow on its way to the composter itself. A small garbage can with a lock-on lid or a 5-gallon bucket stationed on your deck or patio are perfect for this.

A common myth about composting is that you can speed it up. Composting works best slow and steady. Don't try to rush it. I have made smoking-hot batches of compost dozens of times, and each one took a lot of work. The results I got from pushing the composting process to go faster were no better than compost dug from the base of a slow-rotting pile or the ground floor of a stationary composter.

No composter can make compost in three weeks. It takes 10 weeks minimum, and that is if you know your way around composting, you have warm weather, a good composter and a balance of materials to put in it. Slow speed is good and natural for compost. You don't have to fight it, and fancy equipment can take you only so far in speeding it up anyway.

Another myth is that composting is a productive process that yields a good return of the finest soil amendment a gardener can have. Certainly, compost is valuable stuff, but the truth is you do not get very much of it. You can drop six months' worth of potato peelings, bygone bread and salad greens into an enclosed composter and harvest only enough compost to plant two tomatoes. Composting is a reductive process. You get back less volume than you put in. But so what? The more important purpose of home composting is to capture and recycle organic waste before it leaves your yard. Enclosed composters make this easy.

A final myth is that compost requires regular mixing and turning. True, a well-mixed mass of evenly moist compostable stuff is more likely to rot quickly than unmixed pockets of this or that, but you only need to turn compost occasionally. If you are patient, you need not mix and turn at all, though I have found that magic happens when I lift my stationary composter to move it to a new place and then go back and fluff through the old material with a digging fork. Two weeks later, the rough compost has ripened to ready, and I get to have a compost harvest day. That always feels like a party.

Compost Tea

You do not drink compost tea, but your plants will love you for it. Compost tea adds the needed microbes to create a truly diverse and dynamic soil. Brew a bucket of tea to delight every plant in your home or out in the garden. It is fun and easy to make. Simply add water and a little organic molasses to top quality compost, potting soil or planting mix, and off you go! To make good compost tea, the more aged the material the better. If you can add some worm castings and seaweed extract, you will have so many nutrients that your plants will explode with vigor. If you want to kick it up a notch, add a little liquid organic fertilizer.

Here's how to do it. Prepare two empty 5-gallon buckets. Fill one with water and let it sit for 24 hours. This allows the chlorine gas to evaporate. Fill the empty bucket with about 1 gallon of composted organic material and 1 ounce of unsulfured molasses (extra food for the microbes). Fill it with the de-chlorinated water to about ¾ full. Stir the soil and water well until it is dark and completely wet. If you have an aquarium pump, you can insert the pump hose into the bottom of the bucket, turn it on and let it brew for 2 to 3 days. Stir the brew with a stick occasionally to help mix the soil and separate the microbes from the solid soil particles. Apply the strained tea with a standard pump sprayer both to the top and bottom of leaves. The bottom of the leaves is where the "stoma" openings are located. (Stoma is Greek for "mouth.") Here the solution can absorb best. Or apply it directly to the soil. Do not throw the solid material away. Add it to the soil as mulch around any plant in the garden. Use the tea immediately after you brew it. The microbes will die shortly after the oxygen source is removed. That's it. Tea is fun in the sun. Sit back and watch your plants grow.

Mulch, The Final Layer

I believe strongly in mulching. I have practiced it for many years for both my home vegetable gardens and on the Dr. Earth farm. In my experience, mulching brings many benefits. It keeps the soil moist, friable, easy to cultivate and helps regulate the soil temperature away from extremes. Mulches also help to keep ground moisture from evaporating. They help to regulate water by reducing evaporation-respiration. They also protect the soil from sunburn and protect the available nutrients. They minimize soil erosion due to wind and rain. Additionally, mulches create an environment hospitable for a bio-diverse set of microorganisms, which supports fertile soils. Finally, mulches act as a carbon reservoir and keep rainwater from splattering mud on your plants and walkways. This makes your garden look nice, too.

Mulch is like an artist taking the final brush stroke to a masterpiece painting; it completes it. Besides making a garden look good, mulches also have many functional attributes. Mulches help to suppress weed seeds from germinating, which ultimately means less work later weeding the garden. I have tested almost every kind of mulching material available. They all have some benefit to the garden, some more than others. For example, partially decomposed hay is far better than coarse, freshly baled hay. Composted grass clippings are more effective than raw green clippings. The same holds true for leaves and all yard wastes.

I have worked in many community gardens with limited budgets and resources. I used to know a young Guatamalan gardener named Martha in the Vernon section of Los Angeles. She taught me that newspaper, cardboard or even carpet with holes drilled in it makes for effective mulch. Not pretty, but they work. These are all options you have available to you. Although some may be unsightly in the garden, they are all effective.

For attractive, dark brown, organic mulch use a good planting mix or compost. It makes a huge difference and gives it that finishing touch, the final stroke of your gardening project to make it clean and attractive. Generally, put down mulch about 3 to 5 inches thick in your vegetable garden and around the base of all fruit trees.

Building a nutrient-rich, healthy garden soil with mulch will greatly benefit the garden, especially if it is organic compost or planting mix, rather than straw, newspaper or carpet. As the organic materials slowly break down, they contribute to the nutrient density of the soil, build humus reserves, conserve water and help to build friable soil structure.

PART 2

PLANT HEALTH

Chapter 12

GETTING TO KNOW YOUR PLANTS

{

For 200 years we've been conquering Nature. Now we're beating it to death

-Tom McMillan

}

The Simple Mechanics

I must have chlorophyll running through my veins. Over the years, I have had the pleasure of educating thousands of gardeners on plant biology. As soon as I began Healthy Garden, Healthy You, I knew I had to write a chapter simplifying how plants function and absorb nutrients, and how this relates to us in our daily lives. If you understand the simple mechanics of plants, you will be the best judge of why plants respond in a certain way and how to grow them to their fullest health potential.

This chapter demystifies some common questions. Basic understanding of how plants function makes you a better gardener. If you are a better gardener, you can grow healthier plants.

Plant Benefits to Humans and Other Life

A lush blanket of vegetation, a living, green and diverse blanket covers our earth. This living green cover enables other life forms to survive and thrive. Plants and animals need each other to exist. Plants evolved among earth's first living things. Early in geologic time when oceans began to recede, many aquatic plants evolved into terrestrial plants that supported animal and human life on land.

From their beginnings as microscopic, single-cell organisms, plants have been linked to all life on earth. Plants form the biosphere, a thin shell covering the earth's surface where plants and animals exist. Our reliance on plants has helped humans evolve from primitive surroundings to modern, sophisticated civilizations. Our ability to pass knowledge from generation to generation has taken us out of the primitive, hand-to-mouth existence of the early hominids and accelerated us into prosperous and progressive people. The ability to create art and express our early thoughts of survival, agricultural findings, mathematical equations and scientific data on paper made from plants has given us a progression of knowledge across many generations. Plants are the raw material of much of our created world (clothing, homes, furniture and medicines plus much more) and are essential for survival and the quality of life for all mankind.

Plants clean the air; they exchange the oxygen we breathe for the carbon dioxide we exhale. They use the energy of the sun to make foods that sustain all animals. From the soil, they draw micronutrients, minerals, nitrogen, phosphors, potassium, calcium and iron that are crucial for our existence and health. Plants absorb many of their nutrients from the atmosphere, water and soil in the form of gases, such as carbon, hydrogen and oxygen.

Roots are not the only way plants get the nutrients they rely on. They also absorb carbon dioxide through their leaves to help cleanse the environment. Sunlight energy falling on their leaves creates sugars such as sucrose, fructose and glucose through the process called photosynthesis. Plants also absorb nitrogen gas that has been fixed from the atmosphere. Nearly 80 percent of the air we breathe is nitrogen gas. Nitrogen is essential for protein synthesis in plants, because it is a main constituent of the molecules of most amino acids that form into proteins.

Plants have thousands of microscopic openings located on every leaf for absorbing carbon dioxide and water laden with nutrients. They absorb these gases and liquids through pores in their leaves called stomata. (The word comes from the Greek word stoma, which means mouth.) Stomata are found mainly on the underside of the leaves. What they absorb they transport where needed within the plant itself. The stomata close up during the night (when no photosynthesis occurs), on hot days when plants might lose too much water and dry up, or when wind threatens to dry the plant.

The earth supports approximately 400,000 different kinds of plants, all very diverse in their forms. One third of all plants do not have roots, stems nor leaves as we know them. About 150,000 plant species never produce flowers. An almost equal number of plant species do not grow from seeds but come from dust-like particles called spores. Although the vast majority of plants manufacture their own food by photosynthesis, mushrooms, molds and other fungi rely on foods created by green plants for their sustenance, as do animals. (Some biologists include these unusual, non-green species in the plant kingdom.) Most plants spend a lifetime anchored in one place; yet simple single-cell plankton can swim to different locations in the waters where they live.

The largest group in the plant kingdom consists of about 250,000 species called angiosperms. (Their name shows us their seeds originate inside containers we call fruits. In Greek angeion means vessel; sperma means seed.) These flowering plants are the garden-variety plants most common in suburban landscapes. They supply almost all the vegetable matter in our diet and produce the world's hardwoods. They are the most sophisticated of plant forms and are best adapted to survive in a wide range of climates and terrain.

The second most abundant plants are gymnosperms, plants that produce seeds in the open spaces of cones, such as between the flap-like parts of a pinecone. The Greek words gymnos (meaning naked) and sperma (meaning seed) describe this form of development. (We get the word "gymnasium" from ancient Greek. Their athletes constructed their Adonis-like bodies in the nude, hence, "gym.") Gymnosperms include all the conifers: cedar, redwood, juniper, cypress, fir and pine and the largest living things on earth, the giant sequoias.

How can we know that a potted rose bush is living, while a petal from a rose from the same plant pressed between the pages of a book is dead? From appearances, all the seeds in the seed packet in your drawer are also dead.

When the petal was a part of a living plant, its cells engaged in a complicated chain of chemical reactions grouped together under the term metabolism. As long as a cell or an entire creature is alive, it shows some form of metabolic activity (movement or growth). When metabolism stops, cells die. And when cells die, if they are not replaced, metabolism stops.

How Plants Function
Plants grow in proportion to the amount of light, water, minerals and oxygen they receive. Genes determine a plant's lifespan; one year for annuals, two for biennials and indefinitely for perennials. (If you ever notice the term indeterminate used on tomato plants, it means the plant will continue to grow until environmental conditions, such as cold weather, become a limiting factor.)

When it receives plenty of fertilizer, careful watering, optimum sun energy and thinning (removing plants that compete for available nutrients and light) a plant can be pushed to its limits of leaf and flower production.

The plants we grow for food and flowers remain anchored in one place throughout their life. Soil buries half of a plant's body, the root system. This hidden half of the plant is where nature's magic happens. Above-ground shoot systems (stems and leaves) occupy a bright, sunlit and airy world. This is where the other half of the growth occurs. Roots and shoots grow in opposite directions, but each part has a role to contribute to the song of life. Root growth and shoot growth are brilliantly coordinated and complement each other, with energy reserves and raw materials shared equally by the two halves. When daily or seasonal environmental changes affect one part, the other must respond to support its "other half." A plant can only fulfill its fundamental basics of life, such as reproduction, cellular metabolism and growth, through the precisely controlled interactions between roots, stems, leaves and flowers. This is the bright, beautiful, harmonious song of plant life in full bloom across the earth.

A plant's ability to multiply and grow while we busily lead our lives seems magical and amazing. At the right time of year, you can leave a tomato garden over a three-day weekend and when you return all the tomatoes that were small and green on the vine have become a beautiful, healthy, robust red harvest of produce for you. All this happened while you were busy living your life. We need plants more than they need us. We should feed them and nurture them to the best of our ability as they do for us when we consume them.

Chapter 13

∞∞∞

FERTILE SOIL: THE ESSENCE OF HEALTHY PLANTS

{
The best time to plant a tree was 20 years ago.
The next best time is now.

-Chinese Proverb
}

If the soil is healthy, common sense tells us, so is the plant that grows in it. If you take multivitamins, exercise and sleep well, you are most likely to be healthy. Soil is similar to people. Fertilizers are the vitamins, wind and rain are the exercise, and sun and shade are the rest. Organic fertilizers take a strategic approach aimed at feeding the microorganisms in the soil rather than the plants directly, which is how synthetic fertilizers work. You might ask, "What's the difference if my plants grow?" By fertilizing, or feeding, the soil, you enable it to build nutrient reserves that plant roots can tap into any time as needed. Feeding builds good soil structure, creates pores for roots to extend their reach, helps suppress disease and supports biological diversity. Feeding also helps maintain a neutral pH to support humus formation that adds minerals and micronutrients to a living soil.

Compost and Manure

A well-made compost functions similarly to a well-made organic fertilizer, except it is not nearly as potent in nutrients. Compost is simply the remains of once living organisms that have been degraded by microorganisms. Compost usually consists of organic materials such as yard wastes, plant trimmings, leaves, grass trimmings, soil with microbes and various wet kitchen scraps other than meat. Applying this composted substance to your soil will help provide great tilth, microorganisms, nutrients and nutrient stores.

Part of the beauty of compost is the nutrients from the organic matter in it are released slowly. Compost is so nutrient rich it often meets the needs of a plant for one year or more, although you do not receive the maximum growth and health potential if you apply compost only once a year. Plants grown with healthy and diverse compost will absorb a slower, steadier and more diverse set of nutrients than if they receive synthetic nutrients. Natural compost leads to healthier, disease-resistant plants packed full of nutrients. Caution: Avoid compost made from bio-solids or sewage sludge. Many organic experts warn against them, because they are linked to heavy metals and human pathogens.

Adding compost to your soil is an excellent way to build it up, especially if the soil was nutrient deprived in the past. Where I grew up in Los Angeles, asphalt lots and industrial yards were redeveloped for residential lots as land values increased. The soil under these new homes had been deprived of organic matter and nutrients for many years. If you live in a similar area, amending the soil with compost is one effective way to prepare your area to support healthy growth. Applying a premium home made or store bought compost benefits a soil in any stage of maturity and helps to establish any edible garden. To get safe, effective compost for your garden, look for a trusted nursery or professional grower who can advise you on how to boost your soil's fertility.

Manure, or animal waste, is another effective but risky way to spread nutrients into your soil. Fresh manure has a substantial effect on soil fertility for agriculture. However, I do not recommend using it in a home garden. Raw manure may release ammonia, which is detrimental to plant health. For this and other reasons, manure needs to be composted for a long time before you use it in your garden. Once composted, though, manure is a nutrient-rich material to mix with your soil. Never use the waste of a carnivore (meat eater) such as a cat or dog, as it can carry harmful pathogens. If you raise rabbits, sheep, chickens, horses or cows, these manures are great. Just remember to compost them before you apply them to the garden.

Organic Fertilizers and Soil Amendments

These materials consist of natural ingredients that the beneficial microbes in a living soil digest as food. Popular ingredients include fish meals, feather meal, alfalfa meal, cottonseed meal, bone meals, kelp meal, seaweed extracts, blood meal and liquid animal manures. The meals and extracts contain organic matter and nutrients, while the bacteria and the symbiotic mycorrhizal fungi convert the nutrient sources into usable forms plants can absorb as needed. Also, fungi extend the reach of plant roots to acquire more nutrients.

Organic fertilizers have a much lower chance of leaching through the soil and contaminating the water table. With organic fertilizers, nutrients are physically bound into larger pieces of organic matter lodged in the soil and available so that microbes can free them up for plant use. There is nothing mysterious or magical about organic fertilizers. They simply give you a way of working with nature rather than against it. The objective in using them is to recycle organic matter back into the soil rather than discarding it and relying on chemicals. In fact, the organic process is much less mysterious than the methods of the chemical grower.

A program of organic fertilizers involves far more than just growing plants without chemical fertilizers and artificial sprays. Using organics is a life choice and commitment that recognizes the complex, successful workings of nature in maintaining life for hundreds of millions of years. Sound organic cultivating principles closely follow processes found in the natural world. Also, do not think that using these principles leads to lower yields or quality. In fact, with organics you are likely to increase both. Organic methods also support habitat for wildlife while insuring the fruits and vegetables you produce in your garden are safe, nutritious and free of chemicals. You also reduce the possibility of the harmful effects of chemicals on infants and children.

The soil teems with millions of microorganisms that release nutrients required for healthy plant growth from organic matter. Rather than feeding plants directly, organic fertilizers feed the soil with natural materials that allow your plants to draw on a humus reservoir of nutrients as they need. Plants grown this way are stronger and more resistant to pests and disease. Organic fertilizers work and persist for many months (unlike the short-term affects of chemical fertilizers) because they become a part of the living soil.

You can find a number of different organic fertilizers and amendments at your local nursery. Some are formulated to support the nutritional needs of particular plant categories such as vegetables, while others take an all-purpose approach good for a variety of plants. Fertilizers are generally tested and proven for a specific application. I recommend choosing a selection specific to your types of plants: vegetable fertilizer for vegetables; fruit fertilizer for your fruit trees. In any case, organic fertilizers and amendments are geared for the slow, controlled release of plant food. They are perfect for preparing the soil for upcoming seasons without having to worry about nutrients being wasted or washed away.

Chemical Fertilizers

Chemical fertilizers feed plants directly and do not address the soil, because they are in a form that plants can absorb immediately. While direct plant feeding sounds attractive, it adds no beneficial attributes to the soil. In fact, over time chemical fertilizers can deplete the soil of nutrients. The gardener treating plants only with chemicals uses the soil simply as an anchor to hold plants in place. While this approach appears to have good short-term results, in the long run it has disastrous consequences. When organic matter is not replaced in the soil, beneficial organisms die out, the soil structure breaks down, and the soil becomes hard, airless and unproductive. Attempts at "force-feeding" plants result in soft, sappy growth, which is prone to attack by a host of pests and diseases.

When plants are forced to grow with chemical fertilizers, they become weak. As plant cell walls develop, they do not have enough time to produce two important compounds, cellulose and lignins. These substances strengthen protective cell walls. As cells are forced to duplicate and grow quickly, the amount of cellulose and lignin decreases, making the plant tissues much softer and more attractive for pests to attack. If you were an insect, would you rather bite into a soft head of butter lettuce or chew on a piece of wood? Insects prefer tender, soft growth.

Chemical pesticides are also often used for short-term pest control. Unfortunately, these pesticides also kill the natural predators of the pests that attack plants. Eventually, the problem gets worse as nothing is left to kill the "bad bugs." Stronger, more toxic pesticides then have to be used, setting in motion a hard-to-break, vicious cycle: Plants and soil weakened by chemicals need more chemicals to protect them from pests they resist naturally when well nourished.

Problems with Chemical Fertilizers

Chemical fertilizers feed plants with nutrients directly. This inhibits, and in some cases, kills off microbes within the soil. In addition to wiping out organisms, nutrients added as soluble fertilizers can be lost inefficiently through leaching away or conversion to an unusable form such as nitrogen gas. Chemicals washed away during rain or irrigation can pollute ground water, streams, lakes and oceans. In addition, commercially synthesized chemical fertilizers do not have the beneficial soil microbes that feed the plants certain bio-chemicals such as vitamins and antibiotics.

When soil becomes unbalanced through chemical alteration, certain micronutrients and heavy metals, such as iron, magnesium and aluminum, become more soluble in the soil and can be toxic to plant tissues. Unbalanced soils also reduce the productivity of bacteria (nitrogen fixers) making nutrients less available. Chemical fertilizers also decrease a soil's ability to hold onto positively charged nutrients, which allows water to more easily wash away nutrients. An imbalance of soils locks up other micronutrients and makes them unavailable to plants while concentrating harmful molecules in the soil. All this can lead to further deterioration of the soil by chemically deteriorating humus and organic matter reserves.

Adding petrochemical synthetic fertilizers drives up the salt concentration in the soil and changes the pH, which can adversely affect plants. More importantly, chemical fertilizers only feed for a short time. Organic fertilizers feed continuously, because the microbes do not digest all of the organic fertilizer immediately.

Chemical fertilizers reduce the soil aggregation properties of microbes and sacrifice good tilth. Conversely, organic fertilizers support water retention, reduce runoff and support long-term soil health.

Neglecting living organisms in the soil by treating plants with chemically synthesized fertilizers and pest sprays may eventually lead to the extinction of all living matter in commercial soil. In the future, we may become completely dependent on synthetics to get any yield at all. Many gardeners and consumers regard this cycle as unsustainable over time. They have devoted their lives, farming practices and backyards to restoring and preserving biological diversity in soil.

The Answer: Feed the Soil Not the Plants

Feed the soil, not the plants! When we feed our plants and not our soil, we lose all the benefits from microbes. When we feed the soil, we actually feed the microbes in the soil. Microbes make nutrients available for plants. You feed microbes by adding organic material. If you give plants a synthetic chemical fertilizer, you feed only the plant, not the soil nor the microbes. Soil has supported plants and given them nutrients since long before we invented other fertilizers, so why not feed the soil and preserve the natural biological interactions that support plant survival and growth?

Remember: healthy soils equal healthy plants that equal healthy animals and humans. It is that simple.

Why are people generally indifferent to the tiny life all around us? Perhaps we modern people ignore microorganisms, because we have a strong bias against all microscopic life. Now that we understand the germ theory of disease, and appreciate the many health improvements that came from it, we have become "biophobic." Are we prejudiced against anything alive but so small we cannot see it? Do we think anything microscopic and alive must be bad for our health? Do we take for granted what we cannot see? This is a dangerous bit of blindness.

True, some bacteria and viruses threaten our health. But the vast majority of tiny life is either neutral or helpful. Much of it is even essential. Our lives would be impossible without the essential bacteria and fungi in our guts and in our soil. Without microorganisms we could not have penicillin or yogurt (to name just two.)

The large-scale, corporate food industry sees organic gardening as a major enemy and touts the benefits of genetically enhanced crops instead of first enhancing the soil organically to make crops more healthy and nutritious. Think about it: If everybody grew their own food and were healthy, we would not need giant monoculture and commercial farming. Pharmaceutical companies would generate much less revenue. You would need a medical doctor only if you had a broken bone. It all comes down to corporate manipulation, control and money.

Buy heirloom seeds and transplants. Grow everything you can. What you cannot grow, buy from someone you trust. If you're an attorney, CPA, architect, nurse or have a 9-to-5 job in the middle of the city with no time or space to garden, barter your services with an organic produce farmer, chicken farmer, cattle rancher or neighbor who grows the healthiest organic tomatoes. A few words from you could be worth a fresh basket of healthy fruit or vegetables. I do this all the time. I have not bought a tomato from the market in more than 15 years. As my father, Lou, says, "Every little bit helps." Please consider these ideas to ensure your health and the health of your loved ones.

Chapter 14

ooooo

THE 16 NUTRIENTS PLANTS MUST HAVE

{

I would feel more optimistic about a bright future for man if he spent less time proving that he can outwit Nature and more time tasting her sweetness and respecting her seniority.
                                        -Elwyn Brooks White

}

This chapter is a reference tool. Use it to review to clearly understand the nutrients plants must have for their growth. Sixteen basic nutrients are required for crop development (plus hundreds more we know are needed in minute amounts). Commercial agriculture tends not to address these trace nutrients. The oversimplified commercial approach is like taking a multivitamin with only an emphasis on vitamin C or calcium. Conventional agriculture tells us that sixteen basic nutrients are all that is needed for plant growth

I recommend well-rounded organic fertilizers, soil amendments, aged manures and composts for healthy plants and soil on a regular basis. You never know how much of any one nutrient is needed at a certain time of year, or time of day, for that matter. For example, nitrogen requirements can vary hourly depending on the time of day, soil temperature or the amount of photosynthesis a leaf is producing at the height of the solar index, which is from 10 A.M. to 4 P.M.

Long-lasting organic materials are great sources of nutrients and are a safe way to ensure that all nutrients are available anytime a plant needs them. I favor ocean-based fertilizers, because they are loaded with nutrients, well beyond the basic sixteen needed for crop development. All the nutrients plants use are equally important, yet each is required in vastly different amounts. These differences have led to the grouping of essential nutrients by the relative quantities in which plants require them, namely, primary or macronutrients, secondary nutrients, and micronutrients.

Macronutrients

The macronutrients, required in the largest amounts, are nitrogen, phosphorus and potassium (referred to by the chemical shorthand N-P-K.) Recall from Chapter 9 the importance of knowing your soil's pH, because many of these nutrients may never make it to your plants if the pH is out of balance.

NITROGEN (N) - Needed to produce amino acids, the building block for proteins and genetic material. Essential for plant cell division, vital for plant growth, directly involved in photosynthesis, necessary component of vitamins, aids in production and use of carbohydrates and affects energy reactions in the plant. Nitrogen enables the plant to trap energy from sunlight.

Deficiency causes thin stems, yellow leaves, slowed growth and yellowing where plants should be green.

Excess causes an imbalance in metabolism. Flowering and fruiting can be delayed, with fruits ripening unevenly. Bud and blossom drop, low fruit production. Fruiting and flowering plants may not develop any fruits. May also inhibit the uptake of trace nutrients. Makes plants more susceptible to insects that love young, tender growth.

PHOSPHORUS (P) - Needed for genetic material, cell membranes, root development, seed number and size. Facilitates the use of energy, involved in photosynthesis, respiration, energy storage and transfer, cell division and enlargement. Promotes early root formation and growth. Improves quality of fruits, vegetables and grains. Vital to seed formation. Helps plants survive harsh winter conditions, increases water-use efficiency, hastens maturity.

Deficiency causes purple leaves beginning underneath, halted roots, slow growth, poor fruit and vegetable production.

Excess Toxicity is rare but possible if phosphorus fertilizer is over applied.

POTASSIUM (K) - Needed for carbohydrate metabolism, the break down and translocation of starches and cell division. Influences the uptake of calcium, sodium and nitrogen. Increases photosynthesis and water-use efficiency. Essential to protein synthesis. Important in fruit formation. Activates enzymes and controls their reaction rates. Improves quality of seeds and fruit, improves winter hardiness, increases disease resistance.

Deficiency leads to flabby stems, halted growth, burnt leaf edges and vulnerability to disease.

Excess leads to deficiency in other needed nutrients, because the plant will take up extra potassium before nutrients like magnesium.

Secondary Nutrients
The secondary nutrients are calcium, magnesium and sulphur. Most crops need these three secondary nutrients in lesser amounts than the primary nutrients. People are giving them more prominence in crop fertilization programs as they learn that N-P-K fertilizers alone cannot fulfill plant requirements.

CALCIUM (Ca) – helps regulate access to plant cells similar to the ones needed for nitrogen uptake. Used for continuous cell division and formation. Involved in nitrogen metabolism. Required for enzyme activation and cell reproduction. Reduces plant respiration, aids translocation of photosynthesis from leaves to fruiting organs, increases fruit set and stimulates microbial activity.

Deficiency causes all growing tips to halt, curls leaves, and causes cell membranes to disintegrate, producing thin cell walls and blossom end rot.

MAGNESIUM (Mg) – needed for the chlorophyll molecules that put the green in plants. Also used for enzyme activation. Improves utilization and mobility of phosphorus. Increases iron utilization in plants and influences earliness and uniformity of maturity.

Deficiency causes yellowing of lower leaves and, in some cases, lower crop yield.

SULPHUR (S) – an integral part of amino acids needed to build proteins. Contributes to the development of several enzymes and vitamins. Aids in seed production and promotes nodule formation on legumes. Needed in chlorophyll formation.

Deficiency causes younger leaves to yellow.

Micronutrients or Trace Elements
Here we cover only a few micronutrients and their importance. We know many more exist in the soil, either as minerals or as organic materials. We do not understand them fully, although we know plants need them all in minute quantities.

Micronutrients include at least iron, manganese, zinc, copper, boron, molybdenum and chloride. These plant food nutrients are used in small amounts, but they are just as important to plant development and the success of a healthy garden as the major nutrients. By making all micronutrients available to your plants naturally, you have the "multivitamin" available in the soil ready for your plants to absorb. This is the best and safest way to grow healthy plants. They are especially important because they work as activators or enablers of many plant functions. Proper pH insures many of these nutrients are available to your plants. *(See Chapter 9 for more on pH.)*

IRON (Fe) – important for nitrogen fixation, chlorophyll synthesis and used in other enzymes and proteins. Deficiency more likely in alkaline soil. Causes yellowing between enlarged veins and short, skinny stems.

MANGANESE (Mn) – needed for synthesis of chlorophyll, assists in vitamin, carbohydrate and nitrogen metabolism. Deficiency more likely in alkaline soil. Stops new leaf growth and pale color, mostly between veins.

ZINC (Z) – essential component of various enzyme systems for energy production, protein synthesis and growth regulation. Needed to produce plant growth hormones. Greatly benefits seed and grain production and maturation. Deficiency displays yellowing and mottling of leaves. Plants also show delayed maturity. Not mobile in plants, so zinc deficiency symptoms occur mainly in new growth

COPPER (Cu) – Important for reproductive growth. A catalyst for enzyme and chlorophyll synthesis. Aids root metabolism and helps in using proteins. Deficiency symptoms generally appear on young plants. First symptoms are yellowing of youngest leaves with slightly stunted growth. In extreme cases, leaves die after becoming shriveled, twisted, broken and ragged.

BORON (B) – important for all growing tissues. Exists in cell membranes. Needed for nitrogen fixation, protein synthesis, starch and sugar transport, root growth, water uptake and transport. Deficiency more likely in alkaline soils. May lead to growing points dying and cells being disrupted.

MOLYBDENUM (Mo) – Important for nitrogen metabolism and protein synthesis. Needed to convert inorganic phosphates to organic forms. Deficiency occurs mainly in acid soils. Can cause pale, deformed, thin leaves.

CHLORIDE (Cl) – Most soils have enough chloride for adequate plant nutrition. However, chloride deficiencies are reported in sandy soils in high rainfall areas or those derived from low-chloride parent materials. There are few areas of chloride-deficiency, so this micronutrient is not considered in fertilizer programs.

In addition to the 13 nutrients above, plants also require carbon, hydrogen and oxygen. Plants extract these elements from air and water to make up the bulk of their weight. Plants need micronutrients only in minute quantities to function properly. On the other hand, too much of these can be toxic, sometimes lethal, to a host organism. For this reason, avoid applying individual nutrients to prevent an accidental deficiency or over application. Adding and maintaining natural and organic matter (rock powders, seaweed, fish bone meal) is the best way to insure plants receive adequate, balanced nutrition. Natural and organic matter contains balanced amounts of the desired nutrients and can keep any excessive micronutrients from poisoning plants.

Chapter 15

⚬⚬⚬⚬⚬

ESSENTIAL MICRONUTRIENTS

{

*Every sickness, every disease, and every ailment can be traced to a
mineral deficiency.*

- Dr. Linus Pauling

}

When it comes to feeding your garden and your plants' health, do not fall victim to clever marketing campaigns that show beautiful, lush gardens fed by a hose end sprayer with a simple, all-purpose synthetic fertilizer. How healthy are the plants in that glossy ad? A Hollywood set is just that, a set, an illusion, not real life. Everything looks great during the film production until the cameras stop rolling and the crew goes home. In Los Angeles, I worked on many movies and commercials. In Hollywood fashion, we would set up a scene with the best decor for mass appeal in a 30-second commercial. Lights went on. Cameras rolled. Actors smiled. Set and scenery glowed. Two days later, everything was gone or trashed.

A stage set is neither reality nor what you want in your backyard. Do not chase after easy, miracle results. The oversimplification in the marketing of fertilizers promotes applying only nitrogen, phosphorous and potassium. This one-dimensional approach produces visible, short-term benefits and saves money but has long-term negative effects on the soil and overall plant health. The likely result of chemical N-P-K treatment is yield loss and poor nutrition from an imbalanced approach to meeting plants' nutrients needs.

Look hard at your plants' need for micronutrients. They are the catalyst in the soil that makes other nutrients available.

Study Your Soil

This is the time to study your soil, test it, track what you apply and consider buying a nutrient test kit along with a pH meter. Using tests to measure the nutrients in your soil is always a good idea, but not always necessary if you are feeding with a complete fertilizer. Know your soil's pH, since the pH determines the availability of many nutrients. To get the best yields and optimum plant health, keep soil fertility in balance and not cut back on nutrients. Even commercial growers on a strict budget know they need micronutrients as well as N, P and K; years ago they would have just cut out the micronutrients.

Proven Results

Research and development (R&D) play an important role in understanding the importance of micronutrients, especially sulfur, which was once a common soil ingredient from atmospheric sulfur deposited by rainfall. As we have reduced sulfur pollution, or "acid rain," indirect and direct yield response to applied sulfur has increased, especially over the past several years.

Without sulfur in the soil, nitrogen losses can be as great as 30 percent when compared to an N-P-K-only fertilizer. Sulfur also plays a critical role in forming amino acids and proteins and in producing chlorophyll. We have also seen dramatic increases in overall plant health. I have done field tests using simple N-P-K fertilizers against organic, micronutrient-rich blended fertilizers. The results were dramatic and clear. The organic fertilizer meets the micronutrient needs of plants better than the N-P-K-only treatment.

The Natural Cycle

The base ingredient of many organic fertilizers is usually one of the following: chicken manure or dried poultry waste, blood meal, bone meal, feather meal, alfalfa meal, or kelp and fish bone meal. The last two are my favorites and produce healthy plants every time. They are full of both primary nutrients and micronutrients.

The ocean is the lowest part of the earth, where all nutrients eventually deposit. Micronutrients cycle back and are absorbed by simple plankton and higher aquatic plants absorb. Fish consume the aquatic plants, and the larger fish eat smaller fish, transferring the eroded micronutrients from microscopic elements to the large fish we harvest from our oceans. This is why I recommend using fish bone meal as your base ingredient. Fish bone meal is also used in pet foods and in commercial fisheries to help maintain needed nutrients. Eating a diet high in wild caught fish is healthy for us. By contrast, animals raised unsustainably in feedlots, fed a "scientific diet," injected with hormones and antibiotics and restricted in their movements to fatten them produce less nutritious food. While you may not consider these practices inhumane to animals, the negative impact on humans is clear.

Many organic fertilizers use chicken manure as a base ingredient. While this is fine, it is inferior, because it decomposes too quickly and mimics chemical fertilizers in its soluble nutrient availability. Chicken manure is also very salty, which can upset the soil pH.

Other organic fertilizers also use blood meal, bone meal or meat and bone meal as the base ingredient. I believe these ingredients are inferior and do not trust them. Many experts report they have the potential to carry "mad cow disease." Many of these commodity meal ingredients are full of hormones and antibiotics introduced to feed lot animals in genetically modified grains. Be wise about your choices and ask questions of makers of chicken, blood and bone meal.

Ocean Rich Nutrients
I prefer nutrients from the ocean. I like fishmeal, kelp meal and seaweed extract. Fish is full of protein that breaks down and becomes a slow-release source of nitrogen. I also prefer cold-processed kelp meal and the very rich seaweed extract, which contains more than 70 trace minerals along with important growth hormones that strengthen plant cell structure. Kelp and seaweed contain amino acids, enzymes and carbohydrates, both simple and complex. They also enhance seed germination and increase the uptake of nutrients. Sea plants are full of micronutrients and potassium, an essential element for overall plant health and stress relief.

Research and Balance
When I am not writing books or gardening, I research different micronutrient blends and crop mixes. I strive to formulate blends that contain a naturally high percentage of micronutrients such as sulfur and zinc. Small amounts of zinc are critically important to plant health. Getting the right specific balance of a wide range of micronutrients is the key to developing any organic fertilizers and amendments.

Micronutrients are important in many different situations. Soil can be depleted from over gardening or farming. Micronutrient replenishment with organic fertilizers increases crop production, quality of produce and yields healthier fruits and vegetables. The process supports the viability of beneficial soil microbes and mycorrhizae, growing the "good" or "healthy" bacteria for human and animal health. Micronutrient-rich fertilizers can help you save money, reduce fertilizer costs, save on energy use and decrease your carbon footprint. Applying more does not always give more benefit. Getting the balance right is the key to success (just as taking one multi-vitamin is good for you while taking the whole bottle can have adverse effects). Get the balance right!

Chapter 16

⌒⌒⌒⌒⌒

HOW AND WHAT PLANTS EAT

{

In wilderness I sense the miracle of life, and behind it our scientific accomplishments fade to trivia.

-Charles A. Lindbergh

}

Plants consume their food primarily through their roots, and the majority of the nutrients are absorbed through microscopic root hairs. We discussed mycorrhizal fungi *(Chapter 6)* and stomata openings on the leaves *(Chapter 13)*, both of which assist plants in absorbing nutrients. This is why a great soil structure is so imperative; it gives the roots regular access to the needed nutrients in a soil that is heavily laden with organic materials. Root hairs also ensure a slow and steady supply of all needed nutrients on a regular basis for all fruits and vegetables.

The perfect formula for root expansion combines a well-constructed loamy soil with balanced pH, soil that can breathe with plenty of air space, organic humus reserves, microbial diversity and activity, mycorrhizal proliferation and spongy organic soil particles for water retention. Microbes help break down organic matter into forms of nutrients that plants can absorb and use for growth. The living portion of the soil, the probiotics, makes the nutrients available consistently all the time, especially when plants can use them the most. This is usually temperature related. The warmer the weather, the more nutrients a plant needs. In warmer weather, microbes are more active in the soil, releasing the needed nutrients from the organic materials.

When nutrients are stored in and on soil particles, they are conserved for plant roots to use as needed, rather than leeching through the soil to the ground water where they cannot be absorbed by the microscopic root hairs. The greater the soil capacity to store nutrients, the more the roots can feed as needed. As the roots burrow wider and deeper, they absorb more nutrients, which allows plants to grow and produce more fruits and vegetables. The cycle becomes self-perpetuating: better soil, more root mass, larger plants, more absorbed nutrients, producing healthier, nutrient-dense fruits and vegetables.

How and What Do Roots Consume?

Plants retrieve nutrients mainly from water within the soil. Eroding rock and degrading organic matter also make nutrients available in the soil. Microbes decompose organic material but roots do not directly consume microbes, just the nutrients that microbes leave behind. Imagine "microscopic manure" as plant food.

The major nutrients required for healthy plant development are discussed in Chapter 15. Avoid manually adding too much of any one nutrient. You need a chemistry degree to be able to measure out specific nutrient requirements to get it just right. Also, you would need a laboratory analysis of the soil or the leaf tissue if you were to add any one specific nutrient. As long as the soil has a balanced concentration of all needed nutrients, the plant's roots will absorb them in a continual process. Plants absorb needed nutrients through microscopic doors on the root hairs via a process called cation exchange. A plant's cation exchange capacity (or CEC) is a technical discussion beyond the scope of this book. If you want to know more on this subject, consult a good soil chemistry book.

However, if you build a good soil as I have described, you will have a high CEC, and you will not need to know the chemistry. As a backyard gardener, your soil will be healthy and full of life. If you want to grow plants professionally or on a large scale, I strongly encourage you to gain a deep understanding of CEC.

Plants need all the nutrients discussed in Chapter 15. They are absorbed from soil, air and water. Plants use each mineral along with carbon and hydrogen to synthesize compounds such as phytonutrients, vitamins and anti-oxidants. These compounds perform many functions within each plant that help provide structural support, transport fluid, nutrients and assist in metabolism of absorbed food. In general, plants consume macronutrients in large quantities to form root, stem and leaf cells.

Rocks and humus reserves contain micronutrients. Micronutrients support metabolic processes like photosynthesis and the uptake and processing of other nutrients by the plant. Micronutrients are just as important as macronutrients and insure plant processes run smoothly. They support many different functions including proper chlorophyll formation, which affects photosynthesis, which is crucial for activating enzymes and forming hormones. Micronutrients also aid vitamin formation, regulate metabolism and cell growth, promote the efficient use of nitrogen and thus protein formation, and simply allow plant cells to engage in photosynthesis.

Depending on the plant species and the micronutrient, a lack or surplus in one of these nutrients can cause major development problems and in some cases death. For instance, a boron deficiency is a make or break situation. By the time one can see the deficiency, it is too late. Also, over applying these micronutrients can poison plants, since they are needed only in very small quantities.

Sometimes deficiencies can go undetected by the human eye, while something inside the plant is not properly functioning. For example, the plant cell wall may be too thin to protect it. This causes a plant to be more susceptible to pests or disease. If a plant is deficient in any of the essential micronutrients for a long period, noticeable symptoms develop *(as discussed in Chapter 15.)*

Manually applying micronutrients to the soil may be a mistake given our limited knowledge of how micronutrients affect plants. As their name implies, micronutrients are needed only in minute amounts. They promote optimum growth only in a small range. For example, the range in which boron is either deficient or over-concentrated and toxic is only a few parts per million. For this reason, safely applying boron requires precision beyond the average gardener's abilities. In addition, even a small excess in one micronutrient can cause a deficiency in another, since these elements interact.

Macronutrients are needed in larger quantities. Introducing too much of a macronutrient through over fertilization can create deficiencies in micronutrients. For example, too much potassium leads to too little manganese absorption. Managing all the hazards is difficult. Fortunately, there are ways you can work around these hazards.

Little Things Matter

Micronutrients may be more important for healthy, strong, pest- and disease-resistant plant development than the major N-P-K nutrients receiving the most attention in recent decades. Raw organic material contains a variety of micronutrients that can be preserved naturally in the soil. Organic matter contains molecules that electromagnetically "grip" the nutrients and prevent them from leaching through the soil and beyond the reach of plants. I stress the importance of micronutrients in the soil, because they are the building blocks for healthy plant material.

Walk down the vitamin aisle at your local grocery store and notice the many options you have for supplementing essential nutrients. You can purchase a single-ingredient vitamin, such as vitamin C, a vitamin complex such as a B complex or a multivitamin that has a bit of everything.

All vitamins are good and necessary. It makes sense to take vitamin supplements, because we do not get enough vitamins in foods that are grown commercially in nutrient poor soils. However, multivitamin supplements do not contain phytochemicals, which may be as essential as vitamins and minerals to maintaining good health. Phytochemicals are beneficial compounds, such as antioxidants other than vitamins and minerals, like beta-carotene, lycopene and sulforaphane found in a number of vegetables. *(See Parts 4 and 6 for more on these.)*

Research on these beneficial phytonutrients is still in its infancy, but some evidence points toward health benefits. Industrially processing freshly harvested plants probably causes us to lose many phytochemicals and their potentially beneficial effects, such as resistance to disease. Processing is like cooking the nutrients right out of fruits and vegetables. We know that the more we alter anything from its natural state, the less nourishment it gives us. For this reason, doctors recommend eating plenty of raw salad.

Plants contain more vitamins, minerals and phytochemicals than one supplement can contain. Because nutrition is a relatively new science, researchers are still unsure which nutrients, plant compounds and ratios work best. The content and balance needs also differ between men and women. Supplementing will not fully compensate for lacking a well-balanced diet of many different fruits, vegetables, carbohydrates and proteins. Even if you grow and consume as many fruits and vegetables as you can, you may still want to supplement with a well-rounded "bioavailable" multivitamin for extra protection. I do. The essence of growing a healthy garden is to maximize the nutrient density in those foods, but we live in a polluted world. If you ever eat out or travel, you will never be able to grow every ounce of food you eat.

Chapter 17

∞∞∞

THE IMPORTANCE OF PLANT HEALTH

We see so many good reasons to grow plants organically for our health. First, the taste is far better than any retail or conventionally grown fruits or vegetables. Corporate agriculture has commoditized our produce for the sake of profits not taste. This loss of quality in favor of profits has been demonstrated in hundreds of different types of food fairs, taste comparisons, farmers markets and your local supermarket. Organic produce is more appealing and flavorful because of the variety and abundance of available nutrients it absorbs.

Second, and most important, organically grown plants are nutrient dense; they have every nutrient available to them as they grow and develop. This nutrient density is the quantity and quality of nutrition plants contain from having consumed all their needed nutrients. You could say people are well nourished when they eat fruits and vegetables from plants that were well nourished themselves.

A third distinction between organic and artificially fertilized plants is the bioaccumulation of toxins in chemically treated plants. This is a fancy way of saying plants grown in conventional soils pumped full of synthetic fertilizers, pesticides and herbicides are detrimental to a living, healthy body. Toxins accumulate in our bodies as we age and consume more contaminated food. The older a plant, animal or human becomes, the more it will accumulate metals and other toxins in the body. Eating organic produce from your own backyard garden is your best insurance against accumulating toxins in your body.

The fourth reason to grow organic is to promote a better environment. When you grow your backyard garden in a healthy, organic way, you contribute to environmental health on an interconnected global level. If you consume healthy foods and apply only natural and organic soil amendments and fertilizers, you have made a conscious decision to care for the environment. These actions have a far greater reach than you might imagine. When everybody employs organic methods, the benefits become global.

The Healthy Cycle

Plants need a naturally well-balanced and dense variety of nutrients for healthy growth and to yield their fullest potential. Healthy plants strive to remain top competitors for their sustenance. Their well developed, more robust roots, stems and leaves are naturally more resistant to pests and diseases. If you minimize weeds in your garden by removing them by hand, you allow your fruits and vegetables to compete against and prevent other, non-desirable plants from becoming established. This ensures your desired plants absorb all of the nutrients.

Most importantly, healthy plants pass on essential nutrients to the next generation of plant growth. After a plant dies, do not put it into the garbage. Instead, do one of two things. Either compost it or turn it back into the soil to allow microbes to digest it and release nutrients the living plant once consumed. Living organisms break down the dead plant into a plethora of nutrients for future plants grown in that soil. This is how nutrient dense plants lead to healthier soil for the next generation. Ideally, this positive loop continues until soils can sustain healthy plant growth with minimal use of fertilizers. There will always be a deficit, simply because as something is always being taken out of the soil, even in minute amounts, whatever is lacking must be replenished. Nutrients are like a bank balance. When you pull money out of your account, you have to make a deposit to restore the original account balance. Whenever you borrow from the soil, you need to reinvest in it.

Conversely, if you directly feed plants water-soluble, synthetic fertilizers that contain only primary macronutrients and micronutrients, the soil account is depleted without being replenished. This depletion undercuts the living soil organisms that degrade organic matter. This practice may eventually lead to the complete depletion of microbes, leaving nothing in the soil to digest dead plant matter and excrete nutrients for new plants. Plants grown this way then have to rely on nutrients applied as fertilizer, with much lower nutrient density. A plant grown in oversimplified N-P-K fertilizer cannot match the nutritive quality of a plant grown in nutrient rich organic soils. Without a constant supply of organic nutrition, plants have no way to obtain trace elements for strong healthy growth. Consequently, they will not be able to contribute as much to the overall nutrition of the consumers of the plants, the animals we consume and ultimately us.

Healthy plants provide a high concentration of nutrients to the food web. All living things benefit from healthy plants, starting with the microorganisms that live in the soil. Life benefits every time we work a healthy plant into the soil and till it under. The next generation of plants benefits because the soil they are grown in is healthy and contains an abundance of nutrients for its continual growth. Animals are healthier because they are consuming healthy plants. Ultimately, humans are the greatest beneficiaries of this cycle, because we are the highest on the food chain. The entire cycle simply translates to human health.

The Global Garden

The healthier the plant, the more carbon dioxide it uses, which leaves less in the atmosphere to contribute to the greenhouse effect and global warming. Through plant respiration, more oxygen goes into the atmosphere so we have better air quality. Plants use CO_2 and provide us with the oxygen we need for motor functions and metabolism. Every time you choose to make a healthy decision for yourself or your family, chances are good that the environment will benefit from it. Even if you did not grow all of your food, and most people in modern countries do not, you can help the health of the environment and further perpetuate your own health. When you buy organic produce from a farmers market, you get your produce via a truck that transported it over a short distance As a result, feeding you requires less fuel and creates less pollution. When you buy a packaged product in a store, (tea as an example), even if it was grown in India, if it was grown organically, you have helped the environment since chemical fertilizers or pesticides were not applied. When you apply an organic fertilizer or soil to your backyard, you aid the recycling of organic materials that would have been thrown away. Ask your neighbor for his leaf litter, and build a compost pile in your backyard. I grew up in an urban setting and still managed to maintain a regular compost pile. I even added chicken manure from the few chickens I raised in the middle of the city. There is no reason not to compost unless you live in an apartment.

Consider the popular phrase, "Think globally. Act locally." Global health starts with human health. If you care for yourself and your family and make conscious choices daily, if your garden is healthy and you care for it naturally, you have just made a global environmental impact.

Chapter 18

∞∞

WHY GO ORGANIC?

> *If you have health, you probably will be happy, and if you have health and happiness, you have all the wealth you need, even if it is not all you want.*
>
> *-Elbert Hubbard*

Organic gardening gives me the comfort of knowing I have adopted a healthy lifestyle on a journey towards a long and healthy life. The true organic gardener becomes familiar with the soil, plants and animals, getting close to the environment. He is also inquisitive and pays attention to detail. Nothing gets by him, as he has a keen eye for health.

Adopting organic methods has become confusing, because we lack a true definition of organic gardening. What do we mean when we say something is organic?

Stipulations on the Term Organic

There are a few stipulations to make in defining organic. To chemists, organic refers to the presence of a carbon molecule. Most gardeners get confused by the terms natural and organic. Technically, all natural materials containing carbon are organic, but not all natural materials are organic. Sand particles are completely natural but are not derived from a living source. Sand never contained carbon as an element, so it is not organic. All things derived from a living source that contained carbon meet the definition of organic. You and I are organic by definition, because our every living cell contains carbon.

Organic gardening refers to a smaller plot grown for personal use. With this in mind, you may do anything you want to your plants without breaking any laws or policies. You can freely apply synthetic pesticides to your strawberries and say you grow organically without any legal repercussions. You might fool your neighbors, but you can't fool your body.

Organic growing is gardening or cultivating intended to bring food to the market place. All organic produce grown and distributed throughout the U.S. must follow strict guidelines set by the USDA (U.S. Department of Agriculture) or private certifying agencies like the C.C.O.F. (California Certified Organic Farmers) and OMRI (Organic Materials Review Institute). These groups make sure farmers are not using anything that would be considered unsafe for human exposure. Each farm must be certified organic through a process that lasts for a defined period. Growers who misrepresent and sell their produce to others may face prosecution for fraud.

To qualify as organic, produce must not have received or been exposed to synthetic (non-organic or non-natural) herbicides, pesticides or fertilizers as well as any ingredients from genetically modified organisms (GMOs). *(See Chapter 19 for a full discussion of GMOs.)* Organic versions of these treatments do exist and must be compounds extracted from plants or other natural resources. These compounds do not have to be naturally produced in the local environment but may come from distant locations. (Some exceptions to these rules allow the use of synthetic chemicals. Where extreme environmental conditions make it difficult to get a significant yield, the USDA has allowed organic certification in the presence of some synthetic chemicals, saying the chemicals it allows do not affect the health of humans, animals or the environment.)

Organic From a Distance
With refrigeration and efficient transportation networks, commercial agriculture supplies our grocery stores with all the produce we can imagine, whether organic or not. Some is grown locally; some across the nation; some imported from other continents. (The National Sustainable Agriculture Coalition says much of our produce travels 1,500 to 2,500 miles to get to the table.) Thus, we can buy many produce items all year round. You may ask, "What enables a farming operation to say it is organic? How does that change the treatment of our food?"

Organic gardeners generally agree on avoiding synthetic pesticides, fertilizers and genetically modified organisms. Outside of those general conventions, you can find a variety of gardening strategies. Some organic gardeners are quite strict, believing that an organic plant cannot receive any type of nutrient treatment other than what naturally exists in the local area. Others take a more liberal approach by treating the soil, feeding the foliage, and even introducing treatments that control temperature and light availability.

Unless you know organic practices and techniques, you cannot know the effects, positive or negative, the plants you grow will have on people or the surrounding environment. It helps to understand how and why "organic is good" before you assume it. Otherwise, it is easy to fall into a trap of uncritically trusting everything that someone somewhere says is organic.

My View on Organic Practices

I see organic gardening, growing and farming as a beneficial cause that generates more good results than bad. A conventional farm that adopts even some organic methods for the sake of marketing its produce is better than one that adopts none at all and continues to farm with artificial chemicals. Truly, every little bit helps.

Many progressive people who follow organic practices want to conserve the beautiful biological diversity of our planet that allows humans and animals to enjoy a comfortable and healthy existence. However, some organic practices are not necessarily beneficial to humans, animals or the environment. Saying "Natural is good" is an oversimplification similar to saying a synthetic pesticide that gets rid of bugs or weeds is good or that genetically modified organisms are good because they give the farmer a better crop. When we understand the effects of our treatments, we can properly apply them to yield benefits while avoiding the adverse effects. Most important is to educate yourself on what goes into your body. We are what we eat, and what we eat has consequences for our health.

What Does Organic Growing Mean to Me?

By now my approach should be clear: To build soil naturally, I rely on supporting beneficial soil organisms. I feed the living soil organic materials using compost, planting mix and organic fertilizers. These provide my plants nutritive sustenance for strong and steady growth. Nutrient-dense plants are full of flavor and have positive effects on the environment and human health.

I allow no synthetic chemicals of any kind in my garden. Government agencies allow many synthetic chemicals on a "certified organic" farm that I would not let within 100 feet of my home. No synthetic pesticides, fungicides or herbicides allowed! My goal is to maintain a safe environment for my family and pets to enjoy.

Here is the rule I live by: If I can't quickly identify the ingredient on the label, I don't use it. (Years ago I heard a health advocate say, "If you can't pronounce it, don't use it. If you can't spell it, don't eat it.")

I attempt to recreate the indigenous conditions plants grew in naturally before human involvement. (After all, if it grew and reproduced, it had all it needed.) If I grow something not native to my area that requires treatment, I use the safest possible organic methods with ingredients I can easily identify.

I avoid harmful organic practices and urge you to educate yourself on any ingredient you wish to use. I have said taking one multivitamin is good, but swallowing the whole jar is bad. This rule (more than the right dose is too much) applies to organic gardening as well. Too much of a good thing can be dangerous. Growth in nature is based on a balance in soil organisms and nutrient cycles. Shoveling a bunch of organic matter, microbes and treatments into dirt may harm the environment. Also, if the balance is off, (a lack of some nutrients and an excess of others) plants will not grow well.

For example, too many applied microbes in an organic fertilizer make it act like a synthetic fertilizer. The excess microbes digest the organic fertilizer too quickly. Infusing too many microbes with an organic fertilizer makes the soil lose nutrients well before the plant roots can absorb them. Similarly, if you use inferior base ingredients, such as chicken manure or dehydrated manure, (which naturally break down very fast) this combination creates a fertilizer that works destructively too fast, similar to a chemical fertilizer.

Inadequate and unwise products such as these come to market from the drive to make profits off people's ignorance and misplaced trust. Many unethical companies try to outdo each other by asserting they have more microbes in their fertilizer blends, making them better for your garden. This is deceitful marketing at its most cynical.

Organic growing follows nature's perfection and beauty. While people are clever and inventive, Mother Nature outwits us with her experience and perfection. I love life and seek to work within the guidelines nature has provided. In trying to push nature to its limits, more is not necessarily better. I want organic farms and my garden to promote human and animal health by producing nutrient rich foods while doing no harm.

Why Choose to Grow or Eat Organically?
Growing everything organically benefits your health by minimizing your exposure to unnatural chemicals. Your minimal to zero use of synthetic chemicals and pesticides also helps reduce the level of toxicity all around us. You also help protect vulnerable species that are not the target of pesticides. (Pesticides and other synthetics intended to exterminate certain pests do not affect only their target species. They also can injure or kill others in the process, including livestock, pets and humans, further reducing the essential biodiversity in our environment.)

Of the tens of thousands of chemicals agriculture and industry use in the U.S. each year, only a few hundred are tested for safety. For example, the pesticide DDT was banned in the U.S. in 1972 only after considerable damage had already been done. DDT is still produced and exported for use in foreign agriculture, and we are vulnerable to exposure since it infiltrates some foods we import. Therefore, buying organics from overseas may also bring health benefits.

I advocate leaving our food pure and simple as the most important choice we make several times a day. Avoid additives such as preservatives and colorings. Food processors use tons of synthesized chemicals to fabricate the taste and appearance of what we eat. Read the label and buy from a trusted source or grow it yourself.

Organic methods also support animal health. We can raise animals without synthetic hormones and antibiotics and feed them nutrient-dense organic food. Besides the nutritive qualities of organic meats, this is the most humane way to raise animals. They can enjoy their time under our watch playing in nature rather than being confined to inhumane cages for the sake of fattening them up.

Whether you eat produce that is commercially grown organic or homegrown, you can better support environmental conservation if you understand which practices create and maintain soil health and fertility. Feeding the soil feeds everything that comes out of it, plants, animals and, ultimately, humans. Organic gardening is all about creating and maintaining the natural circle of life existing between growing plants, soil and living organisms. By applying nutrient packed organic matter (compost, organic fertilizers, soil amendments and seaweeds) and eliminating synthetic chemicals, you enable microorganisms to do what they do best: break down organic matter to enrich the soil that surrounds the roots of our food plants.

The heart of organic practice is feeding the soil without using artificial fertilizers or pesticides. It is also the first step in preventing the loss of microbes and minerals, crop contamination and water pollution.

We can grow plants that are highly resistant to diseases and pests without using modern chemical treatments. While organic control is more labor-intensive, the long-term health of the environment and people is worth it.

My ideal is to stimulate the desire for everyone to develop a "green thumb" and grow organic produce at home. Not having to travel to the grocery store only to face a choice among inferior veggies is terrific. Yet, I understand this may not be practical for people living in small rented spaces or those who work 50-plus hours per week just to make ends meet. And shopping at the grocery store is more practical for people who have many other interests.

Even if you shop regularly at a supermarket, you can still support the values and ideals that organic stands for. Converting to organic farming from less sustainable, less healthy commercial practices requires an enormous investment risk in both money and time. You can support and motivate more of the people making these conversions by purchasing as much organic food as you can afford from local markets. While organic food costs a bit more than non-organic, the short-term cost is more than balanced out by the long-term gain of conserving our soil and providing pesticide free produce to support our overall good health. As we demand and support more organic foods and products, even large-scale companies will have to respond and make changes to serve the market demand. They will adopt healthier practices provided we vote with our wallets. By the sources you choose to obtain your food, you are voting for how you want your food produced.

Chapter 19

GENETICALLY MODIFIED ORGANISMS (GMOs)

> *Not one man in a thousand has accuracy of eye and judgment sufficient to become an eminent breeder. If gifted with these qualities, and he studies his subject for years, and devotes his lifetime to it with indomitable perseverance, he will succeed and will make great improvements; if he wants any of these qualities, he will assuredly fail.*
>
> *- Charles Darwin*

A genetically modified organism (GMO) has had its DNA decoded and manipulated to create something different than what has developed naturally. The technique used is called genetic engineering or recombinant DNA technology. Creating GMOs involves taking DNA molecules from inside the cells of different organisms and combining them into one molecule to create a new set of genes. These new genes are then inserted into the cells of a plant or animal to produce characteristics the recipient never had.

For example, scientists can take a trait of a bacterium such as *Bacillus thuringiensis* (Bt) and genetically insert its DNA into another organism to create a new molecule. They then insert that novel gene into living plant cells such as corn and soybeans to create a completely new set of genes and a food plant with modified characteristics.

Why is this a problem worth our concern? We have no idea of where this may lead. Even the strongest supporters of genetic engineering admit there is great uncertainty concerning these processes and their consequences. As the reports of almost all research results in our popular media say, "Further research is needed."

Besides the unknown consequences, many people are troubled by the ethical problems of "playing God." When you decode the DNA of a living organism and manipulate it to create a new and unique being, an ethical debate is inevitable. Bioengineering has been called the final frontier. The scientists doing this work, however well intentioned, have been accused of tampering with the natural evolution of all living things on earth. These new plants, sometimes called transgenic plants, are highly valued by many conventional farmers and people in poor, Third World countries, because they require fewer people and less money to produce, are often more durable and disease resistant, and may forestall mass hunger and starvation.

Who could be opposed to all those benefits? No one, but the question is not whether GMOs are good or bad. The problem is the mass distribution and marketing of GMOs when so little is known about their impact on our health and the environment.

Throughout most of human existence, we have evolved alongside the plants we have grown in natural ways. In the 1990's, genetically modified (GM) foods were introduced to the marketplace. GM foods changed our relationship with plants significantly. GM products typically are those commodity crops such as soybeans, corn, canola and cottonseed. These plants are everywhere, and a plethora of foods now contain some ingredient from GM production.

The real issue is not legality but ethics. Seventy-five percent of all processed foods in the U.S. contain some GM ingredient. Eighty percent of soy and forty percent of corn is genetically modified. GM products are here, but no regulator required anyone to tell us. Food packagers are not required to disclose if a GM ingredient is present in their products. If genetic modification is completely safe, there should be no objection to a labeling requirement. Perhaps only rebellious, resistant consumers can force GM product labeling.

I am not against modifying and improving on what Mother Nature gave us. I love and respect the brilliant work of Luther Burbank, for example, who worked carefully for many years to produce hybrid plants with just the right traits before releasing them to the public for mass consumption. (According to a wikipedia.org entry, Burbank created more than 800 strains and varieties of plants during his 55-year career.) I am sure he would have wanted no part in genetically modifying plants, which I imagine he would consider "cheating" because it avoids the hard work and research usually invested to make a plant best fit for consumption.

I am all for improving a plant's productivity and health potential provided we do not harm the ecosystem. But genetic modification goes far beyond hybridizing two different plants within a species to create a new and improved variety.

While I support developing and using hybrid varieties, I also believe we must all grow heirloom varieties of fruits and vegetables while they are still available to us. An heirloom plant is one grown in earlier periods of human history before large-scale industrial agriculture began the widespread use of hybrid species. (People disagree on the definition of heirloom. Some say 50-100 years old. Some say when hybrids became dominant in U.S. farming after World War II, which ended in

1945, we no longer had true heirloom plants.) We should foster heirloom seeds and plants as good stewards of the environment and to maintain what is left of our food biodiversity.

I enjoy growing several kinds of tomatoes every year. Most are heirlooms, but I experiment with a few hybridized varieties, too. I appreciate the tireless hard work of horticulturists in their efforts to bring new and improved varieties to market. Still, this is simply helping nature create in a shorter time what she might have eventually developed on her own. For example, taking pollen from one plant and using it to manually pollinate another is the breeder's way of speeding up a natural process to achieve taste, sugar, nutrient content, color, disease resistance or other desirable characteristics. As a gardener, you should always focus on growing heirloom varieties first. However, growing some hybrids is safe for human health.

Biodiversity should concern us all. We can potentially consume about 80,000 different edible plants, yet only 200 to 300 are offered in the supermarket, including the spice rack ingredients. These relatively few plants make up about 90 percent of our food. This lack of diversity makes our food supply vulnerable to even slight changes in our environment. This is another example of giant agribusiness narrowly pursuing high profits at the expense of our health and safety.

The coexistence of GM plants with conventional and organic crops has raised significant concern in many European countries. There is separate legislation for GM crops and a high demand from consumers for the freedom of choice between GM and non-GM foods. There are requirements to separate foods and feed produced from GM plants from conventional and organic foods. European research programs continue to investigate appropriate tools and rules. At the field level, biological containment measures to segregate GM and non-GM agriculture include isolation distances and pollen barriers. I believe there are only a few winners from what I just described, namely, the conglomerate biotech companies, giant agribusinesses and attorneys who represent both. Attempting to regulate and contain genetically modified foods instead of simply banning the process seems to create political confusion when what people want is a delicious, healthy meal at the end of the day.

Altering Evolution

Normal plant evolution occurs through natural selection. Plants with specific characteristics in their genes can retain nutrients and survive under a variety of environmental pressures like high winds, poor air quality, extreme temperatures and rainfall. Plants that are naturally adapted to the difficult conditions are able to survive. Other plants within a species that lack the traits needed to survive those pressures do not reproduce. Eventually their less-favored traits perish out of the species.

By choosing gene combinations in plants and repeatedly breeding those combinations for crops, we interfere with natural selection and alter natural evolution. The fundamental basis of organic gardening is balance. Living organisms evolve over long time periods as their environmental conditions change. If we throw off the evolution of plants in one environment, everything that interacts with the plants, such as predators or organisms with a symbiotic relationship, may be thrown off balance as well. It might take us thousands of years to know the full environmental impact of "playing God" by tampering with the natural evolution of a plant or animal species.

To understand what practices are best for mankind and the natural world requires knowing many fields of study. Genetic modification and its implications are too new to have been well studied. What we can say with confidence: The effects on plant, animal and human health are largely uncertain. Throwing off the balance of nature carries high risks, although much more research must be done to determine the net effects of GM products. Because of the relentless corporate drive for profits, biotechnology companies spend money on researching how they can bioengineer animal and plant species, not the bioethical or long-term health implications for animals and humans. Therefore, the call and pressure to step back and take the long-range view must come from the organic and environmental communities and health conscious consumers.

Genetically Modified Plants in Agriculture

Among the concerns over GMOs, people worry that genetically modified plants are spreading those genes to their wild relatives outside the agricultural operation. Such spreading genetically modifies all plants. This will continue as more genetically modified acres are planted. Many people are studying how to prevent the gene flow between crops and neighboring relatives. The agribusiness companies say they are working to grow GM plants in areas with neighboring crops from completely different species. They assert these efforts act as a hard control for the spread of GM products into the wild or domesticated crops, but it is not an effective control in many environments.

Another concern arises over neighboring agricultural operations growing the same plants with different strategies. One field may use GM products, while another may not and still another might be organic. What prevents the field with GM products spreading through wind and other natural forces into the traditional field or the organic field?

We need more regulation of genetically modified crops in certain systems that have a high risk of spreading their GM properties. Present regulations include creating buffer zones between crop fields and prohibiting growing GM plants in places where their relatives exist as wild neighbors. Additional containment efforts involve genetic modification to change the plant's breeding season. This is a scary thought. In order to control the spread of GM plants into the wild or neighboring operations, more modification is made. When does it end? What effects do more and more modifications have on plant health? When does our intervention stop? I suspect "never" as long as genetic engineering and agribusiness firms control both the law-making process and the flow of research money.

Positive Effects of GM Plants

I am not so extreme that I cannot acknowledge the benefits of something I disagree with. GMOs do carry benefits and have value. If they did not, companies would not develop them and farmers would not buy and use them.

For example, improving plant growth and crop yields might mean less land would be needed to produce the same amount of food, leaving more room for the natural ecosystem.

More specifically, GM seeds may enable us to use fewer chemicals. Because synthetic chemicals like pesticides and herbicides have direct negative effects on soil health, ground water, non-targeted insects, birds and wild plant populations, anything that reduces the need or demand for chemicals is a step in the right direction. Making plants resistant to pests or diseases through genetic modification can reduce the need to spray thousands of gallons of harmful chemicals onto the land. Genetically modified herbicide-resistant crops enable the grower to use less toxic herbicide and therefore reduce the detriment caused to living organisms that interact with the plants.

Scientists are also creating GM plants that are more resilient to environmental pressures like nutrient depletion, lack of water or unbalanced pH. This will help plants to survive and provide higher yields for poverty-stricken countries. For example, scientists have created certain nutrients within foods by adding the gene to rice that codes for a precursor to Vitamin A. Half of the world consumes rice, and the resulting crop helps avoid a Vitamin A deficiency in locations where foods rich in Vitamin A are scarce.

In the future, genetic engineers may be able to breed organisms to help restore soil nutrients and structure bioremediation. GM products might improve the shelf life of fruits and vegetables, decreasing waste and increasing the amount of food available. These are some possible net benefits of GM foods.

Negative Effects of GM Plants

GM plants and products present many bioethical questions. The final frontier of God's divine code has been hidden in the genetic makeup of the DNA double helix molecule. The moment we cracked the genetic code and began altering it, we began to play God. While this is not a book on ethics, a thoughtful person cannot ignore ethical questions.

Using pesticides and GM plants with the Bt gene could lead to an increase in resistant pests through natural selection. We can kill off all but a few insects that carry the resistance to our treatments, but then the survivors may proliferate and create a need for a different treatment. What do we do then? We could genetically modify plants further and run the risk of repeated failure.

Even though we see more GM plants, herbicide sales continue to rise. Increasing use of herbicides adversely affects soil biota, herbivores and birds. These living things interact with the GM plants sprayed with herbicides. A similar problem occurs with using herbicides. We always find a few weeds that are resistant to treatment. This resistance enables the survival and redevelopment of the species. There may be other environmental effects of having all-resistant pests and weeds in the environment. It is completely unnatural for there to be no vulnerable species that eventually die off through natural selection.

The potential negative effects of consuming GM plants fall on many living organisms, from bees eating pollen to rabbits eating wild greens. The inserted genes may destabilize some generation of a GM plant somewhere in its genome, causing a mutation that leads to unhealthy consequences. No one knows what is going to happen in a few years or a few decades to modified plant genes. They could mutate into an uncontrollable form that might be completely unhealthy for human consumption. By inserting a gene into what is thought to be an inactive portion of the genome, we may inadvertently turn on or off another gene, causing long-term destructive effects. It is common knowledge that GM plants have a different protein molecule than their native cousins. How will that molecular difference affect the health of the animals we consume, or even more importantly, our health?

In short, we do not fully understand the net benefit or harm of GMOs to environmental, animal and human health. And that full understanding may be far into the future. Scientists still need to conduct thorough investigation on the effects of each type of genetically modified plant.

I believe financial motives are too strong for most people and companies to resist. If we leave research to the developer or patent owner of a GM crop, the findings will always be skewed in its favor. I do not say there is no place for GM foods or technology, but I do believe we need more testing by independent organizations who have no financial stake in the findings. Many more years of testing will be required before I feel safe.

In the meantime, what should responsible gardeners do? Buy and grow as many heirloom varieties as possible. Keep the gene pool alive with biodiversity. Do not buy foods from the market unless you know they are free of GM ingredients. Stay attuned to developments in GM processes. You can raise and buy food the natural way. We evolved without GM foods, and I am sure we can continue to thrive without them.

Chapter 20

∞∞∞

THE ABILITY TO RESIST PESTS AND DISEASES

{
To feel keenly the poetry of a morning's roses, one has to have just escaped from the claws of this vulture which we call sickness.
- Henri Frederic Amiel
}

Pest control starts in the soil. If your soil is healthy and you have diseases under control, plants are far less vulnerable to attack by pests. Also, biodiversity supports healthy soils that keep diseases under control.

Most plant pathogens are fungal. If you limit or remove the environment that fungus loves by making it less favorable, you minimize their ability to thrive and destroy your garden. For example, dark and damp soil with overhead sprinkler systems is the perfect environment for fungus. If there are ample fungal-feeding organisms present in the soil, many of the fungal spores will be eaten before they begin to grow and spread. Well-aerated and evenly moist soil cuts down on anaerobic conditions to help control fungal pathogens and discourage denitrifying bacteria. These conditions simultaneously minimize nitrogen loss from the soil. In Chapter 5, we discussed probiotics, which also help control fungal pathogens in the soil. This all goes back to biodiversity and a healthy balanced soil.

Healthy plants naturally resist pest and diseases in two ways. First, the thicker a plant cell wall, the more it resists infection and insect attack. Secondly, a weak and susceptible plant transmits an electro-magnetic signal in the same frequency range for destructive insects, calling them to come and eat it. Plants grown organically naturally develop steadily and thoroughly as they have access to a more diverse reservoir of nutrients. As a result, they will be stronger and more resistant to pests and diseases. Biodiversity is the key factor. The living variety of organisms in the soil, both micro and macro, helps regulate fungal pathogens and insects. Beneficial nematodes, mites, and mycorrhizal fungi are all great for fighting pest and disease problems.

Controlling pests and diseases is far more important for farmers because of the sheer volume of produce they handle. Pests thrive in the grand opportunity that exists where they can eat or lay eggs in hundreds of acres of plants. The home gardener, with a much smaller crop, has much less concern for large colonies of pests settling into the garden permanently, especially if he grows a wide variety of fruits, vegetables, herbs and flowers.

Plants do not naturally grow to the standards of perfection (no spots and perfect complexion) we see in a supermarket produce section. Rather than trying to eradicate all weeds, diseases and pests, we can manage them in a way that is non-toxic, sustainable and gratifying. Some diseases and pests, however, are quite abundant and cause problems for gardeners. You have many different treatment approaches other than using commercial chemicals. Don't be misled to thinking high yields and quality demands exterminating all pests, diseases and weeds with chemicals. By taking an organic approach, you can manage the complex functioning of nature that has sustained life for hundreds of millions of years. With organic methods, you can support a diversity of life in your garden.

Approaches to Managing Pests and Diseases

The first step is to grow strong and healthy plants. Not all conditions warrant the use of insecticides or fungicides. If just a few caterpillars or slugs are crawling around on the leaves, you can physically pick them off the plants. As we have said many times, overuse or misapplication of pesticides and fungicides seriously disrupts the biodiversity in the soil and affects the phytotoxicity of the plant itself. Also, pests can become resistant to the treatment. You then need to apply even more chemicals to achieve similar results. Repeatedly applying more toxic chemicals perpetuates an uninhabitable environment so toxic that no life can survive in it. Consider some alternatives.

Natural Chemical-Free Methods

Natural methods manage and prevent harm to plants by pests or diseases without resorting to sprays. The first step is to identify the disease or pest and when they are active. Then we can devise a way to minimize the damaging effects. Here are a few.

Remove pests by hand or rinsing. Some pests crawl along leaves, eating them or using them to lay their eggs. Catching and removing pests early, while requiring more labor, can prevent exponentially escalating problems. Some pests, like slugs and snails, are more active on damp nights, while others are active during dry sunny days. Some pests can be rinsed off plants with a powerful stream of water. Attachments that hook up to your hose are designed to blast bugs off foliage.

Removing pests by hand or rinsing is better than spraying, especially near ponds, streams or lakes, since pesticides can injure or kill aquatic life.

Remove badly infested or diseased plants to minimize spreading to healthy neighboring plants. Put infested or diseased plants in a closed plastic bag and remove them from your property to minimize contamination.

Install barricades. There are a few different types of barricades. If you want to protect smaller plants from birds or animals, construct a small frame around the plant and enclose the area with mesh netting. You can also cover groups of fruits like apples or pears with pantyhose or tights to stop insects or birds from feeding on your freshly ripe fruit. Placing cut-off plastic bottles around smaller plants will help protect and warm up the soil around the roots to promote microbe activity. Row covers made from material with small holes can protect entire rows from birds, beetles, bad worms and maggots. Cabbage maggots like to lay their eggs in the soil right around plants. You can deter them by placing a collar made of cardboard or some other fabric around the stems. This causes females to lay their eggs on the collar where the eggs will dry out before hatching.

Pheromone traps can attract pests to monitor when they will be most damaging. Pheromones are gaseous chemicals that insects and animals use to communicate with each other, locate plants or find a mate. For example, by trapping certain insects, you can determine the best time to apply a pesticide to stop the offspring from causing plant damage.

Sticky traps used in various locations can stop pests in their tracks. Non-flying insects travel up and down plants such as trees. Placing a sticky band around, but not touching, the tree trunk will keep these pests from reaching their destination. You can also place other sticky bands around containers to stop bugs like ants or earwigs. Traps can be hung above plants in greenhouses to capture flying pests. This step indicates the extent of the invasion. Additional controls may further deter plant damage. Other traps such as half-full cans of beer can be buried at soil level near plants to attract slugs and snails. They fall in, get drunk and drown.

Repellents usually deter birds, deer, rodents and moles by using bothersome smells, tastes or noises these animals don't like. Soaps, oils and noise repellents are available at some nurseries. For getting rid of moles or gophers, try this trick. At your local barbershop, ask for some cut hair they normally sweep up and throw away. Place the hair in the rodent's hole. Gophers and moles will perceive a human is down there with them and be repelled from your garden. Buried hair also breaks down into nitrogen-rich fertilizer.

Biological Pest Control Tactics

These involve recruiting the help of pest predators or spraying pests with living organisms. Remember biodiversity checks and balances, but if the balance is off, you can use these techniques

Releasing pest predators like ladybugs and praying mantis are a good, safe approach. Planting flowers and other shrubs around the garden can attract and provide shelter for pest eaters such as birds, frogs, toads, bats and certain insects. This is called companion planting.

Having a small body of water, like a pond, nearby will provide a breeding ground for creatures like frogs and toads. If you add pest predators, avoid following it with an insecticide, which can kill off the predators and be a waste of money. If you must spray, do it first, and release predators a few days later.

Beneficial microbes -- Bt, or *Bacillus thuringiensis* -- are a great and safe way to control lepidopteron larvae, or caterpillars, as they are commonly known. This is considered one of the most effective ways to get rid of leaf-chewing pests. Different treatments have environmental conditions under which they operate best. For instance, Bt is less effective when applied in direct sun. Caterpillars feed only in warm weather, so apply Bt when it is warm, but not in direct sun to maximize its potential. Early morning is the best time to apply.

Botanical sprays use essential oils like cinnamon, clove, mint, rosemary, eucalyptus and wintergreen oil to kill and control a wide variety of pests. These substances kill by blocking chemical signals that control body functions. Basically, the substances immobilize insects. Botanical oils are completely derived from plants and break down in the environment quickly to harmless substances that do not persist or cause environmental damage.

Garlic extract is also a great option to repel pests. Garlic fools pests into thinking they are on the wrong plant so they move to another from sheer confusion. Most pests smell receptors are located on the bottom of their legs. When they land on a plant that has been sprayed with essential oils or garlic, it smells different from their target plant, and they move on to neighboring plants.

Chemical Approaches

Use these as a last resort when nothing else has worked. If you have a biologically diverse garden, you may never need a toxic chemical to control pests or disease. However, if you do use chemicals, read the label carefully and never over apply. More is not better.

I do not like chemicals around my home. The very nature of using a chemical on the healthy garden defeats everything we have discussed. I don't recommend any specific chemical treatment. If you choose a chemical treatment, remember that pests develop resistance to pesticides, requiring stronger and more frequent applications to be effective. Toxic pesticide use may be detrimental to the environment and severely disrupt the balance of living organisms in the soil. Pesticides are also severe pollutants of ground water, lakes, rivers and oceans. While more detrimental on the large-scale farm, backyard pesticide use can also damage the environment.

To Spray or Not to Spray

Unfortunately, in some cases we don't have a choice between using chemical treatments and letting nature take its course. If you must spray to save the garden, employ one of the methods discussed above. When infestation grows out of control, the only quick way to get rid of pests may be to get out the extermination sprays to salvage plants. Fortunately, some well-developed treatments have minimal side effects when used properly.

Any chemical agent controlling insects and disease should be used as a last resort and in modest amounts. Repeatedly using the same treatment leads to pest resistance. Avoid it by switching treatments. Pay close attention to the plant toxicity of each method to avoid killing the plants you want to salvage. Never spray a plant with any treatment in direct sunlight. Even the safest of treatments can be harmful if applied in direct sunlight.

Treating plants is sometimes like treating people. Often a physician will treat a symptom rather than diagnosing a cause. A doctor can tell you to take a pill to mitigate a symptom, or he can tell you to watch your diet and exercise to prevent heart disease. The same symptom and disease relationship holds true for plants. If the soil is healthy and full of bio-diversity, you can prevent disease instead of treating symptoms.

Chapter 21

∞∞∞

BIODIVERSITY: THE KEY TO ABUNDANCE

{

I don't think much of a man who is not wiser today than he was yesterday.

-Abraham Lincoln

}

Biodiversity and human health are bound together. In the natural living garden, biodiversity is the perfect model for health, not only for the soil, but also for all life that comes from it and into contact with it.

Biological diversity is under threat from the growth of our human population, unsustainable resource consumption and the drive for sustained economic growth. None of these consider the value of biodiversity. We see habitat loss at an alarming rate, genetically engineered pollutants drifting and infecting indigenous species and pollution contributing to global climate change. Our lives have become so mono-cultured and sterile that our choices dwindle every day.

Intensified agricultural systems reduce biodiversity. Only a few insect species might make up 95 percent of the dominant species on a mono-cultured farm. The loss of our natural ecosystem is largely a result of agricultural transformation. Spraying to kill insects throws the entire ecosystem off balance. When farmers focus exclusively on growing one species of plant year after year, that also upsets the natural balance. We can help prevent losing all of the natural biodiversity starting right in our backyards. Local action equals global benefit.

The Supermarket and our Backyard

About 80,000 plants are edible. The next time you are in a supermarket, count how many fruits and vegetables you see for sale. At most, you might find 100 to 200 choices. If you include the dried spice rack, you might find up to 300. This lack of choice alarms me. We are being denied choices every day by giant corporations that limit what we can eat for the sake of their profits. If an edible plant does not look pretty, travel well or have a long shelf life, it does not make it to market for us to choose.

I am not opposed to business making a profit. I own a large company that promotes the organic lifestyle and depends on profits to sustain itself. However, I think we need an ethical element in how consumers choose companies to support. I want all businesses to profit from being creative and innovative, which I strive for in my own business.

Economic manipulation has diluted the variety of tastes in life. Perhaps as consumers we need to ask for more than what we see in front of us. Maybe we assume 300 plant varieties are enough. I want choices for my family and myself. I have invented more than 150 products over the years. My customers have choices as to what works best for them. I want you to have the same freedom of choice our ancestors had before monoculture hit us like a tsunami and narrowed our choices of food.

Life, even garden life, can be exciting and unpredictable. We don't live in a vacuum; neither should your plants. Why kill all life in the garden for the sake of a perfect leaf or flower? Don't feed a living soil with a dead synthetic fertilizer. It adds no value to the soil food web. It's boring and in the long term depletes the soil and nutritional value of the foods we eat.

Plants, like animals and humans, seek variety. Plants thrive in wind and rain, through days and nights of different length, and in hot and cold temperatures at different times of the year. All life should be diverse and plentiful. Abundance comes through natural evolution without tampering by human hands.

Modern Technology Can Have Adverse Effects

Diversity is a major factor in preventing pest and disease build-up because of the way in which organisms interact. When any one species becomes dominant in an area, predators move in to take advantage of the bounty. Eventually, predators reduce the dominant species and restore the balance of nature.

In the past, farmers relied on natural methods of agriculture, because that was all they knew. Chemicals were not available to them. Now it is possible to grow crops as monocultures. Pesticides have given us a way to control competition. This unnatural form of agriculture has created a range of unintended problems. We can learn to restore the natural balance by planting a diverse range of plant species in our gardens. Plant diversity naturally reduces pests and diseases.

A bio-diverse garden has global impact. You start by building the life in soil that teems with micro- and macro-organisms. Then you plant as many heirloom varieties of plants as possible. After harvest, give those seeds away to as many food lovers and gardeners as possible on condition that they do the same. The next year grow a completely different set of heirloom plants. Do it all over again until you can savor and taste every possible kind of plant you can get. Now, it might take a lifetime before you can grow and taste all 80,000 edible plants. Wouldn't it be great to try? This is how biodiversity can make a comeback. It's also putting soil to work like a highly trained athlete. With the associated health benefits you and the environment receive from promoting biodiversity, you might even save the plant that contains an agent that could cure cancer.

Diverse is Good, Variety is Better, Freedom of Choice is Best

Heirloom plants are varieties handed down through decades or even centuries from one farmer or gardener to another. For roughly 12,000 years, human civilization has been based on agriculture and horticulture. During this time, thousands of genetically unique strains of fruits and vegetables have been selected and bred by farmers and gardeners. They represent a genetic heritage that is disappearing from commercial horticulture. Large-scale factory production demands that plants conform to strict guidelines to fit into mechanized systems. The conventional farmer today grows crops with the greatest profit potential. A few giant companies control the majority of our food except for a handful of organic growers who choose rich biodiversity over cheap standardization. The backyard gardener can help create an environment that will benefit all of us.

Heirloom varieties celebrate genetic diversity. Their greatest strength is that individual plants within each crop mature a bit earlier or are more resistant to pests and diseases or contain greater nutrient density. Such characteristics are a great advantage in the organic garden, where the produce does not have to fit into a narrow commercial model.

Fortunately, many gardeners recognize the value of maintaining genetic diversity for future generations. Around the world, various non-profit organizations store seeds or enable gardeners and farmers to swap seed and vegetative material of heirloom plant varieties. Look into a seed bank to obtain heirloom varieties. Grow them and step back into time with your taste buds. Enjoy the full bloom that biodiversity offers.

The Vital Roles of Herbs and Flowers in the Garden

Introducing a wide range of herbs and flowers into your organic garden has many benefits. They help attract an increased range of birds, insects, lizards and other animals. Insects and birds act as pollinators for your fruit and vegetables, giving you increased yields. Many of these creatures also help control pests. Inevitably, there are also some negative consequences, such as birds feeding on fruit, but the diversity you create will be an insurance policy. If one food crop is decimated, a host of others crops can replace it.

Herbs often have aromatic oils that give their foliage and flowers a characteristic perfume. Herbs such as pyrethrum and garlic create organic remedies for pest and disease problems. Such plants also release oils into the surrounding air and soil, thereby helping to repel pests from your garden naturally.

Diversification is a great insurance policy in everyone's garden. A great new drug discovery could come from a wild flower you received from a complete stranger from a seed bank or an heirloom tomato you traded at your last garden club meeting.

PART 3

ANIMAL HEALTH

Chapter 22

PET SAFE GARDEN

Your pets can also enjoy the natural environment and produce from your garden. If you intend to grow healthy fruits and vegetables for your family, grow enough to feed your pets, too.

Design your garden with pet safety in mind. Most fruit and vegetable plants are not toxic. Common plants like squash, zucchini, cucumbers and melons are safe for animals. The majority of herbs are safe, too. All outdoor pets have access to fallen fruits (apple, plum, cherry, apricot and peach) with seeds or pits. Although seeds and pits of these fruits contain cyanide, the amount is minute. In addition, most pets do not chew the fruits thoroughly, so the seeds are not usually broken open when ingested. The seed will more likely cause a foreign object obstruction in the animal's digestive system (also needing urgent care) than cyanide poisoning.

Still, a few common plants pose health risks. Onions, chives and garlic contain compounds that in large quantities can cause sudden hemolytic anemia. The leafy part of the potato plant and the green part of the potato skin contain compounds that are toxic in large quantities. Cyanide in fruit seeds and pits can cause fatal seizures. Grapes may cause kidney failure in dogs. Moldy green walnuts are also toxic. Baby's breath, common in many flower arrangements, can be quite toxic.

Visit a good garden nursery for a detailed list of plants that can be grown in your region as well as those not suitable for pets. Many pets accidentally consume harmful plants every year and need emergency treatment by a veterinarian. Chemicals (fertilizer, pesticide and herbicide) are a far greater and more common threat to your pets than the plants you grow. This is another reason, among many, to go organic.

Many nurseries and pet stores offer effective, safe alternatives to chemicals for controlling nasty insects and garden pests. Increasingly, consumers demand higher standards from manufacturers to provide safe, long-lasting pest control treatments that support the growth of organic crops with pet health in mind.

Why an Organic Garden is Safer for Pets

Organic gardening materials (fertilizers, composts and insecticides) pose little health risk to your pets, because they are plant-based or animal-based. Because many of us want to harvest the most produce we can, we may try to completely control all insects, especially when we see pest damage to our crops. Think about the consequences of your actions. Is it worth harvesting all of a crop if you run the risk of poisoning your pets?

I prefer to let Mother Nature take a portion of my crop to ensure the safety of my pets. Gary Poznick, a biologist friend, gave me wise advice when I was a young gardener more than 25 years ago: "Grow more than you plan on harvesting if you want to do it naturally. Remember that all living things need to eat, too. If you want 100 percent of your harvest, then grow 120 percent." This approach to planning fits with the fundamental foundations of organic gardening, which are biodiversity and balance.

I get peace of mind knowing everything I apply to my garden will not harm my pets or my family. If you must apply an insect control, choose the least toxic, environmentally friendly option. For example, diatomaceous earth or citrus sprays are excellent for controlling fleas and ticks in the garden where pets may play or run. These sprays are effective, have minimal side effects and are the least toxic pest control option for organic gardeners. (Do not confuse the diatomaceous earth used in swimming pools with the one you need to control insects in your garden.) As discussed in Chapter 21, botanical sprays are effective as biological controls. Remember: Never over apply. Even safe alternatives to chemical pesticides are broad-spectrum killers that can affect beneficial insects. Spare all the non-destructive life you can, because biodiversity is the most important principle in growing a healthy garden.

Make Sure Your Plants are Pet Safe

The ASPCA (American Society for the Prevention of Cruelty to Animals) offers a complete list that identifies both toxic plants and those they consider safe. Visit www.aspca.org to learn more. Also, ask your local nursery about plants that potentially could harm pets.

I have grown thousands of tomatoes over the years, but my dogs and cats have never eaten any. Still, green tomatoes can cause a toxic reaction in dogs and cats. In rare situations, dogs are attracted to eating grapes, which are also not good for them. Be careful if you grow avocados, as some pets love them and have had toxic reactions. Plants such as rhubarb, garlic and onions consumed in large quantities also can cause an adverse reaction.

Your backyard is your pets' kingdom. Outside in the fresh air during warm spring and summer days, animals love to roll in the dirt, pardon me, "the soil." (Give your cats an outdoor litter box to keep them from using your garden or kids sand pit for that purpose.) Quite often pets, or even children, will destroy plants. Many varieties of ornamental plants naturally attract pets that want to eat them or at least sample them. Their natural curiosity often leads them to taste plants that can sometimes produce irritating and even toxic effects. If you observe your pets acting strangely after being in the garden, call a veterinarian immediately.

A few plants to consider avoiding are mentioned below. Most of the time your pets will avoid these plants on their own. However, if you have a curious puppy or kitten and are not sure of their behavior patterns, you may want to rule out some of these plants for your garden.

I consider these plants potentially toxic to your pets: trumpet vine, Japanese yew, castor bean, Jerusalem cherry, lily of the valley, precatory beans, foxglove, azaleas, ferns, hydrangeas, lilies, oleander, rhubarb, sweet peas, all green fruits and the nightshades (tomatoes, potatoes, sweet pepper and eggplant). My own pets have never gone after any of these plants. Still, if you plan to grow any of them, locate them in an inaccessible part of the garden. You can also install a fencing structure around the plants.

Common Sense Pet Safety

Lawn and garden chemicals pose the biggest threat to your pets, so avoid them. Reach for safe alternatives like those discussed in Chapter 21. Always store chemicals out of reach of pets and kids. A locked garage or storage shed is best for storing potentially harmful substances.

If you must kill or control insects, here are some alternatives to chemical spraying. Try to wash off the leaves and vegetables with a strong blast of water. If the problem persists, try soap and water or other organic methods. Soap and water are safe for getting rid of soft-bodied insects such as aphids. Add a teaspoon of dish soap to a gallon of water and use it in a garden sprayer. The soap is an irritant to many insects and can help break down the protective barrier of their external skeleton.

Mowing the lawn can also pose a threat to pets. Pebbles or sticks can fly in the air as the mower cuts the grass and strike a pet. This could cause your pet great pain and discomfort not to mention an expensive visit to the veterinarian.

Always read product labels for anything you use. (This practice goes beyond pet safety and garden materials. You should adopt this philosophy with everything you buy.) Keep your pets inside or at a safe distance when you apply any treatments, even organic ones, to your lawn or garden.

Before you plan your garden, visit the "hard goods" section of your nursery for treatments that address potential hazards to pets. With a little planning, you and your pets can have a safe, beautiful and nutritious garden that will be a joy to everyone.

Chapter 23

∞∞∞

THE RIGHT NUTRITION SAVES THE DAY
(AND THE KITTENS)

{
The problem with cats is that they get the exact same look on their face whether they see a moth or an axe-murderer.

-Paula Poundstone
}

I would love to rescue every homeless dog and cat from every shelter or owner who is abusive or neglectful. I see so much suffering in the eyes of abandoned animals.

Unfortunately, even owners who dearly love their pets can unknowingly neglect them through poor nutrition. Fortunately, your garden and kitchen scraps can serve as sources of good pet nutrition. A little creativity at the super market blended with some organic store bought pet food also can help.

Consider a story of how nutrition can make a difference in pet health. I had a beautiful cat at my home and was quite content with her. When I moved into my new office, a six-acre property belonging to a family member, I "inherited" 24 cats abandoned by the previous tenant.

I signed up for the huge job of taking care of my relative's property, (an abandoned water park/amusement park with a huge empty pond, four swimming pools and several fruit trees) because I believed it needed the kind of attention only I could give it. I was also running a large company, trying to change the world by advocating for natural and organic garden methods and home grown foods, and writing this book.

Just what I needed on my plate was to rescue 24 cats! With no time on my hands and all the responsibility in the world, I still felt a duty to the welfare and health of my newly adopted pets.

Lives Saved Through Nutrition

All 24 cats greet me everyday when I drive up to my office on the property. It warms my heart to know they eagerly wait for me every day. They know the "man with the good food" is coming. It's like a scene out of National Geographic or a wildlife documentary film. I park my car about 150 feet from the building. As I head toward my office, the cats crisscross in front of me to the point where I can hardly walk. They always meow and look up at me with such anticipation while endlessly rubbing the sides of my legs. They make my morning a joy with their unconditional love.

While all the cats were beautiful and special in my heart, I especially loved two of them, Tony and Wade. I had to bring them into the warm office since winter was just around the corner, and they were very sick kittens. About 8 to 10 weeks old, they each weighed about 1 pound. They both had eyes almost swollen shut from an infection. Both were definitely the runts of the litter. The other kittens, easily twice their size, were forcing them away from their mother's milk and the food I put out for them. These small, undernourished kittens were obviously in trouble.

I could not bear leaving these two to the fate of death by competition and natural selection. I had to intervene, separate them from the others, and bring them indoors. Doing so was hard on the kittens and me. They seemed so sad to be taken from their mother, but their illness was well beyond her means and ability to help them.

The Visit to the Veterinarian

I immediately took Tony and Wade to the veterinarian to get a professional diagnosis. The veterinarian prescribed some eye cream and nasal infection drops and asked me to bring them back in a week.

"How about their diet?" I asked.

"Feed them anything you have available," he said. "It doesn't matter what kind of pet food you give them."

"Why?"

"All pet foods are pretty much the same. Any kitten food is good enough."

When I began to tell him the importance of micronutrients to human health, he looked at me like I was speaking a foreign language. I eagerly told him about my professional background. "I know nutrient rich soil is the foundation for healthy plants. Healthy plants provide maximum health potential for the livestock we raise and eat. What's the difference when it comes to our pets? Why can't a healthy diet be the foundation of good health and recovery for my kittens?"

His diagnosis was bleak. "Too much damage has already been done. These kittens will both likely develop blindness in a short time."

When I questioned him again about supplements rich in micronutrients and essential fatty acids to boost recovery time, he simply said it would not matter. "All pet food is the same."

I was stunned at this response. I was caring for 24 cats. The two that I chose to adopt as personal pets were not going to live a normal, healthy life. I followed his instructions for the eye cream and the nasal infection drops, but I was determined to prove his nutrition ideas wrong. I disregarded everything he said about cat food.

I put Tony and Wade on a probiotic diet loaded with kelp meal, brewers yeast, super green powder supplements, omega-3 fatty acids from fish oil and digestive enzymes. I used boiled organic chicken breast that I make for my family. I used no seasonings, not even salt; just boiled the chicken in water and began to formulate my homemade concoctions. (Dr. Sue Chan, one of my chief experts on animal nutrition, advises me to avoid pet foods with "by-products" in them. Consult books specifically on homemade pet foods to learn more on this subject.)

After one short month on what you might call "Dr. Earth's Emergency Cat Rescue Diet," my sick kittens grew to almost the size of the others. As I write this chapter, both Tony and Wade sit at my feet looking up at me, bellies full, eyes clear and glowing with health.

I have always known nutrition is the foundation of health in all organisms, animal or human. In this instance, I applied the same nutritional techniques to animal health that I apply to my own health and got good results. I used everything I learned over the years from living an organic lifestyle, applying my understanding of functional foods (super foods), bioavailable supplements, mineral nutrients and probiotics to the needs of my kittens. Intensive attention to nutrition brought Tony and Wade back from near death. I doubt I would have gotten this kind of wonderful result if I had resigned myself to the gloomy outlook and limited knowledge of nutrition coming from the vet.

Natural Nutrition For Every Pet

Pet health is similar to human health. We are both mammals. Though pets prefer an all meat diet, they are omnivores the way we are. Dogs are classified as true omnivores and cats are classified as true carnivores. But you can look at any cat food label to see it contains mostly vegetable matter. Therefore, I conclude cats, dogs and humans are all omnivores. You can get your dogs and cats to eat vegetables if you mask the vegetable content with meat. This balance of vegetables and meat offers the maximum health potential for your pets.

Many would argue with me and say that a dog's or cat's digestive system has not evolved enough to digest vegetables. However, digestive enzymes assist in making those nutrients available from the vegetables we feed to pets. The digestive enzymes are catalysts for breaking down and extracting all consumed foods, especially those rich in proteins, lipids, carbohydrates and fiber.

I want to do for pets what growing a healthy garden has done for the health of my customers, readers and friends. I have dedicated a large part of my life now to pet care by rescuing them directly and by sharing my knowledge of animal nutrition. I ask people not to buy pets. I advocate rescue and adoption. I hope that you adopt this philosophy as well.

My kittens and other cats have inspired me to continue learning about animal health. I have always been aware of the nutritional benefits of organically grown animals for human consumption. I have begun to focus my knowledge and learning toward pet health. The science of human and pet nutrition is the same. Everything comes down to understanding and delivering an animal's nutritional requirements.

Much prepackaged dog or cat food is unnatural for our pets, unless you buy high-quality, organic pet food. The generally higher price for such products is justifiable. If the manufacturer blends the food with premium ingredients, it is worth every penny. You either pay now for the good food, or you pay later for the vet bills and the grief of losing your pet prematurely.

Commercial pet foods do not take into consideration a modern, domesticated pet's nutritional requirements. They also hardly consider evolution. To guide you on how to custom blend a natural dog or cat food that your pets will enjoy and thrive on, I have enlisted some help.

The Expert Panel

Over the years, I have done extensive research on animal husbandry and read many books on the subject. I have yet to find a simple book that explains how a garden can aid pet owners interested in better pet nutrition. I work with several biologists at the University of California at Davis. These experts in wildlife rehabilitation and animal biodiversity are near the Dr. Earth ranch in Winters, California. Before I wrote this part of the book, I wanted to make sure that I explored every available resource and the latest technology in animal health. I also worked with a local veterinarian, Dr. Sue Chan, who runs a non-profit pet organization that focuses on educating and helping both people and animals. When necessary, she also rescues animals from cats to horses and everything between. Dr. Chan says, "If you change the diet and environment of your pets, you will see an immediate difference." I do, and you will, too.

My conclusions on pet health are the same as on plant and human health. Pets are only as healthy as the nutrition you provide for them. A healthy garden is one of the steps to having a healthy pet.

Chapter 24

ooooo

PET FOOD FROM YOUR GARDEN

{
Properly trained, a man can be dog's best friend.
-Corey Ford
}

Every animal deserves to be as healthy as possible. The best way to support your pet's health is to take control of their nutrition. I feed animals everything that I would make for my own family. I make my food myself from good, clean produce right from the garden, supplemented with meat and other goodies from the supermarket.

For most companies in all industries, profits are the primary driving force. Yes, companies need to make a profit to stay in business. However, I question when food producers become solely profit-driven to the point that their decisions are potentially detrimental to health. Those who provide any living being with food should be held to the highest standard. Since we are what we eat, what happens when profit comes at the expense of human and animal nutrition? To maintain balance between private profit and public good, a regulatory agency can impose labeling requirements, conduct inspections and enforce laws to insure basic food safety.

Safety is one thing, but legislating optimum nutrition is probably impossible. Why take a chance that your health and your pet's health might suffer in order to add to a commercial producer's bottom line when you can have complete comfort in knowing your food is safe and full of nutrition because you grew it and prepared it yourself? (If you decide to make the transition from conventional store bought pet food to home made pet foods, make it gradually to prevent upsetting your animal's digestive system.)

You may have heard or read you should not feed your dog bones. I agree it is dangerous to feed your pets leftover drumsticks. These bones can splinter and choke them or become lodged in their intestine. However, the bone itself is full of nutrition.

Most of your conventional dog and cat food comes from bone meal or fish bone meal. The pet food industry uses many of the suppliers we use to make Dr. Earth fertilizers. Pet food companies buy the same ingredients I do. Dr. Chan says "raw beef bones" are OK to feed your pets as opposed to cooked bones, because they are dense and not brittle. They also keep your pet's teeth clean.

The Blender Method

Buy a blender at a garage sale and make it your pet food blender. All chicken and soft bones are fair game for the blender method. If you season your cooked chicken dinner, as most of us do, run the leftovers under hot water in the sink to remove all the seasonings before you serve them to a pet. (Seasonings can cause diarrhea and completely throw off your pet's digestive system. Some might say never give them garlic, but I do. It has worked well in my experience. I think it carries great merit in moderation and is good as a parasite control.)

Become the ultimate recycler by taking all unseasoned chicken scraps, excluding the drumsticks, and throw them into the blender. (Always discard the drumsticks. They pose a threat to your pets unless pulverized by an industrial blender.) All other bones are acceptable. Pour hot water or unseasoned meat broth in the blender to about a quarter full. Then add the bones left over from dinner until the blender is about three quarters full. Seal the blender tight and blend at full speed for several minutes until you have a smoothie and all chicken bones are finely chopped. Add a few vegetables from the garden, and you have the ultimate food for pet health.

This is great for either dogs or cats. Do this regularly and you can recycle for your pet's benefit most of the food you do not eat provided it is rinsed or unseasoned. This is one of many approaches to making good pet food.

Using the blender technique allows you to mask the vegetables you want your pet to consume. The vegetables will taste like blended meat. When you use chicken or meat broth as the base, you can entice pets into eating even more vegetables, since the broth coats the vegetables with the meat flavor they love.

Most people think that dogs and cats are carnivores only, but look in the pet food aisle next time you shop. There are more vegetables in pet foods, such as corn, soybean, wheat, peas and grains, than there are meat by-products. Some dogs, especially German shepherds, are sensitive to corn, while others are sensitive to soy. For this reason, over feeding any one product can create allergies or hypersensitivity, so follow a varied, well balanced diet.

Dogs and cats are omnivores. My cats will eat all kinds of concoctions that I make for them from bones and vegetables. Bones are loaded with beneficial nutrients like calcium and phosphorus. Remember when using a lot of bones in the blender, the calcium may constipate the pets, so add vegetables to any blends for their high fiber content. This will aid your pet's digestion.

Next time you shop at the pet food store, look at the labels carefully. Pet food companies list four basic components: crude protein, crude fat, crude fiber and moisture content. Some foods will show a vitamin profile that has been added, but that is about all a pet food label reveals.

Here is something else to try. Buy the best and cleanest organ meats you can find. Dogs and cats love organ meat. It is inexpensive and creates a creamy texture that they like. Many butchers throw away parts of an animal you and I would not eat. However, your pet will enjoy as a gourmet feast intestines, hearts, kidney, liver and brains. Next time you see your cats catching and eating a mouse, encourage it. Dr. Chan advises that eating the whole mouse, intestines, hair and all is a natural and beneficial diet for cats.

A Gradual Transition to Homemade Pet Food

Start slowly. Observe your pets carefully to make sure they are full of energy, have shiny coats, glowing eyes and regular, normal stools. These are the common things you would observe without a veterinarian. If you are hesitant to dive in head first with home made foods for your pets, start with it twice a week and supplement feedings with your favorite organic pet food. See how your pets do. If they like the food, you can make enough once a week and freeze it for daily meals.

Here's a recipe: In a pot, the one you bought at the same garage sale as the blender, put in the meat, bones and all, bring it to a boil and make a pet stew, meat and water only, no salt or any seasonings. For chicken, let this boil until it is almost falling off the bone. The broth is now the base for your home made pet food, and you will build around this with vegetables and other store bought dry pet food that you trust. This stew is loaded with protein, fat, calcium and phosphorous. The carbohydrates, fiber, vitamins and antioxidants will come from your garden. Since you have cooked the meat well to extract the flavor from it, many of the nutrients may have been lost. This is why you must add supplements to your pet diet to be safe. The broth is important to keep, as this will contain many of the nutrients that have leached from the meat and bones. Also, the broth makes all the foods very appealing for your pets to consume.

Use a different type of meat every time you make this stew. Alternate between chicken, turkey, lamb, beef, fish and even eggs. I used to give our Akita a raw egg occasionally as a treat cracked right on top of his food. He loved it, and it was great for his coat. Just make sure not to give your pets too many raw eggs, as they can cause a vitamin B deficiency if served too often.

Never give your pets unblended, cooked bones, chocolate in large quantities (especially dark chocolate, as it is more toxic), avocados, grapes, mushrooms or any leftover fried foods that may contain spices or seasonings. Remember they are still wild on the evolutionary scale, not nearly as evolved as we are, and cannot digest everything that we can.

Custom Blended Pet Foods

Once you have the base for your pet food cooked in a pot, it is time to incorporate the other healthy ingredients. Add any vegetables from the garden that they will eat raw when mixed with your stew base. If they refuse it, boil it with the stew lightly to soften it. Most dogs and cats like it cooked, but it doesn't hurt to see what they will consume raw at first. Watch for the signs of allergic reactions to any new food you introduce such as itchy skin, ear infection or even chewing on their feet. From the garden, you can add things like peas, soybeans, potatoes, alfalfa, carrots, spinach, finely chopped apples, cranberries, cabbage and garlic. Also add some store goodies like grains such as quinoa, flax seed, oatmeal, brown rice (a must), amaranth, brewers yeast and seaweed, which are full of micronutrients.

Supplements, such as vitamin C, vitamin E, omega-3 fatty acids, all green super food powders and especially probiotics such as *Lactobacillus acidophilus*, are also great for your pets. A combination of good meats and homegrown vegetables from the garden will ensure your pet's health. When you first switch to homemade pet food, try mixing conventional organic pet food into the food you have prepared to help your pet make the transition. Simply add the dry pet food at the bottom of a bowl, and then pour your blended slurry of the homemade foods over it as you would gravy over mashed potatoes. Try this once, and then wait a day before trying it again. As they become accustomed to this new, healthy diet, keep adding more of the slurry and less of the kibble. Over a period, you should be able to give them more raw vegetables and less kibble. The crunchy kibble of pet foods helps clean their teeth and scrape away any plaque build up. This is the value of making a real effort to get pets to eat raw, crunchy vegetables. If they simply resist raw vegetables, keep feeding them the meat and vegetable slurry as their regular staple food. Supplement their routine with some store bought, high-quality, dry organic pet food twice a week just for the teeth cleaning benefits. This will also give you a break from having to prepare food nightly.

Cats love fish. If you have a friend who likes to fish, ask him to bring you the bones and intestines along with the head. You can make a fish stew just for your cats, but it must be fresh or it can cause histamine release and allergic reactions such as diarrhea. If fish scraps are not available, buy canned mackerel or salmon and boil it lightly to make a broth. Mix this broth with grains and vegetables as suggested above. Cooking for a pet does take some extra time, but it's an option that gives your pet natural, preservative-free, additive-free meals. It's also safe from pet food recalls. Nobody cares more about your pets than you do, especially not the commercial pet food companies.

Healthy recipes for pets are easy to make. Just imagine you are cooking yourself a meat meal. Dogs and cats love meat. Prepare the meat with vegetables. Selections range from practical meat in broth poured over brown rice to more exotic, elaborate meals of many grains, fresh vegetables, such as pumpkin or squash for complex carbohydrates, and probiotics with a little kibble added. You can also learn to make biscuits for pets baked in your oven.

Custom pet recipes are also available that meet special nutritional needs such as diabetes or heart problems. When preparing home-cooked meals for pets with special diet requirements, prepare the meal as you would prepare it for yourself. Consider what special nutritional requirements are needed. If your pet is diabetic, prepare a meal low in carbohydrates. Conversely, if your pet has a heart problem, prepare lean meat and a high fiber diet. Adopt the same nutritional guidelines for your pets that you use cooking for yourself.

Kittens and puppies require a little more fat early on. Plenty of grains with sugars will keep them full of energy and feeling alive. Fruits, vegetables and whole grains loaded with fiber keep your pet's gastro-intestinal system working right. Certain fiber contents in such a diet are referred to as prebiotics. The term prebiotic has become popular in the pet food industry. It is nothing more then non-digestible fiber that stimulates the growth of probiotics. Most often, prebiotics are carbohydrates with a high non-digestible fiber such as the veins in leafy greens and all grains like brown rice. The idea is to make sure your pets are getting ample amounts of prebiotic fibers that feed the probiotics in the intestine, releasing digestive enzymes. This will make nutrients more available and soluble for your pets to absorb. Fiber keeps the bowels moving and eliminates many toxins from the digestive system. If you think about it, preparing pet food is almost identical to preparing human food except for all the spices and seasonings that we love.

A regular feeding of quality, well-balanced foods is the basis for pet nutrition, although an occasional treat is fine. You can prepare something special from time to time. Try a little agave nectar and organic milk for your cat or a small amount of peanut butter and milk for your dog. Both dogs and cats love yogurt. Feed it to them in moderation. Yogurt is loaded with probiotics, but it is also high in lactose, which pets are not set up to digest easily.

Chapter 25

∞∞∞∞

HOMEMADE PET FOOD

{

Be it human or animal, touch is a life-giving thing. Has anyone ever had a stroke or a heart attack while cozied up with a pet? I doubt it.

-Robert Brault

}

Commercial pet foods are some of the worst junk on the market. Commercial pet food has been around only about 65 years. Animals did fine without it for much longer. Many of the commercial pet foods available on the market keep veterinarians busy struggling to heal ailments they simply do not know how to treat. The pharmaceutical companies are responsible for many of the illnesses of our pets. All our pets need is a regular, healthy diet.

For centuries, dogs and cats in the wild never received conventional pet food. No one walked around with a bag of food making sure all dogs and cats were fed regularly. By preparing their food today, we can mimic what dogs and cats might have eaten in the wild. Homemade pet food will optimize their health. Veterinary research focuses primarily on the diagnosis and pharmaceutical treatment of disease with little attention paid to nutrition and its role in disease and healing. American pet food companies remind us they have the highest standards in the world, and they probably do, but is it enough?

Bioavailable Food

You can lay down a feast for your pet, but unless the nutrients are bioavailable, they are simply not absorbed. The same holds true with plants and humans. Bioavailability determines the solubility of all nutrients. Holistic veterinarians estimate more than half of pet illnesses can be corrected by some kind of nutritional supplement. If we correct inadequate diets and make vital nutrients available, we drastically improve pet health. With a bioavailable diet and a well-planned nutritional supplement program, we insure digestive enzymes are constantly available.

Before commercially prepared diets became available, pets ate almost anything and everything they could find. Animals ate the majority of their food directly off the ground, which we may think of as less sanitary than a food dish. The ground is loaded with trace nutrients and beneficial soil microbes that inoculate the intestines of animals.

Intestinal inoculation occurs with humans from the moment we are born when we receive our mother's breast milk. Breast milk is loaded with *Lactobacillus acidophilus* which inoculates our intestines. As kids we crawl around on the ground and touch everything. Then we put our hands in our mouths. This is a part of our biological evolution. By getting into everything in this way, we further inoculate our intestines with a wide variety of microbes.

These probiotic microbes then inoculate our mouth and intestine with enzyme-producing bacteria. These enzymes assist in making the food we eat bioavailable.

Many pet owners who are meat lovers believe that dogs and cats are strict carnivores. They believe pets will not thrive on vegetarian diets. Conversely, many vegetarians believe that a vegetarian diet is far superior to a meat diet for their pet. I believe you should have both meat and vegetables in your pet's diet. Pets need lean protein and nutrient rich fruits, grains and vegetables. Whole foods are an excellent source of vitamins and minerals. You might ask if a pet's digestive system is so far behind on the evolutionary scale, how can it digest vegetables? Digestive enzymes make this possible, and you should incorporate them into all pet foods.

You can buy the same digestive enzymes at the health food store that you buy for yourself. Our dogs and cats inherently have the digestive enzymes to effectively digest protein in food. We want to assist our pets in digesting grains, fruits and vegetables, since these foods are rich in fiber and carbohydrates. Dogs and cats have short digestive systems, so they need our help with digestive enzymes to absorb the maximum level of nutrients from the food we give them. Buy digestive enzymes rich with cellulase and amylase. They will help in the bioavailability of a diet rich in vegetables. Most animals including humans do not produce cellulase in their bodies and cannot use most of the energy in plant material.

Preparing homemade pet food may not be for everybody. It takes much work to constantly make sure your pets get a good variety of appealing foods they enjoy eating. This chapter is primarily for those who cook for themselves and don't mind making a little extra for their pets. For me, this is easy. I show up at the office a little early to take care of my 25 cats with a little something special every morning. (Yes, 25. I already had one when the 24 came with my relative's property.) I enjoy it and find it therapeutic. I love to experiment with different pet foods weekly to better understand their nutritional needs. I believe nutritional education should be ongoing, as new things are discovered every day. You can get help and support with this by subscribing to a pet magazine or joining a pet club.

The beauty of life is the never-ending quest of learning. When I attended Daniel Murphy Catholic High School, one of my favorite teachers was Brother Albion, a wise and pious Dominican friar who changed my way of thinking forever. Brother Albion took a special liking to me and gave me special attention that shaped my morality and my ethical understanding of our purpose in life. He was full of knowledge and experience. Brother Albion used to tell our eleventh grade ethics class, "Heaven is never-ending knowledge."

I have always known that food can make a huge difference in my health. It is logical that food will have an equal impact on pet health. In addition to working with Dr. Sue Chan and learning much about her work on her rescue farm, I have traveled throughout the United States to meet farmers, gardeners and medical doctors. I have had extended talks with many people who have raised every kind of animal, from indoor kittens to herds of cattle grazing naturally on hillsides. One message was always consistent in these encounters: You are what you eat. Therefore, I conclude pets are also what they eat.

My message here is simple. Stop eating junk food and start eating good food if you want to be healthy. Medical doctors encourage us to consume less processed food and more natural raw green foods to maximize our health. If we have pets that we love like family, we should definitely do the same for them.

Good Food is Clean Energy

How does the quality of food make such a difference in a pet's health? Food is fuel and energy. Life does not exist without it. Nearly every living organism is nothing but energy. To feed all their living cells on the microscopic level, we must give our pets foods that will provide good, clean energy. Energy keeps all living things moving.

Although commercial pet food is convenient and contains some energy burning fuels, they are often lacking in enzymes and provide only basic nutrients that sustain life at the most basic level. Conventional pet foods can sustain life for many years, but are they the best for the health of your pets? How bioavailable are they? Most pet food formulas are simple and contain cheap fillers. They are not as healthy for your pets as fresh foods from your garden or foods you cook for them. Also, commercial pet food ingredients are heated to high temperatures to kill off all pathogens. Unfortunately, the process also renders nutrients in the food much less viable and bioavailable. Ask yourself: Would I eat the products I feed my pets?

Would I feed these products to my children day after day, year after year, for their entire lives? The answer is simple. Common sense says we must have a wide variety of fruits, vegetables and meats in order to live a long, healthy life. You do not need a veterinary degree to see this.

Before processed commercial pet foods, animal lovers shared their foods with their dogs and cats. When I was a boy, we scraped everything into a big bowl and took it outside to feed our dogs. With the exception of all chicken and turkey bones, we fed them everything from our table. My mom washed the seasonings off the scraps, but everything else we fed to our dogs. We fed them large steak bones, chicken carcasses, even pasta and vegetables. They lived long and healthy lives. I don't remember my parents ever taking our dogs or cats to the veterinarian for anything except neutering and spaying.

All animals on our planet evolved over years with good health by eating specific types of foods native to their environments. Their food requirements varied with the physiology of each type of species, but one thing remained common to dogs and cats. They need protein. While dog food and cat food are different, you can easily prepare homemade dog and cat food using similar ingredients. We know certain supplements contain vital nutrients, enzymes and amino acids that you can add in lesser or greater quantities to achieve a desired result for your dog or your cat.

Evolution has helped dictate dog and cat digestive systems for at least 120 million years. The ancestors of the animals we now domesticate were once savage killers. Our pets have teeth and claws that were obviously designed to catch, rip and tear living flesh. Their eyes are strategically placed in the front of their heads so they can focus on prey. Most grazing omnivores have eyes on the sides of their heads so they can be wary of a dog or cat preying on them.

Dogs are more scavengers than cats. Nevertheless, before domestication, both dogs and cats struggled and survived on a diet that consisted mainly of protein from consuming other animals. Yet, dogs and cats are not pure carnivores, nor should your pets eat a diet of only lean proteins. When making dog foods or cat foods, remember to use all the parts. They love the skin, the organ meats and the connective tissue (sinew). Most importantly, feed your pets vegetables, too.

Raw Food

In recent years, a passionate debate has raged on feeding pets raw food. I have yet to talk with any two people who completely agree on this subject. Some viewpoints are extreme and contend all foods must be raw. Others take a more moderate approach and feed raw foods to pets occasionally for nutritional benefits.

With such contrasting beliefs regarding raw or partly raw foods, many pet owners are confused over which direction to go. I believe both raw and cooked foods are good and each has a place in providing maximum nutrition for your pet. I believe your pet's diet should be similar to yours. We should consume meats and cook them lightly to make the nutrients more bioavailable. (There is a fine line between overcooking it to the point that most nutrients and digestive enzymes are burned away and heating food enough to kill any potential pathogens.)

I love sushi and eat it all the time without any problems. I also have eaten steak tartar (raw ground beef) many times when I was in Europe with no illness or side effects. Why can't pets eat only raw food? They can, as long as it is fresh from a trusted source. I have spoken with many veterinarians who believe remarkable good comes from eating a raw diet exclusively. Their conviction comes from experience with pets that were sick and full of conventional food toxins consumed for many years. Many biologists say raw foods aid newborns and promote greater health and normality in later years. This theory makes sense, since the majority of nutrients are most available in their raw state. In general, the less we alter the natural state of any food, the more likely it will contain the maximum nutrition.

Chapter 26

∞∞∞

BACKYARD ANIMALS AND STORE BOUGHT MEATS

{

I like pigs. Dogs look up to us. Cats look down on us.
Pigs treat us as equals.

-*Winston Churchill*

}

Consuming animal meat is a reality and a part of most people's lives. The majority of animals and humans consume meat. If the essence of this book is to discuss and shed light on being healthy through what we eat from our garden, we must also discuss how we raise or "grow" animals for consumption.

Most of the animals we consume for meat are not raised in humane ways. Today, animals are more than likely to be strictly confined, fed genetically altered grains and pumped full of hormones and antibiotics. If you like to consume meat, it is also helpful to understand nutrient dense fruits and vegetables we have discussed in the last 25 chapters. Feeding animals with organic, healthy produce in open spaces will ensure the healthiest meat possible for consumption. If you raise your own animals for consumption, give them a healthy diet, sunshine and the freedom to roam. These conditions will reward you through the healthier food they ultimately provide you. Unfortunately, commercial agriculture has discovered short-term profit in confining animals to unnatural environments indoors or in pens and stalls.

Many people cannot or will not raise their own animals for food. You may live in an apartment and only have room for a few container plants on your balcony. You may have more space but live in a city where domesticating animals is restricted or impractical. You may have no such limitations but not have the heart to butcher anything you raise. It is hard to kill an animal you raised unless you grew up on a farm where slaughtering is just a part of daily life. If you are not going to raise any animals, you will probably buy your meats from a purveyor of some sort; a butcher, a supermarket, or I hope, a local farmer. The choice of meats you bring home and feed to your family or pets determines your health, your family's health, and ultimately the health of the environment.

Healthy Animals Equal Healthy People

Raising an animal in a healthy manner is just as important as growing healthy crops. You must provide that animal with proteins, fats, vitamins, minerals, fiber, phytonutrients, micronutrients and, most importantly, compassion blended with sunshine. Micronutrients are critically important to animals, especially during development so they can grow to their fullest potential and maintain their health. Just as in people and plants, animals need nutrients in differing amounts. Allowing an animal to roam and graze freely ensures it will consume all of the needed macronutrients and micronutrients in a well-balanced manner. Once again, the right balance is the key. If you over feed an animal any kind of nutrient, you run the risk of toxicity. Too much or too little of any one element throws off the balance.

You might wonder: If grazing freely is a great way to nourish livestock, why don't the large commercial farms and ranches do it? It is not because penning animals in huge warehouse-like barns and pumping them full of growth hormones and antibiotics is "better." Rather, this factory-like arrangement saves time and money. More animals can be raised faster at lower cost per pound than the traditional, healthier way. We have inferior, factory-produced meat in our grocery stores and butcher shops, because it is efficient to produce, and because not enough of us— yet—have insisted on something better for our health.

I keep writing about balance. The essential meaning of organic is balance. While the scientific meaning of organic relates to the element carbon, the essence of the organic method is balance. Balance is the key to the health of every living organism on earth. Even antibiotics (which mean "against life") have a place in our lives when needed. When used as a last measure to save lives and relieve pain, the role of antibiotics is also to restore balance.

Micronutrients

In animals, micronutrients play critical roles in activating key enzymes and coenzymes. Coenzymes facilitate communication between enzymes by transferring individual molecules or larger chemical groups from one enzyme to another. Enzymes present in each animal cell play a major role in catalyzing reactions, which enable the proper functioning of many glands and organs. Enzymes are catalysts for many functions including metabolism. Deficiencies in micronutrients can cause detrimental effects to animal growth, productivity, fertility and overall health.

Some farms administer micronutrient treatments underneath the skin of the animals in containers that allow slow controlled release. In this fashion, animals theoretically can receive any one or combination of micronutrients to optimize their growth. For example, pigs receive iron subcutaneously (just beneath the skin) to promote optimum growth and prevent an iron deficiency, which is common in developing pigs. Therefore, it can be a lifesaver in certain situations. In others, it allows farming corporations to raise livestock in overcrowded areas with GMO byproduct foods that lack proper, well-balanced micronutrients.

Micronutrients From Your Backyard

Generally, we can provide livestock with most, or even all, of the nutrition and micronutrients they need. It starts with the soil. Livestock need diets based on energy consisting of protein, carbohydrates, minerals and vitamins. The relative amounts of needed micronutrients differ between and within species depending on factors such as season, energy output, pregnancy and stage of growth. Most commercial livestock receive a diet of commodity grains such as corn, wheat and the ubiquitous protein-providing plant, soybeans. Other elements, including cottonseed, feathers, blood, meat, bone, kelp, fish meal and supplements, are added to livestock feed to give the animals what they need.

Wouldn't it be nice if all animals received a complete set of micro- and macro-nutrients by consuming plants they ate when their species evolved? How simple that would be. Just let them roam and graze. The nutrients are right there in the environment. Why supplement it? The problem is animals are fed crops that are nutrient poor, because they were grown in nutrient poor soils. This directly affects animal health and growth.

This loops everything back to soil health. If the food fed to all animals is grown in healthy soil, the plants will contain ample micronutrients that adequately meet the nutritional needs of all animals including the livestock intended for human consumption. In theory, soils are the multivitamin. They contain diversified and complete nutrients needed to feed all living things on earth. The less we artificially supply nutrition to animals, the better. The ideal, safest approach is to consume animal meat raised on healthy plants harvested from healthy soil with no need for artificial supplements. Artificially administering any nutrition should be a last resort considering the risk of nutrient deficiencies or toxic concentrations. Also, the research on the proper micronutrient densities in animals is not conclusive. We do not know the best concentrations to add to animal feeds. Conversely, healthy plants grown in healthy soils naturally have the proper ratio of micro- and macronutrients. This relieves us of the concern of any inadequacies of purchased supplements.

By now, I hope you understand and can appreciate how complex, yet subtle is the science of nutrition. To do carefully controlled studies in the real world outside of a laboratory, where you change only one thing and see what difference it makes in order to get absolutely clear conclusions, is harder than it sounds. This helps explain why we so often read of contradictory studies and recommendations concerning human health and nutrition. Sometimes the best advice is the simplest and most natural: Choose a wide variety of foods grown in the healthiest, most natural soil, and cook them as little as you need to make them appealing and digestible.

In a sense, deficient soil leads directly to the need to add supplementary nutrients in livestock feed. Micronutrients are just as important for animals as humans. If we can deliver the right combinations of micronutrients to all livestock, whether grown in our backyard or on the farm, we will contribute to the health and welfare of both animals and humans.

Healthy Feed, Healthy Livestock

Buying organic, grass-fed beef is the healthiest option. Cows did not evolve eating corn or grains. When I eat at a restaurant and see a menu that specifically offers beef that is "100 percent grain fed" I know the management has not done their homework. To accept that grain-fed beef is a consumer benefit is to fall into the marketing scheme of the feedlot producers. This ploy has been designed by the agribusiness giants to deceive us into believing that grain-fed beef is better and contains more nutrients. The suggestion is false. Corn is not what cows evolved eating as their primary food. They are much better at digesting high fiber grass and plants than high starch grains. Eating large quantities of grains like corn causes cows' stomachs to be abnormally acidic and could cause a condition called lactic acidosis. This disrupts stomach functioning and can make cows more susceptible to bacterial illness. If continuously fed grains until slaughter, cows can develop an acid resistant version of the harmful bacteria E. coli. This further perpetuates an acidic environment that invites a host of diseases that weaken the animal's immune system, requiring more nutrient supplements and corrective treatments to keep the animal healthy.

Here's how it works. Cows are put in small feedlots with no room to graze or burn any fat. Next, they are fed corn and other grains to fatten them and promote a marbled texture that makes the meat tender and seemingly desirable. This combination of growth allows the farmer to take the cow to slaughter in half the usual time while improving his profitability. The consumer is not told that most of the animal's diet is GM corn and other GM ingredients. Even more troubling is the fact we are also not told that these cows are fed other animals including other cows in the form of blood and bone meal. Even worse and more disgusting, some people speculate feedlot cows may be fed domesticated animals in the form of "meat meal" that may contain the carcasses of dogs and cats. The subject is highly debated and deserves further investigation if consumers are to comfortably support any particular brand of pet food.

Those who run modern agricultural operations suggest farming has become more civilized in our time. For these large-scale producers, gone are the days when a cow roamed the fields and ate grasses that naturally grew without applied chemicals. However, local suppliers of free range and organically raised livestock do exist. In fact, these businesses are making a comeback and are becoming profitable, because people are willing to pay a premium for clean-quality, GM free beef that is raised humanely.

Free-Range Chickens

I love to see chickens scratching the soil looking for bugs to eat. This is the way nature intended them to live. Birds are a great complement to any garden. They are beautiful and have great personalities if you watch them carefully.

When I was a child, I raised chickens at my grandparents' ranch. There were no cages or confinement of any kind. The chickens roamed freely, then returned to roost at night. This model of raising chickens works well and accomplishes many things. Chickens receive a wide variety of nutrients. The free movement of the chickens helps keep the garden or farm free of pests. Chicken manure and beneficial nutrients are distributed back into the soil, creating a mini ecosystem throughout the yard or farm. Most importantly, free-range chickens do not require antibiotics or hormones, because they are not stressed from confinement. Because they are not slaughtered quickly, they do not need fatty grains for rapid growth. Gradual growth is the humane way to raise these animals.

The chickens I eat are exclusively free range, organic and free of antibiotics and hormones. I raise them myself, when I can, on the Dr. Earth ranch. This is the sustainable and humane thing to do. Good practice leads to nutrient rich meat and eggs. If you intend on raising a few chickens, make sure to give them plenty of room to roam so they do not decimate your garden. Raising chickens in close quarters can lead to parasitic loads. I recommend a good book devoted to small animal farms to make sure you completely understand all of the variables. A local feed store can suggest one of the many books available on the subject.

Free-Range Living and Bioaccumulation

Many farmers adopt ethical and sustainable practices in raising their animals, because it is more profitable. More farmers are starting to support sustainable methods in something of a return to the past. Sustainable farmers are keeping cows on traditional grasslands, allowing grazing on native sustenance. They are also no longer implanting growth hormones and feeding antibiotics to animals.

As a result, cows raised this way are left to develop at a more natural pace with low stress. They end up healthier.

With healthier cows, farmers don't have to invest in initial antibiotics or other costly and unhealthy preventative measures for disease control. In general, these cows also require less treatment for illness than if they were fed concentrated corn. Cows in a high output regimen endure much more physiological stress that is correlated with a higher susceptibility to infection and disease. While pasture raised animals produce less milk and leaner meat than feedlot animals, farmers can make up the difference in reduced overhead costs and a higher sale price for healthier meat.

Pasture raised, grass-fed meat contains less bioaccumulated environmental contaminants than grain fed meat. Since we consume these animals for food, we want to make sure they are exposed to the least amount of treatment as possible. Bioaccumulation is a problem for humans, since we are highest on the food chain. We consume just about all things, both clean and toxic. Substances accumulate and are stored in our organs, such as our liver, muscle and fatty tissues and bone marrow, causing many health problems. The cleaner and less toxic the foods we consume, the less we accumulate any environmental toxin. That is why environmentally aware nutritionists advise eating only small amounts of tuna meat. They also suggest eating smaller fish. Some fish accumulate heavy metals such as mercury, lead or zinc. Bioaccumulation in the tissues of larger fish occurs over their longer life span. Larger fish have bioaccumulated toxins of the smaller fish they eat. This explains why shark meat is downright toxic.

Grass fed cows tend to bioaccumlate fewer toxins and contain more "good" fats like omega-3 fatty acids. The beef also has much higher vitamin concentration. These cows are eating grasses that are nutrient rich and dense. If you are what you eat, it follows that you will be less healthy consuming most feedlot animals. If these animals are fed monoculture grains that are synthetically farmed with simple N-P-K fertilizers, chemical pesticides and genetically modified crops in nutrient deficient soils, what kind of nutrition do you think you will get from eating them?

Environmental Contamination
When animals are raised through intensive farming such as feedlots or cages, they deposit large amounts of manure in a concentrated space. After a short time, the manure must be collected and transported away from the area. To cut transportation costs, the manure is often dumped as close to the feedlot as possible. As a result, the surrounding soil is overloaded with concentrated nutrients that are not absorbed for plant growth. The concentration can cause ground and water pollution. Conversely, when animals are raised outdoors on pasture, manure is spread

over a wide area of land. Instead of becoming a waste management problem, the manure is a welcome source of organic fertilizer to support the growth of more pasture grasses. This is a natural cycle.

Bioethics and Our Food

I studied theology and ethics extensively at a Catholic preparatory high school in Los Angeles. I took away an appreciation of subtext in these studies as I reached adulthood. I have good insight into the underlying meanings of language and can read the meaning beyond the literal words.

I often sense that in modern religious teaching, especially Catholic and Protestant, animals do not have a telos. Telos comes from the Greek for "end," "purpose," or "goal." This belief that animals do not have a purpose or goal may explain decisions to treat animals without higher regard. It becomes possible to disregard the screams and cries of monkeys, dogs, cats and all animals as they are literally dissected without anesthesia. We explain it away as the mechanical response of a soulless body responding without self-consciousness to a physical stimulus. As their living tissue is being dismantled, can animals not feel on a higher level? If they do not have a telos or self-consciousness, are we justified to do as we wish with them? This form of thinking baffles me. It should confound every thinking person, whether they love animals or not. It should give discomfort to vegetarian and carnivore alike. There is no need for such suffering. You don't have to be an animal lover to understand this.

If animals possess no purpose of their own, many modern religions find it easy to conclude animals cannot suffer. On this basis, humans can infer that the "purpose" of animals is to serve human needs, especially our nutritional needs. Confinement, unnatural environments or experimentation become means to the justifiable end of advancing the human race.

This is a philosophical discussion that has evolved over the last few hundred years. It requires much more detailed coverage than this book can offer. However, ethics are a valid consideration, whether buying meat or simply making a pet food purchase. What you buy helps support the methods by which it is produced.

Animals are used for all kinds of testing. Many products now carry "cruelty free" labeling. Buy these products when possible. Many large companies do not operate with the highest ethical standards. Others revere profit over all else and have no concern for animal suffering. In such a context, animals are manipulated not unlike an automobile part might be adjusted to achieve speed or cost savings.

Do the agribusiness giants believe these animals don't suffer, because they have no telos or purpose beyond serving human needs? Or can they take the justification a step further? Can they assert the animal's purpose is not only to serve nutritional needs but the more deeply selfish desire for profits among owner/stockholders? This self-serving thinking is not for the modern ethical person.

I do not suggest we all stop eating meat. I just want animals raised and slaughtered in a humane way.

Genetic engineering plays a role in animal cruelty as well. Some animals are born with intentional deformations as part of bioengineering experiments. The bioengineer knows the animal has no way of being born normally. This situation creates a major ethical concern and debate. The bioethics of genetically modified animals might be saved for an ethics book. For now, be alert to the realities of modern bioengineering companies and the giant agribusiness companies. Many people support their businesses unknowingly. These are some of the practices they engage in to pursue profits. The fact that an animal is intentionally altered and manipulated genetically and suffers as a result appalls me. The best we can do as conscientious human beings is to create a better environment for all animals that we keep and love as pets and animals we intend to consume. Support farmers who share your beliefs. Consumers are the final decision makers. We vote with our pocketbooks when we decide not to spend in support of companies with no ethical standards.

In fairness to the many brilliant, dedicated minds in the field of bioengineering, I do not believe bioengineers are evil people who intend to make animals suffer. Many study this field because they think they develop new technologies to help mankind, feed the hungry, eliminate disease and make the world a better place. I do not condemn bioengineers. I simply want the freedom to choose – or not to choose – genetically modified foods.

PART 4

HUMAN HEALTH

Chapter 27

HEALTHY GARDEN, HEALTHY YOU!

{
Let food be thy medicine.

-Hippocrates
}

The three pillars of health have been known for thousands of years. The ancient Greeks described them best: proper rest, proper exercise and proper nutrition.

We focus here on the nutritional component of health. However, all three components are bound together. Proper nutrition leads to good digestion, circulation and immunity, all benefiting the body's total system. Getting the correct balance of rest, exercise and nutrition is imperative to good health.

Nothing can replace a good night's sleep. Dr. Steve Pratt, author of the best selling books, SuperFoods Rx and SuperHealth, says we need at least seven hours of sleep to maintain good health. Nutrition alone cannot replace adequate sleep. We also need to exercise moderately to maintain and maximize our health. Gardening is a great way to work up a sweat. Look at pulling weeds not as a chore but as a great form of exercise.

Start every day by looking deeply in the mirror. I do not mean a superficial glance when you apply your makeup or shave your face. I mean look deeply inside yourself. Look into your eyes and ask yourself what you see. Do you dwell on any part of your body? What part? Why do you dwell on that part? Could you make a change to correct it if you are unhappy with it?

Take a deep look inside the person staring back at you. You owe it to yourself and those whose lives you touch to do everything in your power to be as healthy as you can be. Every day is a good day, because it gives you another opportunity to be who you want to be and do what you want to do. If you want to make a healthy change for the better, start in your backyard with a good mental attitude and plan to have a great day.

I hope by now I have convinced you that growing a healthy garden can be one of the most rewarding and healthy experiences of your life. The better you understand the benefits of healthy gardening, the more you will adopt it in your life. Make your garden a large part of your life. When people get involved in growing their gardens, their quality of life improves significantly. A healthy garden offers a healthy place for you and your family, a place you can regularly depend on for healthy foods.

If you understand the fundamentals of healthy gardening, you know how they relate to your health. Gardeners are at the forefront of an organic revolution. Growing your own food is one thing you can control to enrich your life and your health.

When you walk through the supermarket, it seems as if every other product claims to promote your health. Yet consider the health problems that plague modern, industrial society: cancer, heart disease, diabetes, stroke, arthritis, obesity, degenerative diseases and premature aging. Research shows these are primarily lifestyle and environmental diseases. That means they come from or are made worse by toxic exposures via our air, water and food (including cigarette smoke, air pollution and chemically tainted food), poor nutrition (too much of what is bad for us and/or not enough of what nourishes us), and lack of vigorous exercise.

Self Analysis

When I set out to write this book, I knew reading it could be a life changing experience for my readers. While bringing such change motivates me, I did not anticipate how much it would change my own life. I now force myself to go through the mental exercise of analyzing everything I do on a daily basis. I start from the moment I wake up and turn on my computer to start writing. I analyze every action throughout my day, whether I am sitting in front of my computer gathering a few special thoughts or doing something to run my business.

I have trained myself to think about what I have learned. In this way, I aim to be the best student of my own teachings. The ideas in Healthy Garden, Healthy You have already changed my life for the better, because they have made me more conscious of my everyday choices.

I have always tried to make the best choices for my daily nutrition. On a typical day, I wake up at about 4 A.M. I drink some green tea, work on the computer until sunrise, shower and drive a few miles to the health food store to drink a fresh squeezed green juice they make just for me. The food choices I make throughout the day give me with the energy to continue writing, running my company and staying alive and healthy. I make a routine of practicing a healthy lifestyle and have developed over many years a kind of nutritional compass, my gut instinct, if you like. I feel intuitively that eating well is the right thing to do.

My own diet is high in fiber, rich with chlorophyll, micronutrients, phytonutrients and lean, fat-free proteins. I prefer wild salmon, organic free-range chicken and turkey, and organically grown, grass-fed beef. These are food choices I make throughout the day.

However, the most rewarding time of my day is when I come home and play in the garden with my family. My time in the garden is priceless. My garden is my sanctuary and place to gather with those I love. In my garden, I feel I am being most truly my best self. I also love to plan my garden. I fertilize and till it. I add all the nutrients to grow healthy fruit and vegetable plants to feed my family. My favorite time of the year is when I begin the harvest. It is the time I can pick the fruits (and vegetables) of my labor of love.

A Little Work, a Lot of Health

I love to work. I work at everything I do, from building my relationships with my family to building my business every day. I love it all. However, my time in the garden is a little different. Gardening is the kind of work that transcends the purely physical world and becomes a spiritual experience. The simple act of working with the soil and nurturing plants goes back thousands of years. It is a very special feeling to know my ancestors did the same thing ten thousand years ago. The act of gardening connects me with them. In a sense, my garden links me to all past and future humanity.

Look at your backyard as you might look at a place of worship, a healing ground or a place of nurturing. After all, churches, houses of worship and meditation halls exist to nurture souls and lift our spirits to connect us to a higher power. What else but a higher power of some kind makes all of biology happen? The garden is like a "natural chapel" in the ways it can heal and connect you to the past and future. Many spiritual men were known to love working in their gardens. And many of the best gardeners I have known or read about were deeply spiritual in some way.

Invest some time every day in your garden. Even if you do not touch anything, just walk in it. Plan your next crop, or think about how your garden can improve your future. This alone is healing.

Few things are as exciting as growing a healthy garden or being a farmer. I am blessed, because I own many acres of land and can raise every kind of plant that will grow in Northern California. Nevertheless, I also was a city boy for much of my life. Even when I lived on an average 60-foot by 150-foot city house lot, my parents and I always managed to grow an organic garden and several fruit trees. I have always grown herbs in containers. I landscaped in spaces large and small with trees that produced edible fruits. I always designated a sizable part of my backyard to my vegetable garden. My philosophy includes believing that if I use water to maintain a garden or any plants, I might as well grow things that I can also eat to provide nutrition for me, my family, my pets and my friends. If I turn a sprinkler on and pay a water bill, l feel I should grow as much edible food as I can. Growing my own food is the essence of healthy living.

None of us is immortal, of course, but many of us reach for a life-extending elixir. Historically, humanity has always searched for the fountain of youth or healing herbs or something else that might enable us to live a very long life free of ailments and disease.

In this age of technology and modern medicine, we have become disconnected from our agrarian roots. Television commercials show images of cows in beautiful green pastures and fields of fruits and vegetables to sell food products. We fall for the imagery and buy. The image manipulation works, because we love the images. Advertisers use this idealized image of farming and rural life to sell us multivitamins, anti-aging skin creams and antioxidant drinks, among other things. What we do not see, perhaps do not want to see, is the factory-farming reality of where and how our food is processed and packaged. Those real images are disturbing. Instead, we embrace the pictures of bucolic open fields, get good feelings from them and link them with being healthy.

Here is the paradox: The more we progress in modern times and see the limits and costs of "progress," the more we reach for the ways we did things in the past. In the last hundred years, as we have moved forward technologically or industrially, we have striven to return to what we did hundreds of years ago. What a paradox: The easier life becomes, the more difficult it is to live. My computer makes it easy for me to gather my thoughts without having to write them down on several pieces of paper. However, it also sends out electronic waves that may not be good for my health.

As we move forward and advance the quality of our life, we expose ourselves to more potential ailments. When we had to run and hunt for our food or work in the fields to gather the fruits and vegetables we ate, we were also leaner. Obesity was less pervasive. Certainly, some people throughout time have been genetically disposed to retain weight, but for the most part humankind was leaner in the past when physical work was more commonplace. Today, stress management is a minor industry and a major need for so many people. Arguably, no one had the time to manage stress when most industry took place in the fields working to grow as a community towards the shared goal of survival. A modern backyard garden can be a gateway to the beneficial aspects of life in the past.

The Future of the Healthy Garden

As I continue to grow and look at those around me, I wonder what I will look like 20, 30, 40 or even 50 years from now. Will I be able to walk on my own? Will I even be here? If I am here, what will be the quality of my life? In this book, I hope to teach you how to be as healthy as you can. I live an organic lifestyle that I want to share with you. I believe from the very depths of my heart if you grow the majority of your own food, you will live a better quality life. You will be freer of ailments, carry less body fat, have glowing skin and experience a more youthful, healthier life. We all want to look good and age beautifully. Your own healthy garden is the most accessible tool to achieve all these desires.

Since I carefully observe every detail around me, my family and friends accuse me of wanting too much control over my environment. Quite the opposite.

Others control everything around me, especially companies motivated solely by profits. This forces me to pay close attention to every detail in my daily choices. My genetic makeup prompts me to observe and be mindful. I love to read labels before I consume anything. I am not so much counting calories as looking at the ingredient list. When I go out to eat, I study the menu and customize every dish I order. I skip the mayonnaise and choose multigrain bread, for example. Paying attention to such details every day is part of who I am. I want to live a long and healthy life, and I hope you do, too. I suspect we share that goal, or you would not have read this far.

Knowledge and Vitality

Most people want energy and vitality. In our young adult years, we feel so full of energy we believe we are invincible. Most young people cannot even imagine not being here. If you are older, you know you cannot turn back the clock to when you were 20, but you can age gracefully and live a good, energetic life. I believe the garden is the tool to help us achieve that lifestyle. Besides helping your vitality, gardening helps you relieve stress through daily exercise and connecting to the natural world, even if your only activity is to pull a few weeds or transplant with a 4-inch container.

Beyond your health, the best part of gardening is the knowledge you accumulate with every season. The better you are as a gardener, the higher and greater becomes your understanding of how all life is connected. The biodiversity in your backyard is a natural laboratory with more specimens in it than any university life sciences department. If you can learn about all the microbes in the soil, the insects that crawl and fly around, the plants you grow, and the nutrition they hold to help you become healthy, it is worth every ounce of energy you exert in your garden. The garden gives you a reason to continue learning and to keep exercising. It also gives you something to anticipate with excitement. If you are already a gardener, you know how I can say, "Harvest time is party time."

A health insurance policy will not truly help you if you become sick. The best policy might spare you the financial burden, but becoming ill is the worst thing that can happen to you regardless of your financial means. You cannot put a price tag on your health. My father, Lou, has always told me, "If you have your health, that's all that matters, because without your health you cannot enjoy life." I always think of my father's words with every choice I make. If you have ever been gravely ill yourself or seen someone you care for get sick, you probably thought to yourself, "I would pay anything so my loved one or I could feel better." Money is not what we value most when we want to restore our health.

Here is how to pay your next health insurance premium in sweat. Dig that hole in your backyard. Plant and cultivate the soil. Start your healthy garden full of nutrient-rich vegetables, herbs and fruits. Do not wait until you have to call on your health insurance policy to get a preventable ailment treated. The quote at the top of this chapter says, "Let food be thy medicine." Your daily choices can keep the doctor away. We all need to have a good medical doctor that we see regularly. However, we should not be routinely going to the doctor when we are already sick. Regularly getting a clean bill of health every time you visit a physician is the ultimate goal. Your garden will help make your visits to the doctor a repeated validation of your healthy lifestyle.

Chapter 28

HOME GROWN NUTRITION

{

There are lots of people in this world who spend so much time watching their health that they haven't the time to enjoy it.
-Josh Billings

}

This chapter gives evidence that homegrown organic produce is far more nourishing and healthful than conventionally grown produce. It compares the two growing methods and gives sound reasons for going organic.

I have been praying for the consumption of homegrown foods to increase all over the world. According to the Edibles Gardening Trends Research Report published by the Garden Writers Association Foundation (GWAF), more than 41 million U.S. households (38 percent) grew a vegetable garden in 2009. More than 19.5 million households (18 percent) grew an herb garden and 16.5 million households (15 percent) grew fruits during that period. Gardening has grown more popular for two reasons: money and health. It makes good financial sense to grow your own food, and a growing number of unbiased scientific studies confirm the superior nutritional value of foods grown organically. Organically grown foods, especially those grown at home, have the greatest nutritional value and positive health benefits when eaten as part of a regular diet.

Nutrient Density

Homegrown organic crops contain a significantly higher amount of phytonutrients compared to conventionally grown foods. Organic produce offers more antioxidants (vitamin C, polyphenols and flavonoids), micronutrients and minerals. Also, when you grow and eat organic food, you avoid or stop exposing yourself to the wide array of pesticides, heavy metals, nitrates and other contaminants in conventional crops. Avoiding contamination and bioaccumulation takes you a giant step closer to good health.

For a long time, I have seen a definite relationship between the methods of chemical fertilization and plant treatment and the poor nutritional quality of conventional crops. Organic produce contains higher nutritional value, or nutrient density, than conventional produce. Furthermore, with homegrown produce, gardeners can exercise complete control to restrict or eliminate contaminants like chemical fertilizers, pesticides and herbicides. Therefore, the organic grower minimizes or eliminates the health risks and diseases associated with consuming mono-cultured food crops that are conventionally grown.

Scientists have known the link between human health and soil health for many years. However, many of the giant agriculture corporations that manufacture chemicals also fund or endow the majority of university experiments and testing. This financial relationship between large-scale food producers and academic research presents bias barriers to achieving objective research results. Companies that support scientific inquiry and research have a financial stake in cheaper, less healthy forms of food production. Scientific trials pointing to or supporting the positive benefits of organic foods, or the detrimental effects of conventional growing and processing methods, pose a financial threat to established agribusiness interests. If you owned or invested in a huge chemical company that makes fertilizers, pesticides, herbicides or genetically modified products, you would not want to conduct testing to prove that what you sell is inferior and poses health risks. I am an optimist not a cynic, but it is simple human nature in a capitalist economic structure that companies will suppress or avoid revealing evidence that undermines their sales and profits.

If agriculture and food research were done with pure objectivity and an attitude of "Let the chips fall where they may," we would have widespread testing and publicity to show which chemicals are unsafe and should never come near our food and water. Chemical treatments would have to be retired. Some conventionally grown crops would have to be redirected for sale (at significantly reduced prices) to poorer developing nations that have weaker regulations.

The public hears little about the disparity in nutritional quality of produce and foods grown and processed by different methods. To be fair, some conventional foods do contain respectable nutritional quality. Some food crops are raised on newer farms where the land has not been overworked for many years. Lands under recently cleared forest and jungle are still raw, pristine and nutrient rich. However, most soils farmed in the U.S. have been depleted by destructive mismanagement methods over many generations. Such land is much less likely to yield high quality produce.

The Taste Test and Nutrition

Have you ever heard a gardener say, "Nothing can beat the great taste of my homegrown tomatoes"? You may also hear complaints (or experience yourself) that store bought tomatoes have little flavor and are full of water. Grocery store produce often does not taste anything like the wonderful fruits and vegetables many families ate from the farms where past generations lived and grew their food.

Why are grocery tomatoes so inferior to home grown? Most tomatoes are picked green, transported and refrigerated unripe to help them stay looking perfect. They are also artificially ripened by exposing them to ethylene gas at the produce distributor. The result is the mealy, tasteless tomatoes you see in the average grocery produce section.

After growing their own, some gardeners decide they cannot go back to store bought tomatoes. They do not always know why the homegrown produce tastes so much better. Perhaps they just thought it was sweeter for some reason. Maybe they noticed less water in their plants or credited that dark compost they had been adding for years. Home gardeners usually cannot identify a purely scientific reason as to why their produce tastes better than what they generally find in the supermarket. Organic gardeners have known what they grow tastes better but they could not prove their produce was better for them. Logical deduction suggests if we feed the soil with clean and pure organic nutrients, we can produce healthier plants. However, not much science was applied to that reasoning.

The science below is simple to understand. Low-quality produce is easy to identify. It has low amounts of total dissolved sugars and low nutrient content. It also does not taste as good or sweet. Dissolved sugars are converted to needed energy when we eat them. Low nutrients and low dissolved sugars equal less available energy or fuel for our bodies. Conversely, plants with high nutrient content will have a high sucrose content, or brix level. (Brix is a measure of the dissolved sugar-to-water mass ratio. This is what we associate with a juicy quality.)

Plants that yield inferior produce are weaker. They transmit an electromagnetic frequency in the same range as destructive insects. These plants are in a way inviting consumption by pests that occupy a lower level on the food chain. The human intervention of chemical pest control prevents a weak and inferior plant from naturally being consumed by pests. Healthy produce, on the other hand, contains a high level of dissolved sugars and thick protective cell walls. These plants do not send signals that cry out, "I am sick" to insects that attack them. Healthy plants emit electromagnetic frequencies that insects cannot identify. This is a natural deterrent for insects to consume otherwise healthy plants. The high dissolved sugar content in healthy plants will convert to alcohol in an insect's digestive system and cause the insects that eat these plants to suffer from diarrhea and dehydration. Insects do not have a liver as we do and cannot digest these sugars, so consuming healthy plants and their sugar content actually kills them. In this respect, healthy plants contain a natural pesticide, namely sugar. Conversely, natural sugar is just what we need for energy, health and long life.

The lesson of this chapter is to trust your taste buds. If a fruit or a vegetable tastes sweet, it probably contains some nutrient density. Even when they contain nutrient density, plants treated with the toxins in fertilizers, pesticides and herbicides often carry chemical residues harmful to human health. Home grown or organic produce is still the healthiest choice.

Bioavailability

Many of the nutritional supplements on the cutting edge of technology get their nutrients from food-based ingredients and adding catalysts such as digestive enzymes and probiotics. These ingredients make nutritional supplements bioavailable. (Nutrients are useless to our bodies unless we can absorb them.)

Whole foods provide us with bioavailable nutrients. Because these foods have not been altered, they have the highest potential to readily breakdown in our body for maximum use and value. This is basic biochemistry. The simpler the molecule, the easier it is for us to absorb it. We should try to derive all nutrition from food, because our body was designed to identify those compounds in their unprocessed form. Nature never isolates vitamins or minerals the way so many supplements are isolated in containers and stacked on a store shelf. Vitamins and minerals in nature are available in complex combinations found in the wide variety of food we eat. Nutritionists know our body does not absorb essential nutrients most effectively when taken as isolated USP vitamins or minerals. (USP stands for U.S. Pharmacopeia, a non–governmental, official public standards–setting authority for prescription and over–the–counter medicines. USP also sets widely recognized standards for quality, purity, strength and consistency in food ingredients and dietary supplements.)

Absorption rates are less than 5 percent in some cases. For example, your system may use less than 50 milligrams of that 1000-milligram pill you took. The rest is eliminated. If you want to supplement your organic healthy garden foods, make sure you use food-based ingredients and not synthetic/USP nutrients.

Nothing mentioned above considers simple processed sugars. Avoid foods with high-fructose sugars as much as possible, because they are completely bioavailable. This may pose a major health risk. Additionally, the calories in high fructose sugars have no nutritional significance for us; they are "empty." Read the label on packaged foods you buy. Many contain high fructose corn syrup, a sweetener substitute for white sugar.

The term bioavailability refers to the relationship between how much of a nutrient you consume to how much you absorb for use in your body. Bioavailability can vary drastically from person to person based on the beneficial probiotics in the digestive tract and the amount of food rich in digestive enzymes a person eats. Other factors affect bioavailability. How certain foods are cooked and how fast a person chews and swallows affect nutrient absorption. Alcohol consumption, metabolic rate, gastrointestinal disorders or disease, age and state of general health all influence bioavailability.

With our desire to look young and healthy, many of us have gone to a low-calorie diet focused on nutrient density and the bioavailability of the nutrients in the foods we eat. The idea is to consume less food but make sure we are absorbing the maximum amount of nutrition from fewer calories. This makes perfect sense and is a logical approach. However, many people still eat junk food and consume cheap supplements in hope that they fulfill the nutritional requirements for a full and energetic life. I understand this reasoning, but healthy food from an organic diet with bioavailable nutrients is still the best and safest way to better health. Simply eating fewer calories and consuming supplements will keep you energized and moving. However, it does not add any long-term health benefits. Also, using supplements requires a complete understanding of how nutrients react in our system for full absorption or bioavailability. This requires study with tests and trials for each individual's unique biochemistry.

To keep things simple, grow as much as you can organically in your backyard in nutrient rich soils. People wanting weight control will be pleased to know that with organic produce you can eat less, because the nutrient density is higher. If you want to take supplements, make sure they are food-based. Complement supplements with synergistic, broad-spectrum catalysts such as probiotics and a wide variety of digestive enzymes. These will help your body extract the nutrients in food to make them bioavailable. Grow organic, eat organic and be healthy even when you eat less.

Chapter 29

ooooo

HEALING COMPOUNDS FROM OUR PLANTS

{ *If you have health, you probably will be happy, and if you have health and happiness, you have all the wealth you need, even if it is not all you want.*

-Elbert Hubbard }

Every plant we eat has hidden jewels. Nutritional scientists used to think we take in just a few vitamins and minerals when we eat fruits and vegetables. However, research is beginning to reveal the added benefits of "phytonutrients" and high fiber in plants. Chlorophyll from green foods supports intestinal health. Soluble fibers in these foods help remove heavy metals from our bone marrow and living cells. This also supports joint health and helps normalize primary hormonal levels in both men and woman. Phytonutrients and antioxidants help us resist age-related illnesses and cellular damage caused by free radicals.

Trauma can come from poor diet, exposure to environmental toxins, a car accident or a genetic disposition to a disease. Trauma causes permanent damage to the extent we cannot fight off the effects with a strong immune system. Homegrown produce supports our immune system by delivering more complete nutrition. When we absorb a diverse set of trace nutrients that support the functions of digestion, circulation, metabolism, detoxification, bone formation, cardiovascular support and blood sugar control, we benefit from stronger immunity to all forms of trauma and stress.

Phytonutrients are Powerful Healers

Consuming plenty of fruits and vegetables takes the guesswork out of finding nutrient balance. Mother Nature is the best chemist we have. Vitamins and minerals, micronutrient supplements, and plant-based super foods are all great, but nature in its most raw form gives the most abundant bioavailability.

Phytonutrients are recently discovered. In the 1990s, scientists first acknowledged phytonutrients, which they now recognize for their disease protective compounds. When you eat fruits and vegetables, your body absorbs phytonutrients which act as nutraceuticals. They support healthy blood vessels, connective tissue, organs and all other parts of the body. Phytonutrients protect us from toxics in the environment and in conventionally grown food we eat. They also help control different bacteria and pathogenic fungi, free radicals and carcinogens. The worldwide nutritional science community is working to understand and connect the disease preventive characteristics of these phytochemicals.

The natural world contains tens of thousands of different phytonutrients. So far, we have identified only about one thousand. Of all these recognized nutrients, fewer than one hundred have been analyzed effectively for their disease preventive properties and nutritive qualities. Perhaps the most beneficial attributes of these phytonutrients is their protective quality against the destructive action of free radicals, degenerative diseases and even the oxidation of our physical body. (Yes, your body literally rusts out over time.)

Phytonutrients in the whole foods we eat control the most basic functions of human chemistry. As free radicals begin to destroy our body and our physical integrity, our bodies rust and deteriorate. Phytonutrients come to our defense, protecting us from disease. They protect cellular membranes from free radical damage. If free radicals cannot penetrate into cells, they cannot oxidize them. Remember the discussion of plant cells in Chapter 12, which reviews cell wall thickness. Cell walls provide structural integrity in plants, defending them from insect attack. Human cells are similar in the sense that the thicker the membrane surrounding our cells, the more structural integrity we have to support muscle mass and skin tissue. This directly translates to tight, glowing skin and a lean, muscular body. Phytonutrients clean the blood. By keeping our blood clean and pure, our bloodstream more effectively controls bacteria and fungi, toxins, environmental pollution and all destructive bioaccumulation.

Everything we need to know about the beauty and benefits of phytonutrients exists in a bowl of salad. Phytonutrients are potent chemicals that can help us make up for lost time nutritionally. Despite the scientific research and advances in understanding human health, we suffer from increasing rates of obesity. We still contend with heart health issues and joint conditions associated with aging. What is the optimum diet? The volume of literature on this subject would require a lifetime commitment to read and comprehend. My instinctive compass tells me to go back to where we evolved more than 10,000 years ago. Raw foods with minimal processed ingredients offer the most simple, safe approach to a healthy diet.

When I was a kid in nutrition class, my teachers explained the six basic food groups and showed us how to separate them, but the instruction never included phytonutrients. Modern science had not yet discovered them. I have always gravitated towards the raw green diet. Consuming raw, green foods seemed to be the most natural and healthy approach to living disease free. Our backyards held hidden jewels we never discussed in nutrition class. A good nutritional advisor can offer you a list of foods with the highest amounts of phytonutrients suited to your age, weight, activity level, sleep habits, stress and living environment. I have included some examples of plants in this book with their phytonutrient properties.

Cruciferous vegetables (so named because their cells are arranged in a cross-like shape) like kale and broccoli contain powerful antioxidants called sulforaphane, which has demonstrated properties to prevent a host of diseases, including breast cancer. In general, the cruciferous vegetables are powerful carcinogen inhibitors, support all the organs that detoxify the bloodstream and increase the bioavailability of other nutrients. Phytonutrients come in all colors including green, yellow, red and purple. By growing the widest color variety of fruits and vegetables in your garden, your crop has a wider spectrum of phytonutrients.

Antioxidants and Disease Prevention

The word antioxidant literally means "against oxidation." This takes us back to the idea of the body literally rusting away from free radicals that oxidize our blood. Oxidation breaks the human body down on the cellular level. If you have ever smoked, drunk alcohol, lived in a city, or painted or remodeled your home, you have been exposed to environmental factors that damage the body on the molecular level. Free radical oxidizers literally rob electrons from molecules in the body and the cellular membranes that encompass the DNA of our genetic makeup. As molecules within our body react with each other, free radicals damage the connective tissue of muscles, organs and complex structures that make up the human body. Molecular disruption by free radicals ultimately leads to the breakdown of the body and creates conditions like heart disease and cancer.

However, antioxidants have the ability to stop this chain reaction by releasing electrons. This neutralizes free radical oxidizers and minimizes damage. For some reason, antioxidants do not become reactive or unstable when they lose an electron. The released electrons from antioxidants combat molecular breakdown in the body caused by free radicals, helping to prevent a variety of degenerative diseases associated with aging. Free radicals can cause cognitive impairment, macular degeneration, cataracts, Alzheimer's disease, immune dysfunction, cardiovascular diseases and a variety of cancers. Nothing will stop the human body from breaking down eventually, but antioxidants help to keep us together longer.

Antioxidants are found in a variety of different foods you can grow in your backyard. These foods help blood circulation and protect the body from free radical damage. As mentioned earlier, the body literally rusts away primarily through the damage of free radicals. Antioxidants over time can affect genetic makeup, the DNA that carries our genetic code and determines our lifespan. For example, the Japanese diet, rich in raw vegetables and fish, has been effective in health and life extension due to the high antioxidant foods they eat. In raw form, such as in sushi, the fish loses none of its nutrients to cooking. The Japanese also drink a large amount of green and white teas that are potent antioxidants. You may not be able to grow these teas in your climate zone, but you can buy them from an organic source.

While antioxidants play a major role in human health, what are they really? It is a collective term for micronutrients, trace elements, vitamins, polyphenols, and carotenoids. The most common antioxidant sources include liver, fish, dairy, grains, nuts, citrus, berries, tomatoes and colored fruits and vegetables. When you visit your local nursery to start your healthy garden, keep color in mind. The wider color variety you choose, the wider the variety of antioxidants in your produce.

The media we watch and hear flood us with messages touting the healing properties of antioxidant foods. This is one time I join the chorus of popular culture. However, most commercial fruit juices and supplements have been processed to a degree that reduces their antioxidant beneficial properties. Nothing can replace a well-balanced diet. The best supplements on earth cannot replace a healthy homegrown meal.

Vitamin A and E are fat-soluble and can potentially be stored in your liver and fatty tissues instead of being used quickly or excreted through your urine, as are the water-soluble B vitamins and C. Taking too many supplements can run the risk of toxic concentration in your system. It is safer to grow and eat a wide variety of fruits and vegetables to ensure that you get the widest variety of antioxidants in a natural form.

Grow it. Eat it.

Chapter 30

◦◦◦◦◦

FIBER AND METABOLISM

{
The longer I live the less confidence I have in drugs and the greater is my confidence in the regulation and administration of diet and regimen.

-John Redman Coxe
}

Prebiotics and High-Fiber Foods

Prebiotics have received much attention in the media for good reasons. Prebiotics are non-digestible, high-fiber ingredients that prepare an environment for the beneficial probiotics in our intestine. Typically, prebiotics are carbohydrates found in the grains and greens, but they can also come from other sources such as soluble fibers. Fruits and vegetables, especially those fibrous vegetables that have thick veins, can promote healthy bowel regularity. It has been said many times, "Death starts in the colon." Over time, eating meats or highly processed foods loaded with simple sugars, preservatives and other processed foods slows down your digestive tract. Without the bulk of fiber, digestion becomes sluggish, causing more toxicity in the body, while metabolism also slows severely.

Eating probiotics along with a high-fiber diet keeps the colon "clean" and working vigorously, as it is meant to. Fasting, drinking high volumes of distilled water daily, and eating leafy greens and other fruits and vegetables high in fiber all promote colon health. The general idea of consuming fiber is to eliminate all waste and non-essentials as quickly as possible. The longer the contents of your bowel sit in your body, the greater the potential for them to become toxic. When digestion and elimination are sluggish, the colon fills with undigested, putrefied waste that can leach back into the bloodstream and make the entire system toxic.

People who eat a lot of meat, potatoes and white bread are at greatest risk of developing colon cancer and other digestive conditions. Diets high in fiber help eliminate cholesterol and sugars that, when left to build up in the body, can contribute to diabetes. The high-fiber foods (fruits, vegetables and whole grains) act like a sponge in your intestine to absorb and eliminate putrefied toxins. These foods literally drag out impurities through elimination.

I eat salad at least once a day. My body depends on it to stay regular in eliminating all other foods that I have eaten, such as meats and breads. We need to clear our digestive tract regularly to maintain our maximum health. We must take the trash out before it becomes putrid and creates a host of other problems. A diet high in fiber also helps reduce the risk of heart disease, high cholesterol, cancer, diabetes and gallstones. High fiber diets prevent overeating, and obviously, constipation. What a relief!

I like to eat vegetables with every meal. It is good for me and makes me feel better. I do not closely follow the often-cited U.S. recommended daily allowance, or RDA. I simply eat as much as I feel I need. If you feel as if you are not eating enough fiber, perhaps take a high bulk fiber product such as psyllium husk. I do this regularly when I feel I need a boost to eliminate foods after going on vacation and over indulging at the buffet during the holidays.

Without high-fiber in your diet, meats and other processed foods tend to accumulate in your colon. In our modern world, we tend to exercise less, eat more processed, unnatural foods and take many synthesized medications. These all lead to bioaccumulation in the intestine and seepage of toxins back into the body. Eating clean, pure organic fruits and vegetables along with probiotics helps eliminate these digestive problems

Fast Metabolism – Lean Body

During my college days in Los Angeles, when I was 19 years old, my friends and I would run out to a Mexican catering truck at 2:30 in the morning. We would eat beef tacos and a beef burrito with all the trimmings. Then we would go right to bed only to wake up and go out for a huge breakfast. I would then down an omelet, hash browns, toast and a smoothie. In an 8-hour period, I probably consumed about 10,000 calories and never gained a pound. Also, we drank beer and ate appetizers before we got to the catering truck, so there were another couple thousand calories with no weight gain.

Things changed quickly when I turned 25. I began to count the calories that I put into my body. I have always exercised, so weight gain was never an issue for me. Now, years later, I can feel the difference in my body. My metabolism, or the rate at which all the processes in my body burn up calories from the food I eat, has slowed as part of the normal aging process. I must carefully watch what I eat. I consume those foods I know will accelerate my digestion and give me energy to keep me active and going strong.

A healthy metabolism turns the food we consume into energy very effectively. Conversely, a slow metabolism, or low metabolic rate, burns food less effectively. Like a bank account, if we take in more calories than we spend/burn, we accumulate the excess as a "balance" of fat. This is how we gain weight by overeating and under-exercising. (We can also gain weight by building larger, stronger muscles, because muscle is denser than fat, but this is not related to overeating.)

We can do many things to accelerate our metabolism and thus burn calories more effectively. Eating healthy foods (with measured, small portions) drinking certain energy producing juices balanced with a good exercise plan can keep you looking great and maintaining a fast metabolism.

If you consult a nutritionist, he may use the term basal metabolic rate or BMR. The BMR measures the amount of energy your body uses when at rest. It includes all the energy you use to do simple tasks like breathing and maintaining your body temperature. Metabolism varies with age, gender, genetics, exercise habits and the type and quantity of foods in the diet. Your BMR is largely tied to a period of about twelve hours after your last meal before bed and when you wake up the next day. During sleep, our organs do not exert much energy. The nutritionist wants to know your BMR because of its relation to your daily activities and schedule.

Because our BMR usually slows down as we age, it is well to do what you can to maintain a faster metabolism. Faster metabolism is associated with low body fat content and a high-energy lifestyle full of vitality. As we age, it becomes more difficult to jump start our metabolism and keep it high. Although aging makes it progressively more difficult to change your eating and exercise habits, you CAN do both. Many healthy, happy exercisers did not make their important lifestyle changes until their 50s and even 60s. It's never too late to do the best thing for yourself.

Here is a quick and simple way to get an approximate number for your BMR. Multiply your weight in pounds by 10. For example, if you weigh 175 pounds, your BMR is 1,750, meaning you need at least 1,750 calories daily to maintain energy for survival. You should eat more than this for energy to move freely and think clearly, but this simple calculation will demystify BMR and give you an idea of the minimum you should consume daily.

To make your life simple without having to count calories, you can adopt a few things into your daily life. Eating the right foods at the right time and getting the proper exercise makes all the difference. Here are some more tips.

Drink plenty of water daily. Drink before, during and after your meals and all day between. Some European studies indicate that metabolism can increase 30 percent after drinking 17 ounces of water.

Drinking antioxidant-rich teas such as green tea, white tea or even a little coffee will speed up metabolism and burn fat naturally. I am not a coffee drinker, because it gives me the jitters, but many have found it to work for them. Just lay off the sweeteners.

Eat plenty of green foods naturally high in fiber and loaded with phytonutrients. Green foods not only speed up metabolism by eliminating the foods quickly, they also help chemically prevent disease. I love probiotics. They digest all the accumulated foods in my system and eliminate them effectively, which also helps speed up metabolism.

I like to eat meat to maintain a strong and lean muscle mass, but the right meat is very important. Try to consume turkey, chicken breast, or my favorite, wild caught salmon. Salmon is not only good for metabolism, it is loaded with omega-3 fatty acids that aid the heart, nervous system and brain. Avoid fatty meats like ground hamburger and anything fried.

Here is another trick I have been using for years. Eat lots of cayenne pepper powder. It speeds up the metabolism and has many other nutritional benefits.

Work up a sweat in the garden. Speed up your heart rate daily to maintain a fast metabolism. Do not expect miracle diets to do the work for you. Avoid synthetically formulated metabolism pills that suppress your appetite. These pills might work in the short term but will disappoint you in the long run.

Every day you have the ability to make a series of choices. Your life is a cumulative summary of those choices. Whether you are overweight at 30 or look great at 70, how you look and feel today reflects the daily choices you made over a lifetime. Again, it is never too late to start making healthy choices. The backyard garden could be the best place to speed up your metabolism through a healthy diet and exercise.

Grow it. Eat it.

Chapter 31

∞∞∞

THE JUICE OF LIFE

{

We drink one another's health and spoil our own.
                                                    -Jerome K. Jerome

}

Concentrated Nutrients

I may have chlorophyll running through my veins, because I drink so much leafy green juice. Much of what I grow and cannot eat, I throw into a juicer. This prevents wasted food and allows the most nutrient absorption for my body. Much of what I have written in this book can be reduced to a glass of fresh juice every day. I have a lean, low-fat body, because I live primarily on green foods. My metabolism is very fast, which allows me to burn fat even when I sleep. You can have great looking skin, high energy levels, organs that function to their fullest potential, bioavailability in consumed foods, antioxidants, phytonutrients, heart health, fast elimination and micronutrients …all if you adopt juicing as a regular practice. I could write an entire book on the nutritional benefits of juicing. (Perhaps I will.)

The great thing about juice is that it delivers so many energy-boosting phytonutrients, vitamins and minerals. I can literally feel a burst of energy running through my body every time I finish my glass of juice. Green leafy drinks are one of the best things for your living body. They feed the cells at the microscopic level. Consider this: You would have to forage for about 10 hours per day and consume more than 7 pounds of green vegetables to get the energy you can drink in 20 minutes with 48 ounces of juice.

Drink your juice as fresh as you can right after it comes out of the juicer, because it begins to oxidize as it goes through the machine. The beauty of juicing is the nutrients are immediately bioavailable. Our bodies do not have to break them down to absorb them. However, because plant cells explode when their membranes are broken through the juicer machine, the exposed chlorophyll and other nutrients are exposed to oxygen that quickly breaks down the beneficial contents. If you use a straw to drink the juice from the bottom up, you receive maximum nutrients and minimum oxidation, because the juice at the bottom is the least exposed to oxygen. Do not put your fresh juice in the refrigerator, because it loses its effectiveness even a few hours later. Simply juice what you can drink in the next 10 minutes. Leave the rest of your produce on the vine or intact in the refrigerator until you are ready to drink what you juice.

Another plus of juicing comes as the abundance of nutrients gives you that full feeling. You will then eat less, because you feel satisfied, not hungry, and your metabolism has gotten a boost. As the day progresses, you can snack here and there. I keep several heads of romaine lettuce in the office refrigerator. I often eat three heads of lettuce a day and never touch anything else at lunchtime. I also keep several organically grown oranges in my backyard available for that afternoon snack. That orange gives me a natural sugar rush and is loaded with vitamin C and antioxidants.

Juicing is a lifestyle and a commitment worth making. Once you make the choice, it becomes an automatic behavior. Instead of coffee, you choose juice and lose inches off your belly. Weight loss is the result of energy you receive by drinking plenty of green juice and staying away from greasy, fatty foods.

I encourage everyone I speak with to treat themselves now and then to a hamburger and fries along with a soda if they crave it. You can safely eat almost anything once in a while. What you eat regularly, day after day, makes the difference in your nutrition and health. You do not have to be a dietary saint, but a regular healthy diet full of energy-boosting vitamins and minerals, and low in fats and carbohydrates helps you lose weight fast. I can lose 5 pounds in a week without exercise and still eat a protein rich meal with healthy greens every night. I have done it many times.

Why would I want to lose 5 pounds in a week? When I have advance notice of another interview on a television garden show, I use a few days of juicing to help me slim down. Something about the television camera "adds" a few pounds. (I always say yes to an opportunity to spread the word about Dr. Earth and the organic lifestyle.) To compensate for the "extra" weight TV adds, I put myself on my recommended diet: only green juice and water throughout the day, then lean, free-range chicken breast with a huge salad at night. This lets me safely lose about a pound a day.

What do I mean when I say "green juice"? I mean whatever I cannot eat from my garden that has a green color. I even juice all the wild dandelions that I pick from my lawn, along with mint from my herb garden, lettuce, zucchini, bell peppers and cucumbers. I throw in a few tomatoes, the most abundant crop in my garden. With my busy schedule, I cannot make juice every day at home. I also do not grow enough to make my recommended 48 ounces a day. Therefore, I rely on my dear friends at my local health food market to make juice for me. There I have access to a fresh daily selection of wheatgrass, a great source of energy and chlorophyll. I also drink kale, broccoli, daikon, parsnip, turnip, dill, cilantro, beets, celery, carrots and ginger. Dandelion is a major body cleanser, especially for the liver, which has more than 400 blood purifying functions. Dandelion, long maligned as a nuisance weed in mainstream thought, is actually a tonic, an elixir, and in my opinion, the closest thing to the fountain of youth.

Grow everything you possibly can organically, so you know what you are eating. We know homegrown produce is nutrient dense. Juicing homegrown produce concentrates those nutrients even more. Even if you drink juices from crops grown conventionally, you will receive concentrated nutrients.

What you cannot grow at home you can buy at the local farmers market or organic produce market. I like to support local growers I know and trust. Supporting them is good for my community and ultimately for the environment, because growers who are close to me use up less fuel to ship their produce to where I can buy it.

I also recommend supporting your local health food store that sells good quality produce. Take a good supplement daily. Drink plenty of green juice and clean filtered water. Avoid soda. Stay away from fatty fast food. Do these things regularly, and the pounds will fly off and doctor visits will confirm your improved health.

One of the best side effects of juicing is looking great with tight, glowing skin. You are feeding your living cells. The organic lifestyle is something you do as a treat for yourself not as a chore. You want the energy you need to live a full life free of ailments. You want your mind to function to its fullest potential. When you have achieved physical health, spiritual health often follows, because you are free to elevate your mind and creativity without being held down by physical limitations. One of the best byproducts of being healthy is confidence. You feel confident every day, because you feel good and look great.

Grow it, eat it, juice it and live healthy.

PART 5

GARDENING BASICS

Chapter 32

ooooo

SIMPLE THINGS YOU NEED TO KNOW

{

Live in each season as it passes; breathe the air, drink the drink, taste the fruit, and resign yourself to the influences of each.
*- **Henry David Thoreau***

}

This book focuses on the large picture of a healthy lifestyle through growing your own food, but it helps to review the basics of gardening. While the information seems basic, especially for the seasoned gardener, even experienced people can benefit from a refresher on the basic information. A novice gardener certainly needs to know the material in this section.

You can succeed in growing your healthy garden no matter what your level of gardening experience. With some forethought, planning and sound information, you can get it right the first time. After all, this is science not magic. My approach is to give you the basics and show you how to garden in a healthy way.

This gardening primer is brief and to the point, lightly touching on what you need to know. If you want more education and preparation before you start, get a comprehensive manual or talk with a seasoned gardener. Good independent nurseries also have knowledgeable staff ready to help you, because it is good business to help aspiring gardeners. Perhaps join a local garden club, as they have some of the best minds and vast experience in your immediate area. Members will have many answers and guidance, and you will likely make new friends who share your interest in both health and gardening.

MICROCLIMATE

Know Your Backyard

To succeed, you must understand your environment and become an expert on your natural surroundings. First, learn the usual dates of the first hard frost and the springtime thaw in your area. What you can plant and harvest depends on when your planting and growing season begins and ends and how long it lasts.

Also, you must know where the sun rises and sets in relation to your planting beds. For example, you need to know how many hours of direct sunlight your plants can receive and where the shadows, if any, fall in the afternoon.

Next you must attune yourself to the annual and seasonal weather patterns in your area. Gardeners love a comprehensive weather report (rain, wind, high and low pressure and temperature extremes) because it helps them plan their activities. Note when seeds germinate and when insects (and which ones) begin to appear.

Invest in thermometers. A good quality soil and air thermometer with high and low capabilities will simplify your life and give you an edge in living with the elements.

Your garden is likely to have small yet important microclimates. For example, hard reflective objects such as statuary or a shadow created in the afternoon might cause a cold pocket. Hot and cold pockets can interfere with a desired plant you have in mind. These areas will not only change daily but will evolve annually as you greet the different seasons. Summer might be bad for lettuce but great for tomatoes. Anticipate these changes when you decide where to grow your healthy garden.

You may have at least four different microclimates around your home:
- A hot side facing South
- A shadowed, cool side on the North
- A warm Western side with afternoon sun
- An ever-changing Eastern side that may be warm or cool depending on trees, high fencing or the time of year

Carefully observe heat and light to know where to create your healthy garden. Position your raised beds, rows or plots to run north and south so plants will receive more sunlight in winter. In winter, too, keep tall trellised plants against the north wall and the shorter plants to the south. In the summer, do the opposite. There is much more to know, but these are the basics of microclimates.

PLANT ZONES
What and Where to Grow
We decide on a plant's ability to thrive in a certain area according to its geographic climate zone. The USDA publishes the most commonly used hardiness zone map, which divides the continental U.S. into 11 zones. The zones are derived from the average annual minimum temperatures, from zone 1 (-50° F) to zone 11 (+40°F). You can find a copy of this map online or at a local library or university. Many independent nurseries have books that clearly describe the different zones. You can also just visit your neighborhood nursery. If you see something there you

like, almost certainly it will work in your backyard. Especially when you grow from seeds, you need to pay close attention to your zone map.

Another good zone map comes from the editors of Sunset Magazine. They divided the United States and Southern Canada into 45 climate zones, considering many variables. It looks at many area temperature extremes, as well as humidity, rainfall, local topography, elevation and even proximity to large bodies of water. However, visiting your local independent nursery and selecting the plants they carry will serve you as well as the very best zone map. Nurseries want to stock and offer plants that will thrive for their customers. Withering plants are bad for business. Your success is also their success.

If you buy seeds and plants from catalogues, invest in a Sunset reference book. Besides the climate zones, these books have a complete description, often with color photographs, of every plant appropriate for your region. These comprehensive books are also fun to browse through to get ideas and inspiration for your next garden project.

SUN AND SHADE

A Defining Factor

To grow plants that produce fruits, make sure you have plenty of sun. Allow at least six hours daily for tomatoes, cucumbers, zucchini, peppers, beans, corn, eggplant, summer squash and cabbage. In general, the bigger the fruit, the more sunlight it must have.

On the other hand, many vegetables and herbs do well in shaded areas. You can grow them with about four hours of daily sun. In these areas, try carrots, beets, chard, cauliflower, chives, lettuce, chicories, radicchio, arugula, basil, mint, parsley, spinach or winter squash. A good rule of thumb: If the plant is a leafy green vegetable, less sunlight is fine.

Here is a small biology lesson. Sunlight creates sugars through photosynthesis. More light creates more sugars. Less light and fewer sugars are fine for non-fruiting plants. Herbs are great for shady areas. Many healthy plants will grow regardless of the sunlight or shade your garden receives.

DRAINAGE

Get the Wet Out

Most fruits and vegetables need a good balance of rich organic materials to grow to their full potential. This means they require plenty of air space between soil particles while also being able to retain moisture. Most garden plants like both air and moisture around their roots in order to drain well. If you can thoroughly wet the soil and have the moisture drained relatively quickly, that is a good sign. If that same soil can stay a medium moist, not sopping wet, for a few days, you have good drainage.

Organic materials usually help make for great drainage. The structure of the soil has a lot to do with the drainage. If you have a good balance between sand, silt, clay and organic materials, you have a solid foundation for good drainage. Good drainage brings good results, including reducing fungal pathogens in the soil, better root development, a healthy aerobic environment and better nutrient availability.

In brief, in sandy soils, water drains too quickly. In clay soils, water drains too slowly. Adding organic materials helps correct and balance both types of soil. Do a simple test to see how your soil drains and whether you have to make changes to correct your drainage. Dig a hole about 1 foot deep and 6 inches wide. Fill the hole with water and let it drain completely. When the hole is empty, fill it again with water to the very top. If it takes more than 10 hours to empty again, you have a drainage problem. The good news is you can fix the problem several ways. You can add organic materials. You can add drainage pipes to direct the water away. You can also grow plants in raised beds. I love raised beds. Read on to learn why.

Raised Beds Elevate Your Growth

I love to grow plants in raised beds for many reasons. They make it easier to plant and harvest crops. Aesthetically, they are beautiful when constructed handsomely with a sense of design and purpose.

Raised beds also give you total control of soil composition. The soil you use to fill the raised bed can be full of life with composted organic materials rich in humus and full of nutrition. Crop yields typically improve a great deal in raised beds. I have seen crop yields increase as much as 42 percent compared to typical planting directly in the ground.

Raised beds also address drainage. They make your garden less dependent on the variable drainage characteristics of your native soil. Even more importantly, the native soil might be poor and have little nutrient value. What if the previous homeowner had no regard for soil health or the environment and dumped his motor oil or other toxins directly on the ground you intend to use? You might be afraid to grow any crops in it except ornamental plants; a raised bed gets around that problem. A raised bed looks great and makes the statement, "I am a professional gardener."

After you build the beds, you may find it easier to start on projects in one bed at a time. Focus on one area every day or weekend so you are not overwhelmed by the entire garden. Beds are easy to weed because the soil is light and fluffy. Since raised beds are knee high, planting causes less back strain. Plants in raised beds do not compact. Because you are not walking on the area where they grow, plants in raised beds grow better with more air circulation.

When constructing your raised bed, you can use brick and mortar or natural looking stones with mortar. I love using hay bales, which look cool and organic. Hay bales form a raised bed instantly and are the perfect height. If you want to frame a wooden bed, use redwood or another hardwood that has not been dipped in chemical wood preservatives. Pressure treated wood is loaded with toxic heavy metals. Do not use painted wood, as the paint will eventually decompose and contaminate your soil. Finally, do not use cheap plastic, instant beds. They look temporary and unprofessional. Unless you live on the go, construct a real bed built to last.

Container Gardening

You can grow enough organic fruit, vegetables and herbs on a 4-foot by 8-foot balcony to satisfy your hungry appetite. Space may be limited in your garden. Perhaps you live in an apartment. Or you may not want to invest a lot of time in a full-scale garden. Whatever your situation, you can still enjoy produce you grow within reach of your kitchen. Using containers to grow organic edibles is rewarding and easy. Container produce can give you nutritious, tasty and visually pleasing organic plants. Nothing tastes better and is healthier than a few fresh herbs, vegetables or fruits from your garden. Put them in a salad within minutes of harvest when they contain the most nutrients and are full of flavor.

Pay close attention to a few important rules, and you will need to invest only minimal time to enjoy an abundance of organic and healthy fruits and vegetables. You must consider five factors before you plant your organic container garden. Considering these variables will allow easy set up, maintenance and harvest of a productive container garden.
- Sunlight
- Container size
- Potting medium
- Fertilizer
- Trellising support

SUNLIGHT

Light is Energy

Sunlight is the most important factor to consider. Too little prevents your plants from converting enough sunlight energy to produce fruit of real value. (On the other hand, some herbs grown specifically for their foliage do fine with less sunlight.) Track the sun and shade patterns in your immediate area to get a good sense of the space where you intend to garden and what plants will do well there.

Here is a simple rule: Fruit trees and vegetables that set flowers (such as oranges, plums, tomatoes, cucumbers, eggplants, peppers, or squash) need a lot of sunlight. Photosynthesis produces sugars that directly feed flowers and help grow fruits of appealing size, taste and nutritional value. A good local nursery has staff people who can help you understand the sunlight you need for the kind of plants you can grow in your region.

CONTAINER SIZE

More Soil Equals More Nutrition

The second most important variable for container gardening is the size of the container. The more soil volume your plants have, the more extensive the root system that can draw on a larger pool of nutrients and water. Available container space directly influences the nutritional value, size and quality of the fruits, vegetables and herbs you will harvest. More is definitely better. For example, tomatoes require a minimum of 15 gallons of soil in order to develop into full size plants with rewarding taste and nutrition. Other vegetable crops can survive in smaller containers with less soil volume. They still benefit from more soil by producing larger, more bountiful crops in a larger container.

The type of container you use can also make a big difference in growth and quality. Terracotta containers are a good choice, because they breathe with the soil and do not fluctuate quickly with extreme temperatures. Redwood is another good choice that also breathes and retains moisture longer. Plastic containers, which come in a great variety of styles, work fine but will require more watering than thicker, denser pots. With plastic containers, you must use mulch to retain moisture. I use mulch with all containers. Plants in small containers will dry out quickly, so keep a close eye on these pots. In general, less plant foliage requires less regular watering. A larger plant needs more water. Pay close attention to all your plants, and water them regularly as needed.

Potting Medium: Premium Quality, Better Nutrition

Soil is the source of life for every living thing on earth. Healthy soil produces a healthy crop. The type of soil or "potting medium" you choose has a large affect on your plants and their ability to produce an abundance of large, nutritious fruits and vegetables. If you have a potting that gives you good results, stay with it. Chemicals are common in many bagged potting soils. Make sure your bagged potting soil contains no chemicals such as synthetic plant nutrients.

Potting soil is different from composts or planting mixes. It can be difficult to formulate. Getting the balance right is the key. You want potting soil to drain fast to prevent root rot, but you also need the soil to hold on to enough moisture to support a healthy transfer of nutrients to the root.

Use some of that compost from your kitchen and yard waste. It makes a good component to mix with the potting soil. A good formula is about 1/3 compost to 2/3 potting soil. Do not skimp on the soil, as it is the only source of nutrition for your edibles. If the soil is poor, the nutrient value will be poor. A plant grown in a container is like a caged animal; it eats only what you feed it. Container plants do not have the luxury of drawing nutrients from the native soil. Therefore, spend a few extra dollars for the best soil available.

Fertilizer Feeds the Living Soil

You must feed the soil that feeds your plant root systems. Chemically fertilized soils are low in organic matter, which helps conserve the soil and its moisture, providing insurance against drought. Soils lacking organic matter are more vulnerable to drought and to extreme climate changes.

Fruit trees, tomatoes and most other vegetables, especially in containers, need a lot of fertilizer to reach full potential. Roots in containers cannot tap into food reserves the way they can in natural soil. Because the plants receive only what you give them in the container, it is especially important to use the best quality organic fertilizer. Feed the roots in your container plants slowly with the best organic fertilizer to harvest the maximum amount of nutrition from your plants. Sea based organic fertilizers are superior and contain the most multi-minerals. You will benefit from these nutrients as you consume your harvest. Healthy soil leads to healthy food. Feed containers every two months throughout the year to maximize the plant's potential. Because the plant is in a confined space, it will use all of the nutrients quickly. Keep container plants on a regular feeding schedule. Rich, tasty and nutritious vegetables are just outside your kitchen. Enjoy.

TRELLISING SUPPORT

Form and Structure with Better Health

Exposing as many leaves to sunlight as possible helps to increase your harvest. Some of your vegetables will not require any support at all, but cucumbers, tomatoes and other vine plants need support to keep them off the ground and growing in the desired location.

Air space between your plants is also important to help minimize fungal diseases. Air space also encourages beneficial insects to do their pollination work more easily by making flowers more accessible.

When you buy your trees or vegetable transplants, ask your nursery professional what he recommends. Some plants may need a stake in the center of the container, while a tomato wants a sturdy cage, and a cucumber needs a grid-like trellis. You can build many of these support systems from scraps around the house. I like a well-assembled product that looks good. Some gardeners prefer a grungy and scrappy look. Plants do not know the difference. Just give them a shoulder to lean on!

WATERING
Wet Your Whistle Just a Little
Every living organism needs water. Most plants are 90 percent water. The task of delivering water from the soil to the plant is considerable. Sixty percent of water is absorbed by plant root hairs. To keep your plants healthy and thriving you must have a good soil with plenty of organic matter to act like a sponge and allow the almost microscopic roots to travel through porous, well draining soil. Organic matter allows the soil to breathe with a good ratio of minerals that holds onto water.

When and how often should you water? No set watering schedule can be prescribed. The only schedule to go by is the one that literally feels right. I have studied many plots of land supporting many different crops. Whether growing an annual vegetable crop or perennial walnut trees that are 30 years old, I have drawn the same conclusion: You have to water when it FEELS right to you.

The best way to tell when and how much water your plant needs (whether in the ground or a container) is to feel the soil. Probe your finger about an inch or two and feel if it is dry or moist to the touch. You can buy a water meter at your local nursery. They work, but I feel closer to the soil and my plants when I touch the soil with my bare hands.

When a reference book says something like, "Water every three days in the summer and cut back to once a week in the winter" I am amazed and disappointed. I wonder: Has the author ever been a farmer and paid attention to the watering needs of plants? The soil type makes a huge difference. Also, the more organic material in a soil, the less you have to water. The hotter the day and the shallower the root system, the more you have to water. I could go on and still not cover all the unique watering needs of the plants in your backyard or in a container. Gardeners should pay attention to soil, weather, dryness and humidity. You must base your watering decisions on observation not rigid rules that may not apply to your environment.

Do not set your sprinkler system solely based on what your gardener tells you. You might need to change those sprinkler timers once a month depending on weather conditions. Otherwise, you may waste water. Best for your plants is to get just the water they need when they need it. Inspect your soil. Look at it and feel it. If it looks and feels dry, you may need to alter your watering schedule.

Watering in the morning gives your plants the entire day to draw the water from the soil as needed, especially on hot days. Water slowly to insure proper absorption. Water deeply so that it does not run off the surface, never making it down into the root zone. Plant roots are sunk down deep in the soil where you cannot see them. Pay attention to shady spots. They need less water, while the sunny areas dry out more quickly and need more water.

Let's Make a Plan

Before a contractor can build a home, the architect must provide a plan, a blueprint that clearly shows how the house looks and functions. The same is true when creating and designing a garden of any size. You must know how to put it together. Some questions to consider and answer intelligently:

- Will you start from seeds or transplants?
- In-ground or raised beds?
- Sprinkler system or hand irrigation?
- Fruits, vegetables or both?
- How will the elements of your garden work together?
- What are the sun requirements for your plants?
- Where will the same plant go next year?
  (Rotate crops each year to avoid plant diseases.)
- What plants are you going to grow in summer, winter or fall?
- What is the best soil mixture for you?
- When will the transplants go in the ground?
- How hardy are the plants you want to grow?
- When should you start them?
- What is the nutrient value of a desired plant?

Remember you are growing a nutrition garden. You will have a health food store right in your backyard. Make sure to invest time planning it.

I love to dream about how a garden will come together. A solid plan brings you that much closer to your dream garden. The possibilities are endless when we put dreams to paper and act on them. When your dream is realized in your garden, your harvest tastes that much better. There are thousands of books on planning your garden. Pick one up and get more ideas. You can never have too much knowledge about your garden and your health.

PART 6

---

100 PLANTS YOU CAN GROW & EAT
FOR HEALTH AND WELL-BEING

Chapter 33

ooooo

GROW IT - EAT IT – LIVE HEALTHY

{
*Happiness is a bowl of cherries and a book of poetry under
a shade tree.*

-Astrid Alauda
}

How to Use This Part of the Book

Here I list all plants in alphabetical order with equal emphasis and not arranged in the usual categories of fruits, vegetables and herbs. Because of the health and nutritional diversity of all plants and their beauty in your back yard, I list plants that meet three criteria:

- Important nutritional value
- Easy to grow
- Easy to find at your local nursery

The essence of Healthy Garden, Healthy You is accessible health through the backyard garden. Any good local nursery can easily understand and guide you to a seed rack, a 4-inch container or a fruit tree in a 5-gallon bucket to get you started. Also, instead of the Latin botanical names that are correct and give an air of proper taxonomic designation, I use the simple common names that Uncle Joseph or Aunt Rosette may have mentioned at Thanksgiving dinner. You can easily remember and repeat the names to the local nursery or farmers market seller to grow or buy that plant with ease and no further reference. You might call this "gardening for the rest of us."

The list aims to cover the top 100 fruits, vegetables and herbs that you can easily find at most nurseries across the United States that will grow in most regions. I list some warm climate plants, such as citrus and avocados, although they may not be practical in Michigan or Minnesota unless you build a greenhouse. You benefit from understanding the nutritional quality and importance of a plant, even if you do not grow it, because you can still buy and eat it.

The list is easy to use and understand. With more than 80,000 edible plants around the earth, even an extensive encyclopedia set and 50 years of research could not cover them all. Instead, the list is practical, because it covers 100 plants you can grow that a good independent nursery will have the seeds or plants for you to buy.

Each plant listing begins with the nutritional value of the plant (its health power and disease prevention qualities) as far as we know it. We can know something is good for us even if we don't yet understand the exact mechanism of how it works. The next part tells the practical details of how to grow it.

Be healthy and grow as many as you can. The rest you can let your local organic gardener grow for you. Remember to buy heirloom varieties as often as you can and avoid genetically engineered seeds. Eat fresh and live long with vibrancy and energy.

General Growing Tips:

1. Rotate plants from the same family every 2 to 3 seasons. Don't grow the same plants in the same plots in consecutive years. Some plants use one or more nutrients more than others. If you keep growing that plant in the same place, the soil may get depleted and unbalanced in nutrition. For this reason, you need a number of beds equal to the number of plant families you grow. If you re-amend the soil before each growth period, this will be less of a problem but is still good practice. While crop rotation is especially important for large farm operations, it also helps the home gardener by breaking pest and disease life cycles, rejuvenating nutrients and reducing weed invasion.

2. Water in early- to mid-morning to reduce evaporation and avoid frying plant foliage. This also helps foliage dry off during the day to reduce the risk of a disease. Avoid getting the soil waterlogged, which also invites disease.

3. Weeding reduces the competition for nutrition in the soil. Remove weeds as quickly as possible so they do not have time to produce seeds. Weeds also attract pests and diseases.

4. Remove dead, diseased or damaged parts of plants as soon as you notice them to avoid compromising the rest of the plant.

5. Prune woody plants by making cuts just beyond a bud and very slightly angled to promote bud growth. Ragged cuts invite infections. Cuts at too sharp an angle or below a bud prevent bud growth. If cutting an entire branch, leave a small portion attached to the trunk to prevent exposing bare wood.

❧ *ALFALFA SPROUTS* ❧

✚ **Health Power:** Health benefits come from phytonutrients not vitamins and minerals, which are in trace amounts except for vitamin K. Nutrient quantity low if eating only a few sprouts in salads or sandwiches. More concentrated dose comes from juicing. Phytonutrients include an amino acid derivative, canavanine, plant estrogens and saponins. Early studies of canavanine suggest it may help fight leukemia and cancers of the colon and pancreas. Abundant plant estrogens may support bone formation and inhibit deterioration. May also protect against many cancers (ex. breast, bowel and prostate). Saponins lower bad cholesterol (LDL) and help stimulate parts of immune system.

⬆ **Vitamin and Mineral Content:**
Vitamins – K, C and traces
Minerals – Copper, Manganese and traces

⊘ **Disease Prevention:** Sprouts or juice may help prevent or reduce symptoms of osteoporosis, atherosclerosis, cardiovascular disease and many cancers.

❦ **How to Grow:** A perennial legume requiring soil with good drainage and pH near 6.5. Can be used as green manure and added to soil as nitrogen-rich organic matter. Many farmers plant these cover crops after fall harvest, let grow over winter and till in spring. Excellent way to maintain soil tilth, organic matter and nutrient content. Other gardeners or farmers work alfalfa into crop rotation plan to help restore soil fertility during part of year. Sow in spring. Till into soil in fall. In warmer climates, sow in fall and till in spring. Sowing for food is fun project. Use sterile, clear, quart glass jar, seeds, cheesecloth or other filter material with small pores for draining, rubber band and windowsill or sunny indoor location. Put tablespoon of seeds in glass jar. Cover seeds with lukewarm filtered water to 1-2 inches above seeds. Secure filter material (cheese cloth or pantyhose) around top with rubber band. Let seeds soak overnight. Drain jar the next day by inverting over sink, leaving only enough moisture to keep seeds damp. They grow best in 70-80°F. Place jar in the dark undisturbed for four days. Each day, remove seeds and rinse with quality water up to three times a day. Drain out so seeds are damp but not soaked. Watch seeds turn white and grow several inches over a few days. After rinsing and draining on day 4, place sprouts on a tray on windowsill or sunny spot. In 15 minutes they turn green and are ready to eat.

✗ **Insect Control:** Jar is protected from pests, which are not usually a problem.

✓ **Tips:** For continual supply of sprouts, start a new jar every few days. Phytonutrient content of sprouts is highest after setting them in the sun and letting leaves turn green.

❦ *ALMONDS* ❦

✚ **Health Power:** Surprising benefit: high fat nut reduces risk of heart disease. Antioxidant Vitamin E, monounsaturated fats, fibers, other phytonutrients together reduce LDL blood cholesterol. Moderate eating (2-3 servings weekly) may help control weight. Also rich in magnesium (improves blood flow) and potassium (needed for neural firing and muscle contraction). When salt is absent, monounsaturated fats, magnesium and potassium prevent arterial plaque buildup, control blood pressure and improve heart performance. Several ounces reduce blood sugar, reducing demand on insulin-producing cells in pancreas. Also provide energy, help prevent gallstones and supply protein for building body structures. Almond skins give flavonoids with Vitamin E to enhance antioxidant action. Like all nuts, especially walnuts, promote good health. Eat a handful a day.

↑ **Vitamin and Mineral Content:**
Vitamins - E, B2 (Riboflavin)
Minerals – Manganese, Magnesium, Copper and Phosphorus

⊘ **Disease Prevention:** Lowers risk of cardiovascular disease, gall bladder disease and diabetes.

❦ **How to Grow:** Grow similar to peaches. Tree spreads 20-30 feet. Dwarf variety spreads half that size. Choose among several cultivars. Consult nursery for which grows best in your location. Most popular is full-size, "all-in-one" cultivar: self-pollinating, high yielding, great tasting. Most popular dwarf is "Garden Prince" cultivar: self-pollinating and small enough to grow in containers. All produce delightful flowers in bloom. Best time to plant is early in year when cooler temperatures prevent leaf growth and tree puts most of its energy into root expansion. Requires lighter loam, nutrient-rich soil with great drainage. Choose plot with full sunlight, few or no late-spring frosts, soil pH 6-6.5. Dig hole deep enough for taproot to fit undisturbed. Soften soil around the hole if needed to give roots pathways to grow and correct drainage issues. Carefully place tree in hole to avoid root damage. Fill with soil dug out while mixing in handfuls of organic matter (planting mix, compost or well-aged manure). Don't add too much or roots will remain in hole, making tree top heavy and vulnerable to blowing down. Mulch a few inches of compost or other material containing humus around the tree (not flush with base). Consider staking first year if tree grows tall before trunk thickens, especially if prevailing winds get strong. Water regularly first year to keep soil moist but not water logged. In dry, warm weather water longer to reach deeper soil. Ready for harvest after fruit surrounding almond, called drupe, dries out and cracks, revealing almond seed inside. Refer to Peaches for pruning after season ends. Three years needed for almond production but can continue for 50 years!

✘ **Insect Control:** Many different pests affect nut trees, none lethal. Encourage resilience by cultivating healthiest possible tree. Control leaf-eating caterpillars by hand or use Bt if needed.

✓ **Tips:** Look to buy tree with straight trunk and slight widening at base. Look for branches well gapped and evenly spaced throughout trunk. When choosing where to grow, avoid location that has history of standing water. During flowering, do not water branches, which interferes with pollination and risks disease.

∞∞∞

❀ *ALOE VERA* ❀

✚ **Health Power:** Used for centuries as a medical treatment. Juice from broken leaves soothes wounds, rejuvenates burns and treats rare skin conditions. Benefits of drinking juice less well known. Great for digestive tract. Helps maintain healthy tissues and promotes slower, more controlled absorption of food. Good source of essential amino acids that help replenish and build enzymes crucial to functions throughout the body. High volume of phytonutrients and vitamins. Antioxidant and antimicrobial properties help protect immune system and major organs from cellular damage. Increases blood circulation, metabolism and detoxification of blood stream.

⬆ **Vitamin and Mineral Content:**
Vitamins – A, B1 (Thiamin), B2 (Riboflavin), B3 (Niacin), B6 (Pyridoxine), B9 (Folate), B12 (Cobalamin), C and E
Minerals – Iron, Copper, Manganese, Calcium, Chromium, Potassium and Magnesium

⊘ **Treatment and Disease Prevention:** Excellent for skin conditions like eczema or psoriasis. May help prevent colon and colorectal cancer, indigestion, irritable bowel syndrome, ulcers and constipation. Juice may help reduce symptoms of joint disorders like rheumatoid and osteoarthritis. Alkaline nature soothes acid indigestion.

❦ **How to Grow:** Popular succulent is great to have during hot, sunny weather. Prefers warm climates and full sun. Choose plant with erect, healthy leaves. In mild climate, plant in a pot and bring inside to the warmest sunny spot indoors or in greenhouse. In warm, sunny weather put outside to help dry up excess moisture. Outdoors, it prefers great drainage and full sun. Amend planting soil with pebbles, compost/planting mix and sand. If soil naturally lacks good drainage, put in a raised bed. In a pot, must have 18 inches minimum depth. Water plants weekly, depending on soil moisture. Water less in humid or moist weather, more in warm, dry spells. Native to warm, dry areas. Tolerates dry weather well. Never over water, which causes root rot. Let soil dry out to 3-4 inches deep where soil begins to pull away from the sides before watering. Remove weeds to maintain proper pH and nutrient availability. Plant is good at foliar feeding. Apply foliar spray several times during growing season to maintain rigidity and spur healthy growth. When harvesting leaf for medicinal use, trim mature exterior leaves at the base. Leaves will not grow back following harvest. After some growth, plant produces baby plants around base. Pluck these out to replant or share with friends.

✖ **Insect Control:** Extremely hardy. No known pests pose serious threat.

✓ **Tips:** Avoid letting suckers (new shoots around the base) establish. They suck the life from the mother plant. Cut them at 3-4 inches in height, repot and water well to spur root growth. Makes a nice gift.

ooooo

❧ *APPLES* ❧

✚ **Health Power:** Many effective antioxidants help decrease oxidative cell damage by free radicals. Contain dietary fiber and helpful phytonutrients called flavonoids, which have many different functions. Some act as antioxidants; some help maintain blood consistency without excess clotting; others help regulate blood pressure and reduce inflammation. Fiber stimulates healthy digestion and helps moderate the bad form of cholesterol (LDL), contributing to heart health.

↑ **Vitamin and Mineral Content:**
Vitamins – C
Minerals – traces

⊘ **Disease Prevention:** Phytonutrients help reduce risk of heart disease, asthma and female lung cancer. Early studies (lab and animal) suggest apples may reduce risk of colon, lung and breast cancer.

❧ **How to Grow:** One of the most popular, widespread and easily grown fruit trees in the world. Many different cultivars. Ask local nursery which cultivars best suited for your climate. Apples are self-sterile and need another variety to cross-pollinate to bear fruit. Growers often graft two varieties of a species onto one rootstock to produce fruit from only one tree. Many flavors to choose among. Different varieties best for cooking, eating fresh and making cider. Many patterns to train trees:

fans, bush trees, dwarf pyramids, espaliers, cordons, stepovers, festooned trees or standard trees. Plant in spring or late fall. Trees prefer sunny, sheltered site with soil pH just above 6. Add lime to raise pH, if needed. Prepare soil by digging hole large enough to accept tree without altering root structure. Amend removed soil and around hole with organic matter and nutrients like aged compost or planting mix. Plant tree in style recommended for particular cultivar. Usually plants are bare-rooted or container grown. Some cultivars need ground stake for support. Water during dry weather and when apples begin to swell. Stop watering when apples begin to ripen. Apples are ripe and ready when a soft lift and twist removes them easily. Avoid bruising apples during harvest if you want them to store well. Discard any with signs of rot or disease. Store healthy apples, one variety to a bag with holes for airflow, in a cool place that will not freeze. During growth season, remove any apples that appear infected or dead. Thin out branches that block light from reaching interior of tree. Enjoy.

✗ **Insect Control:** Apple pests are aphids, wooly aphids, winter moths, coddling moth, apple sawfly and wasps. If pests threaten integrity of entire harvest, effective treatments are same as for aphids and sawflies on apricots. See Plums for dealing with wasps. Female winter moths have no wings and must crawl up tree to lay eggs between autumn and spring. Tie a sticky band around bottom of tree trunk during egg laying period. Wooly aphids cover themselves with wax-like lining, making them hard to remove with sprays. For large quantities building up, cut them out. Maggots inside apples probably come from coddling moths. Hang pheromone traps, which confuse males and keep them from finding females to fertilize eggs.

✓ **Tips:** Apples harvest at two times. Early in summer just before they ripen. Left on tree they get soft and mushy. Harvest later varieties in fall or early winter. Apple trees take about two years to bear fruit. Reapply fertilizer over the roots each spring to stimulate nutritious development. Each winter, pick up fallen leaves to prevent fungus or disease from over wintering next to tree. Note: Eat the skin, which holds the beneficial nutrients. Another reason to grow organic apples with natural, uncontaminated skin.

∞∞∞∞

❦ *APRICOTS* ❦

✚ **Health Power:** Good source of Vitamin A and beta-carotene. Antioxidant properties prevent free radicals from oxidizing the bad form of cholesterol (LDL), a first step in forming plaque in blood vessels. One form of Vitamin A, retinol, essential to light sensitivity. Impaired night vision early sign of deficiency. Good source of dietary fiber to support digestion, elimination and regulation of blood sugar.

↑ Vitamin and Mineral Content:
Vitamins – A and C
Minerals – Potassium, others in trace amounts

⊘ Disease Prevention: Reduces risk of macular degeneration, cataracts, heart disease, lung cancer, perhaps colon cancer. Vitamin A associated with reduced risk of cancer in organs lined with epithelial tissue.

❦ How to Grow: Many types of apricot cultivars; dwarfs and standard. Best depends on climate and space available. Dwarfs grow near 6 feet tall. If fan trained, grow to 15 feet. With minimal pruning, standard cultivars can reach 30 feet. If planting only one tree, use self-fruiting cultivar. Need sunny spot sheltered from wind. Soil should be well drained and fertile, with pH near 6. Prepare soil by working in plenty of organic matter and some plant mix two spades deep in radius as far as you think roots will spread. Be careful not to over fertilize with nutrients, which causes rapid growth and makes tree more susceptible to pests and disease. During growth, thin out branches that crowd the tree. Thinning heavily grouped fruits on a branch increases size of remaining fruits and prevents excess weight on branches. Produces fruit 2-3 years after sprouting. Ready to pick when soft. For dried apricots, pick while firm and split them.

✗ Insect Control: Apricot pests include red spider mite, aphids, birds, sawfly, green fruit worm and peach tree borers. Tiny red spider mites problematic in dry weather, causing yellow spots on leaves and visible webs. Spray leaves regularly with insecticidal soap. Control aphids by planting French marigolds to attract predator ladybugs and hover flies. Also spray off with strong water stream. Repel birds by surrounding trees with netting. Distract birds by planting more appealing mulberry trees. Caterpillar stage of sawfly makes fruit inedible by boring holes. Control sawfly pupae by hoeing around bottom of tree to expose them for birds to eat. If large infestation, spray insecticide like Bt (*Bacillus thuringiensis*) or pyrethrum. Bt also controls green fruit worms. Look for small sawdust-like buildups next to holes. Probe into holes to kill borers.

✓ Tips: When selecting trees, choose one grafted to a seedling apricot rootstock. Generally grows better than ones grafted with other rootstocks. When thinning fruits, pick out central fruit first, as they tend to be odd shaped.

ooooo

❧ *ARUGULA* ❧
(RUGULA, ROCKET OR ROQUETTE)

✚ **Health Power:** Tasty leaves (nutty and/or peppery flavor) contain small quantities of many phytonutrients and vitamins. 4-5 cups give moderate to large dose. Cruciferous vegetable (similar to broccoli, Brussels sprouts, bok choy) helps prevent many cancers. Most benefit comes from phytonutrients. Glucosinolates and sulforaphanes help stimulate enzymes for detoxifying and removing cell-damaging (possibly carcinogenic) chemicals. Carotenes act as antioxidants to protect skin cells, blood vessel cells and others from sun and free-radical damage. Help ward off cancer and cardiovascular problems. Source of chlorophyll, present in all plants. Limited research on this phytonutrient. Some basic studies suggest chlorophyll may protect from carcinogenic chemicals eaten or created during metabolism. More carefully controlled research is needed to confirm link between chlorophyll and reduced cancer risk. Health benefits come from synergy of all or many nutrients with regular consumption.

⬆ **Vitamin and Mineral Content:**
Vitamins – K, A, C and B9 (Folate)
Minerals – Calcium, Manganese, Magnesium and Potassium

⊘ **Disease Prevention:** Regular eating linked with reduced risk of cardiovascular disease, cataracts, macular degeneration, many cancers (lung, colorectal, skin, perhaps others).

❦ **How to Grow:** An easy-to-grow annual. Matures quickly (6-8 weeks). Likes cool weather and plenty of water. Sow seeds early spring and fall. Successive plantings OK through summer in cooler areas; through fall in warmer areas. Choose site with much sun. Soil wants good drainage. Enrich with much compost, manure or planting mix. Sow seeds thinly (1-2 inches apart) in rows spaced roughly 10 inches apart. Water regularly to keep soil moist. Take care not to over water. Ready to harvest when leaves are young and tender. Cut them and encourage plant to grow again. Make successive sowings every 2-3 weeks after first sowing. Watch out for sensitivity to hot weather; makes plant go to seed. Avoid growing during heat waves or plant in partial shade.

✘ **Insect Control:** Resistant to common insect pests and diseases. Susceptible to slugs or snails. Early morning or evening, remove by hand. Or embed cup of beer in soil; lures them to crawl in and drown.

✓ **Tips:** Harvest leaves while young. Older, larger leaves tough and bitter. Works well added to soups and salads or as garnish.

⚜ *ASPARAGUS* ⚜

✚ **Health Power:** Improves digestion by increasing number and health of good bacteria in large intestine that suppress harmful bacteria. Promotes overall health with wide range of nutrients. Amino acid asparagine is a natural diuretic. Used to reduce swelling; may help diminish premenstrual water retention. Contains B vitamin folate (more than 50 percent RDA), a crucial nutrient for normal fetal development during pregnancy. Helps avoid birth defects by helping DNA synthesize and replicate properly. Pyridoxine promotes heart health by lowering homocysteine levels in the blood stream.

↑ **Vitamin and Mineral Content:**
Vitamins – K, B9 (Folate), C, A, B1 (Thiamin), B2 (Riboflavin), B6 (Pyridoxine) and B3 (Niacin)
Minerals – Manganese, Copper, Phosphorus, Potassium, Iron, Zinc, Magnesium, Selenium and Calcium

⊘ **Disease Prevention:** High Vitamin B9 (folate) concentration helps reduce risk of heart disease by lowering high levels of homocysteine in the blood; converts homocysteine to cysteine. Asparagus also has phytonutrients that may prevent growth of many cancer cell lines (notably colon cancer).

❦ **How to Grow:** A perennial plant needing initial investment but offering valuable returns. Choose plot with plenty of sunshine and exceptional drainage. Amend soil with compost or quality planting mix for loam with good air space, drainage and nutrient availability. In heavy soil, work in more compost or planting mix to raise bed slightly. Soil pH should be above 6; add lime as needed. Start from seed or buy plants with one-year-old root crowns from a reliable nursery, saving the first year of effort. Dig a trench 6 inches deep and 1 foot wide, with center raised a little. Soak root crowns in water for 1 hour. Plant one foot apart, making sure to spread roots around the slightly raised center of trench. First year, water well, never depriving plants of water. Each spring, apply more mix rich in organic matter and micronutrients. In fall, mulch around plant with compost or balanced planting mix. Full harvest comes two years from crown stage or three years from seed. Begin harvest in second year (after planting crowns) when shoots grow more than 5 inches. Harvest all but a few shoots by cutting or snapping them just below ground shortly before tip opens. Be careful not to hurt crowns when you cut.

✗ **Insect Control:** Asparagus rust, slugs and asparagus beetles are most common pests. Beetles controlled by hand removing. If seriously infested, spray or dust with rotenone. Avoid asparagus rust (rust-colored spots on leaves and stems) by buying resistant strains from trusted nursery. Slugs controlled several ways. Physically remove and dispose each morning or night. Sink saucers of beer into soil to attract and drown. When plants are still small, cut off plastic bottles and secure over plants. Spread a thin layer of lime or soot around plant to repel slugs.

✓ **Tips:** To preserve soil balance, start new bed every 10 years. (Three years before discontinuing old one to avoid missing a season of tasty, fresh, homegrown asparagus.) To avoid crown rot, do not let crowns lie in bed of water. Slightly raised beds help prevent this.

∞∞∞∞

❦ *AVOCADOS* ❦

✚ **Health Power:** Delectable fruit high in monounsaturated fats (the good ones). These lipids help reduce LDLs and raise HDLs. Also rich in beta-Sitosterol, a natural substance that lowers blood cholesterol level. High levels of potassium in avocados also can help reduce elevated blood pressure. Folate is great for circulatory health and normal neural development in fetuses. Avocados also contain the fat soluble phytonutrients carotenoids and tocopherols, potent antioxidants and anti-carcinogens.

↑ **Vitamin and Mineral Content:**
Vitamins – K, B9 (Folate), B6 (Pyridoxine), C and E (Tocopherols)
Minerals – Potassium and Copper

⊘ **Disease Prevention:** Bad cholesterol and triglyceride lowering effects help prevent heart disease. Folate helps prevent atherosclerosis. Avocados linked to preventing oral and prostate cancers. Carotenoids and tocopherols are fat-soluble and synergistically inhibit growth of these cancer cells. Source of good fats in avocado also provides medium for absorption of these phytonutrients in the intestine, rendering avocado an all-around health promoter.

❧ **How to Grow:** Grow on trees of various cultivars (same plant with slightly different characteristics). Origin is tropical; flourish in warmer climates. Varieties have slightly different tolerances and ripen at different times. Ask local nursery which work best in your climate. Choose several different kinds for maximum production. Plant in spacious location with full day's sun to grow up to 40 feet high. If winter freezes over, plant tree in pot at least 2 feet in diameter and bring into garage during cold months. In milder climates, dig a hole 3 feet wide by 3 feet deep. Tree needs regular deep watering with superb drainage to prevent root rot. If soil is heavy and dense, amend with coarse organic materials to get thorough draining. Sprinkle a few handfuls of plant mix in and plant in the hole. Do not plant too deeply; avocados have shallow root networks. Mulch area generously to extend interval between waterings. Keep soil moist but not wet.

✗ **Insect Control:** Pests rarely hamper fruit production on fully developed trees. Young trees need protection from large infestation. Most common insects: avocado loopers, pyriform scale, dictyospermum scale, avocado red mites, borers and lace bugs. As a last resort only, spray low-toxic, organic pesticides-fungicides: soaps, oils or Bt.

✓ **Tips:** Avocados prone to scab disease. Have nursery staff help choose resistant strain. Pinch terminal roots to keep tree in check. Fast growing; need aggressive trimming to keep nice shape.

ooooo

🐛 *BANANAS* 🐛

✚ **Health Power:** Excellent source and high doses of potassium, vitamin C and fiber at low cost with low sodium, fat and cholesterol. Potassium essential for nerve and muscle functions and to control blood pressure. High fiber promotes healthy heart, lowers total cholesterol, adds bulk to stool and speeds up digestive process. Fiber also helps regulate blood sugars by holding onto carbohydrates in intestine and slowing down absorption of sugar into blood system, which lowers stress on insulin-producing pancreatic cells. Special banana fiber, pectin, promotes normal digestion and nutrient absorption. Promotes stomach health by building strong inner lining and eliminating ulcer-causing bacteria. Bananas have compounds (fructooligosaccharides and short-chain fatty acids) that feed helpful intestinal bacteria.

↑ **Vitamin and Mineral Content:**
Vitamins – B6 (Pyridoxine) and C
Minerals – Potassium and Manganese

⊘ **Disease Prevention:** May help reduce symptoms or onset of atherosclerosis, heart disease, stroke, diabetes, ulcers, breast cancer, and colon cancer. Bananas, like cabbage and other root vegetables, have high concentrations of phenolic compounds that help reduce cancer in animals, possibly in humans.

🌱 **How to Grow:** Many varieties. (If above zone 10, choose cultivar that tolerates cooler temp.) Fruit develops best with long, humid, warm growing season.

Misting leaves morning and evening helps nurture. Choose warm site with dark, highly fertile, well-drained soil and full day's sun. Needs shelter from wind. Plant is self-fertile; only one plant needed to bear fruit. Local nursery usually has banana suckers or baby trees in containers. Plant trees in well-amended soil 10 feet apart (or more depending on how large cultivar grows). Keep soil moist throughout growth, but avoid standing water. Adding fertilizer (compost tea, manure tea or other) helps meet high demand for nutrients. Many suckers sprout from base to create more plants. Prune off all but one or two to concentrate energy for fruiting. Control weeds by hand pulling and laying down compost mulch or other material to retain moisture and deter weeds. Takes 9 months to fully plump up and ready for harvest. Although green, will ripen to yellow. Need little pruning to remove dead plant matter. After harvesting, cut down banana tree, leaving sucker that produced bananas. It develops into new tree to renew growing process.

✘ **Insect Control:** Pests will differ depending on the area where you grow. Banana aphids, spider mites, weevils, rose beetles, flower and red rust thrips, whitefly and mealy bugs. Talk with nursery to see what may cause local problems and how to treat.

✓ **Tips:** After 6 months, when flower opens and male fingers fall to the ground, remove purple flowers and stem about 6-8 inches below last female fingers. (Fingers become bananas.) Growing bananas in cooler climates may be risky, as frost kills growth above ground. To protect from freezing, cut down plant and cover with mulch and sheet of black polypropylene.

∞∞∞

❀ *BASIL* ❀

✚ **Health Power:** Basil known for flavonoids (protect DNA, which creates and regulates cells) and volatile oils (antibacterial action). Some oils even halt growth of drug-resistant bacteria. Volatile oil eugenol may reduce inflammation and pain, such as in arthritis.

↑ **Vitamin and Mineral Content:**
Vitamins – K, A and C
Minerals – Iron, Calcium, Manganese, Magnesium and Potassium

⊘ **Disease Prevention:** Basil contains strong antioxidant beta-carotene. Prevents unstable molecules (free radicals) from damaging epithelial cells including blood vessel walls. Beta-carotene helps prevent plaque build up (atherosclerosis) in arterial walls by blocking oxidation of LDL cholesterol. Lowers risk of heart attack and stroke. Contributes to the prevention of asthma, rheumatoid and osteoarthritis.

❦ **How to Grow:** Grow as an annual where winter snow or frost are common; a perennial in warm, Southern regions. Two types: sweet and bush. Sweet is taller (1.5-2 feet high, more productive, better flavor). Sweet basil grows best in sunny, protected area with healthy soil. Sow seeds in early spring in smaller containers indoors. Prepare soil by working in aged compost, manure or planting mix with plenty of organic matter. Transplant outdoors about one foot apart after last frost. Keep soil moist; water thoroughly during hot, dry weather. Remove flower buds when they appear to stimulate more growth. Harvest younger leaves through summer in quantities needed for cooking. Also dry and put in airtight containers or freeze for later use.

✗ **Insect Control:** Minor pest problems. Prevent Japanese beetles from eating foliage by hand picking.

✓ **Tips:** Save seeds for next year by harvesting stems after seeds ripen. Hang upside down in a closed area. Set cloth underneath to catch seeds as plant dries up and releases them

ﾟﾟﾟ

🕸 *BEANS* 🕸

✚ **Health Power:** Among many varieties, pinto beans are surprisingly nutritious. More fiber than most foods. Excellent at lowering cholesterol, regulating blood sugar (especially for those with insulin resistance) and smoothing out digestion. Crucial contribution to heart health. High content of folate, potassium and magnesium. Folate lowers concentration of amino acid homocysteine. (When elevated in the blood, can seriously damage blood vessels.) Potassium an essential component of nerve cell communication, muscle contraction (especially heart) and blood pressure regulation. Magnesium helps maintain blood flow through vessels by blocking calcium channels. Iron optimizes oxygen attachment to hemoglobin molecules, which transport oxygen in blood. Copper and manganese help protect energy-producing cell bodies (mitochondria) by activating superoxide dismutase, which knocks out free radicals. Copper also needed to form hemoglobin. Vitamin B1 (thiamin) contributes to energy production and healthy brain function by helping produce neurotransmitter acetylcholine. Excellent source of protein at low calorie cost.

↑ **Vitamin and Mineral Content:**
Vitamins – B9 (Folate) and B1 (Thiamin)
Minerals – Molybdenum, Manganese, Phosphorus, Iron, Magnesium, Potassium and Copper

⊘ **Disease Prevention:** Reduces risk of heart attack, stroke, cardiovascular disease, irritable bowel syndrome, diabetes, colon cancer and Alzheimer's disease.

❧ **How to Grow:** Part of the Leguminosae family. Hundreds of different cultivars. You can find a variety that will grow in your location. Two main types: shell beans used for seeds and snap/bush beans grown for their pods. Two types of growth patterns: self-supporting and others (pole and runner beans) that grow on stakes or suspended strings. Most beans grow best in warmer temperatures (about 75°F) and are very sensitive to cooler temperatures. Prefer sheltered sunny site with well-drained soil and lots of organic matter. Prepare rows by amending soil with aged compost or planting mix rich in organic matter. If soil is heavy, use more compost to loosen. For seeds to sow properly, soil should be above 60°F and near pH 6.5. Beans do not easily transplant, but if warm season is short, you may have no choice. Start beans indoors in pots about a month before frost. Sow seeds outdoors about two weeks after the last frost. Place them about 1 inch under the soil and pat the soil down over top. Place bush beans 4-6 inches apart in rows and space rows about 2.5 feet apart. Pole beans are more sensitive to cold. Plan on planting a week or two later and harvesting a week or two earlier. Yield about three times as many beans per area as bush types. Sow seeds 2 inches deep and 10-12 inches apart in single rows spaced about 3.5 feet apart or double rows spaced 1 foot apart. A bean teepee makes nice addition to garden. Water beds evenly and keep soil moist. Letting soil dry out may hurt yields. Bush types germinate in 1 week; pole types in 2 weeks. After seedlings are a few inches tall, apply a thick layer of mulch to retain moisture, deter weeds and buffer the soil against temperature fluctuations. Light application of fertilizer containing micronutrients mid-season produces high yields. Snap beans and shell beans ready for harvest when soft and a little longer than index finger. Harvest all as soon as they are ready to stimulate re-growth. If you see outlines of seeds on pod, you have waited too long. Eat or freeze them immediately to preserve the fresh flavor. Both unshelled beans and those in pods preserve for about a week in refrigerator. To dry shell types, let them sit in pods on plants until pods turn brown and dry out. If weather is wet, cut plant and hang upside down in dry area. Dried beans last about one year.

✕ **Insect Control:** Common pests are aphids, corn earworms, cabbage loopers, corn borers, Mexican beetles and Japanese beetles. Aphids can be handled by interplanting French Marigolds, which attract their predators. Hoverflies and lady bugs eat tons of aphids. Corn earworms grow roughly 2 feet long and grub on bean plants. Not a large threat, but if you get a manually uncontrollable infestation, apply the insecticide *Bacillus thuringiensis* (Bt). Cabbage loopers feed on leaves and eat twice their body weight a day. If they are uncontrollable by manually picking, use an insecticide like Bt. Mexican beetles will ravage the bean plants if they infest in numbers. The first sign is small yellow groups of eggs, which hatch into larvae that look like small yellow caterpillars. Adults look like larger, darker ladybugs. Remove eggs and larvae and smash adults when you see them.

✓ **Tips:** In order to get continuous harvest, successively sow every two weeks until 2 months before first frost. Be careful not to knock off blossoms when watering.

ꝏꝏꝏ

ꙮ *BEETS* ꙮ

✚ **Health Power:** A great vegetable for defending against cell damage in digestive tract. Color comes from betacyanin, which prevents pre-cancerous cell damage. Fiber induces liver production of antioxidants (glutathione peroxidase and glutathione S-transferase) for detoxifying body from damaging, potentially carcinogenic chemicals. Stimulate production of immune cells in animal colon and protect from damage by nitrosamines (created from nitrates) in stomach. Phytonutrients choline and its metabolite betaine correlate with lower levels of C-reactive protein, tumor necrosis factor alpha and homocysteine. All help reduce inflammation and blood vessel damage, loss of cognitive function and insulin resistance. Folate deters blood vessel damage by lowering concentrations of homocysteine and prevents neural tube defects in fetus. Lowers total cholesterol and triglyceride levels, which is great for the cardiovascular system. Magnesium assures calcium absorption in gastrointestinal tract. Calcium helps make healthy bones. Iron essential for hemoglobin to deliver oxygen to all body tissues.

↑ **Vitamin and Mineral Content:**
Vitamins – B9 (Folate) and C
Minerals – Manganese, Potassium, Magnesium, Iron, Copper and Phosphorus

⊘ **Disease Prevention:** Beets lower risk of heart disease, colon cancer, stomach cancer, birth defects, type II diabetes, osteoporosis and anemia.

❦ **How to Grow:** Beets prefer a deep soil rich in organic matter, microbes and nutrients. Work in some aged compost or planting mix to both fertilize and improve drainage. Like other root vegetables, they benefit from raised beds but not needed if soil is naturally deep and worked well. Grow best at 60-65°F. If summer is scorching, grow beets in winter/early spring and fall. Prefer full sun, but in hotter areas, part shade prevents scorching. Seeds come in groupings; one "seed" is a group of 7-8 seeds. When soil is workable, create shallow drills at 1 foot apart or more. Rinse seeds vigorously in a filter or soak overnight to promote germination. One month before the last frost, sow each cluster of seeds 1 inch deep and 2.5 inches apart within the drills. Since each seed is a cluster, thin out seedlings by pulling up roots. Once seedlings reach a few inches tall, thin out to about 6 inches between plants. For continual harvest, sow the seeds successively every couple weeks until weather heats up (midsummer). Keep beds weed free, but be careful not to damage roots. Mulch between plants with compost or other organic matter. Last sowings will be the main crop. Keep soil moist by watering roughly one inch a week or more during hot stretches. Harvest early ones when they are smaller (ping pong ball size) and later ones when they reach baseball size. When separating leaves from beet, make sure not to damage skin. Leave about an inch of the stems on so they don't bleed. Store some undamaged ones for winter in a container surrounded by peat, sand, vermiculite or sawdust.

✕ **Insect Control:** Grown in healthy conditions, usually develop pest free. You may see flea beetles (small, dark creatures that jump up when approached) and leaf miners (tiny black insects that burrow into the leaf leaving yellow tunnels). To rid crop of flea beetles, cut out a rectangular card (plastic or cardboard) and cover one side with sticky material (thick grease works). Slowly run the sticky side of card about an inch above plants and watch flea beetles jump up and get stuck to the card. Leaf miners are tiny black insects that burrow into the leaf, leaving yellow tunnels. Remove the leaves and destroy them as soon as you notice them.

✓ **Tips:** Key to tender beets is to grow quickly and harvest when they reach full size. To encourage growth, fertilize every few weeks with compost tea or liquid seaweed extract.

ooooo

❧ *BLACKBERRIES* ❧

✚ **Health Power:** Blackberries are a great source of antioxidants. Some fall in the groups of polyphenols and anthocyanins, both known to help fight against free radicals that cause damage to blood vessels, heart disease and many types of cancer. Anthocyanins give the deep color. Blackberries are also solid sources of vitamin C and magnesium. Vitamin C, an antioxidant, helps maintain healthy immune system by protecting cells from oxidative damage. C helps reactivate vitamin E, a fat-soluble antioxidant in fatty tissue/liquids. Trace mineral magnesium promotes bone health by increasing the absorption of calcium and the proper functioning of all cells. Great source of fiber, promoting smooth, healthy digestion, regulating blood sugar and lowering cholesterol. Vitamin A protects eyesight, boosts immune system and maintains elasticity in epithelial cells inside internal organs, especially blood vessels.

↑ Vitamin and Mineral Content:
Vitamins – C, K, E, B9 (Folate), A and B3 (Niacin)
Minerals – Manganese, Copper, Potassium and Magnesium

⊘ Disease Prevention: Medical research (but not clinical studies) suggests blackberries in the diet may help prevent cardiovascular disease, lung inflammation, clotting deficiency, diabetes and many types of cancer especially colon, breast and cervical.

🥦 How to Grow: Blackberries have extensive growth range. Varieties grow in the Deep South, while others endure harsh northern winters. Self-fertile, so only one variety needed for fruit. Plant in early spring or early fall. Choose a soil site with plenty of sun. Blackberries prefer deep rich soil that holds lots of moisture yet drains well. Needs pH 6 or just below. Work in plenty of well-aged compost and/ or planting mix rich in organic matter, especially if soil is sandier loam. Dig a hole about 1.5 feet deep and 2 feet wide. Place compost or planting mix in the bottom, followed by the blackberry plant. Refill the hole with amended soil and top off with a couple handfuls of nutrient-dense fertilizer like seaweed extract or bone meal. If planting more than one, separate trenches by about 10 feet. Trim plant down to about 6 inches tall after planting. To train, use wire and two 6-foot posts per row. Place the posts roughly 5 feet outside the last plant in each row. Connect the two posts with the first wire about 3 feet up the posts. Successively place more wires to the top of the posts at 12-18 inch intervals. During first year, regularly train shoots to one side of the post. The following year, train new growing shoots to the other side. This keeps new growth away from the fruiting wood. In late winter, place a mulch layer of compost, manure or other all-encompassing source of nutrients around the bushes. After harvesting fruit, cut the fruit bearing shoots down to the ground.

✗ Insect Control: Blackberry pests are aphids, raspberry beetles, Japanese beetles and birds. See Strawberries for aphid control. Raspberry beetle larvae feed on fruit as it ripens. They are seen when fruit appears damaged. The only way to treat is to spray an insecticide like pyrethrum when the flowers open. Be careful not to use an insecticide that kills bees, which pollinate the flowers. Japanese beetles are a shiny blue-green color about one-half inch in size. Shake them off the plant early in the morning, set out baited traps, and/or apply floating row covers. Floating row covers also stop birds, which can eat a lot of berries in one session.

✓ **Tips:** Make blackberries a part of your fruit intake.

ooooo

❀ *BLUEBERRIES* ❀

✚ **Health Power:** Blueberries top the antioxidant list of major fruits and vegetables. They have more highly effective antioxidants than a glass of red wine. Multiple different vitamins, minerals and nutrients work together to give this fruit many potential health benefits with few calories. Antioxidants (the anthocyanidins) disarm free radicals and prevent damage to the collagen network (the backbone of cells keeping them stable and durable for proper functioning). Also help prevent heart problems, ulcers and vision loss. Protect and maintain proper cell structure in blood vessels. Contain both soluble and insoluble fibers to help control blood sugar spikes, lower cholesterol and support digestion. May increase brain function to improve learning ability and muscle coordination. Adding blueberries to your diet does wonders for your overall health.

↑ **Vitamin and Mineral Content:**
Vitamins – Vitamin C, K, E and others in small quantities
Minerals – Manganese, Iron, Calcium and others in small quantities

⊘ **Disease Prevention:** Preventing free radical damage may help the brain avoid conditions associated with aging, like Alzheimer's, dementia and osteoporosis. Many studies suggest blueberries help deter heart disease, macular degeneration, peptic ulcers, varicose veins and many types of cancer (especially colon and ovarian). Also contain many phytonutrients which help prevent urinary tract infections and digestive system inflammation.

❧ **How to Grow:** Native to North America, aesthetically pleasing and naturally pest tolerant, these nutrient-rich, delicious little nibbles are popular among home gardeners. Aside from preference in taste or texture, soil requirements keep gardeners from growing this super food everywhere. Bushes come in forms that grow short with smaller berries and a tall, higher yielding type with larger berries. Crosses have height and berry size falling between. In warmer climates, rabbit eye blueberries are popular. These grow more than 10 feet tall, sometimes higher than 20 feet, and can yield up to 20 pounds of fruit each. Tall bush berries are most popular in home growing. Blueberries are particular about growing conditions, so initial testing may be needed to find suitable spot. Grow best in well-drained soils with loose loam or sandier base. Prefer slightly acidic soil pH around 4.5-5.5. If soil is basic, lower it by mixing in sphagnum, peat moss or compost made from oak, hemlock bark or pine. Avoid aluminum sulfate, which kills certain soil creatures and changes the taste of fruit. Another soil fix: Grow in raised beds, which are fine for blueberry's shallow root system. Prefer a sunny spot. Since they cannot self fertilize, plant at least two cultivars to yield fruit. Mix in a handful of planting mix suitable for maintaining soil pH per square yard before planting. Plant tall bushes and rabbit eyes 5 feet apart in rows spaced roughly 8 feet apart. Low bush plants should be placed 1 foot apart in rows 3 feet or more apart. Apply a thick layer of mulch around the plants every year. Mulch derived from oak, pine, woodchips or hemlock will help support soil pH. Near the end of winter, add a second application of organic fertilizer (well-aged manure or compost) rich in nitrogen that also supports the acidic pH. Fertilizers with fish bone, seaweed, or cottonseed meal are excellent sources of micronutrients as well as phosphorus and nitrogen. Water regularly to keep the soil moist especially during drought periods, as blueberries dry out quickly. During growth, remove any weak branches or damaged growth to conserve energy and prevent infestations. Keep the bush from growing too thick by removing branches to leave at least a few inches for light and air to get in. Berries are generally ripe and ready for harvest about a week after they turn blue. Tasting is the best way to tell. Leftovers can be frozen for later use. In fall each year, trim the tips of all branches.

✗ **Insect Control:** Home growers have few problems with pests. Cherry fruit worm or blueberry maggot may cause problems by burrowing inside berries to make them inedible. Remove any berries showing signs of infestation or damage. Clear your plot of any rotting fruit before winter. If insects become a serious problem, dust with an organically approved Bt or rotenone. Birds are the largest worry with ripening fruits. Hold them out by constructing a shelter of strong netting with small perforations around the bushes, which keep birds from entering.

✓ **Tips:** Blueberries take 5-7 years to reach full yields, but you can get a head start by purchasing 2-3-year-old plants. Inter-planting blueberries with other species of flowers that attract pollinating insects helps increase chances for pollination. Test to see if ripe (berries come off easily with a slight twist). Easy to grow, but treated as a luxury item in stores because they are hard to keep perfect when shipped.

ooooo

🦋 *BOK CHOY* 🦋

✚ **Health Power:** Bok choy is another crucifer (like broccoli, cauliflower and cabbage) with many beneficial phytonutrients. Also zero fats and low carbohydrate count. Most researched are the glucosinolates and carotenoids. Glucosinolates are a mixed blessing from plants. In high doses, they can inhibit thyroid hormone, which is needed for proper cell metabolism. In moderate amounts, they block cancer cells by directly affecting the cell cycle and protecting against harmful free radicals. Isothiocyanates, some derived from glucosinolates, are other powerful agents preventing cancer cells from forming and proliferating. Bok choy is an excellent source of many carotenoids, especially beta-carotene, an antioxidant throughout the body. Studies suggest beta-carotene lowers cancer risk and is great for the eyes. (More research needed to prove these claims.) Bok choy is especially high in vitamins A, C and K, with some folate and vitamin B6. A and C are antioxidants that protect immune cells, prevent plaque build up in arteries and help preserve elasticity of epithelial tissue (especially blood vessel walls). Folate and vitamin B6 lower blood plasma homocysteine, linked with vessel damage at high concentration.

↑ **Vitamin and Mineral Content:**
Vitamins – A, C, K, B9 (Folate), and B6 (Pyridoxine)
Minerals – Calcium, Potassium and Manganese

⊘ **Disease Prevention:** Bok choy may help prevent heart disease, macular degeneration, cancers of colon, prostate, endometrial lining, lung and pancreas. Potentially reduces risk of many other cancers.

❦ **How to Grow:** Known as Chinese cabbage, requires same soil preparation as other Brassicas (members of the mustard family; broccoli, cabbage, cauliflower) but are more demanding than other cabbages. See one of these entries for soil prep. Choose a site with full sun. Plan to grow them next to other Brassicas in their own bed with extra compost, manure or planting mix worked in. Sow seeds beginning late spring or about three months before the first intense frost. Place seeds two every 8-10 inches in shallow drills spaced 1 foot apart. Later, thin out to leave most prominent seedling every 8-10 inches. Does not store long. For continuous harvest, sow seeds every two weeks. Keep soil moist and weed free. Hoe and water regularly. Crops are ready to harvest 2-3 months after sowing.

✖ **Insect Control:** Slugs, earwigs and flea beetles are common pests. Try to remove and destroy pests by hand. Slugs feed in twilight, morning and evening. If infestation seems severe, try another method. For snails and slugs, embed a cup of beer in the soil. Both will be attracted, slither their way in, get stuck and drown. Earwigs attack by nipping at buds and leaves of plants. Generally, not a problem, but if needed, you can easily set a trap. They don't like daylight. Create a dark environment by filling a pot with dry grass, leaves or plant material and perching it upside down on a skinny post above the affected plants. Earwigs will crawl in during the day. Destroy the plant matter inside the pot every week or so. Control tiny flea beetles by using their instinctive responses against them. Like fleas, they spring up in the air when approached. Create a sticky piece of wood or cardboard by applying grease or other adhesive that will remain sticky. Walk along the plants with the sticky side a couple inches above the foliage. Watch them jump and get stuck.

✓ **Tips:** To get the most nutritional benefit from bok choy, change how you prepare it. When left raw, the glucosinolates are more bio-available. When cooked lightly with a little oil, the carotenoids are more available for absorption. Golden Rule: diversify your diet. Get many different fruits, veggies and other sources of nutrition worked into the weekly menu.

ooooo

🦾 *BROCCOLI* 🦾

✚ **Health Power:** Broccoli is a super food with many vitamins, minerals and phytonutrients that trigger a complex, intricate set of biochemical pathways supporting overall health. High fiber content lowers concentration of low-density lipoproteins (LDL) in the blood and elevated blood sugar, promoting cardiovascular health. Helps promote weight loss. A superior source of antioxidants. Folate helps protect the heart/circulatory system and promote healthy fetal development. Contains sulforaphane, which fights *Helicobacter pylori* bacteria that can cause stomach cancer. Along with isothiocyanate, it also boosts production of detoxification enzymes, which can help rid the body of potentially carcinogenic chemicals. Speeds up metabolism of estrogen, which may help suppress breast cancer. The phytonutrient indole-3-carbinol in broccoli reduces the metastasis of cancer cells and risk of breast cancer. Other beneficial phytonutrients include carotenoids, flavonoids and glucosinolates (which get converted to sulforaphane). Great source of calcium for bone building. Vitamin C, beta-carotene and the enzyme cofactors zinc and selenium help maintain strong immune system.

↑ **Vitamin and Mineral Content:**
Vitamins – C, K, A, B9 (Folate), B6 (Pyridoxine), B2 (Riboflavin), B5 (Pantothenic), B1 (Thiamin), B3 (Niacin) and E
Minerals – Manganese, Potassium, Phosphorus, Magnesium, Iron, Calcium & Zinc

⊘ **Disease Prevention:** Lowers risk of atherosclerosis, heart disease, stroke, anemia, osteoporosis, cataracts, lung cancer, stomach cancer, breast cancer, bladder cancer, ovarian cancer, colon cancer, colorectal cancer, prostate cancer and potentially many more.

❧ **How to Grow:** In the Brassica family, broccoli is one of the most popular, easy-to-grow vegetables. Start from seed or find good local nursery to get disease-free transplant. Broccoli grows best in cool climates where daytime temperature remains below 70°F. Choose soil that has drainage, good aeration and plenty of sun. Place plant where it will not cast a shadow on another that needs the sun, as broccoli can grow up to 3 feet tall. A pH between 6.2 and 7 is good. If higher, lime the soil to reduce. Mix in well-aged compost or manure. Broccoli has high nutrient demand. Add a couple fistfuls of plant mix with alfalfa, fish bone, and feather meal per yard to ensure nourishment. If you start with seeds, sow them about a month and a half before planting outside. Plant seedlings or transplants 20-30 inches apart. Keep soil moist by watering regularly. (Avoid water logging.) Keep soil weed free by pulling, mulching with organic matter or putting down black plastic as last resort.

✘ **Insect Control:** Broccoli is affected by many common pests and diseases. Most significant is caterpillar stage of white cabbage butterfly, root maggots, flea beetles and aphids. A plastic row cover protects from the first three. Use an insecticidal soap or limonene spray to repel aphids. Remove pests when you see them. If physical removal doesn't work, organic pesticide is a must. If caterpillars are resilient, spray *Bacillus thuringiensis* (Bt), an organic agent that is safe for pets, humans and other garden plants.

✓ **Tips:** When harvesting, cut the central shoot first to promote outgrowth of side shoots. This maximizes production of the edible vegetable portion. When cooking, the crunchier the better. If you let cooked broccoli get soggy, most nutrients are lost. To prevent club root disease, never grow Brassicas in the same plot year after year.

∞∞∞

🦋 *BRUSSELS SPROUTS* 🦋

✚ **Health Power:** Brussels sprouts contain phytonutrients that assist a range of functions. Contain sulfur compounds like sulforaphane, which triggers vital detoxification enzymes in the liver. Also an excellent source of vitamins C, A, folate, fiber and other phytonutrients, all promoting healthy skin, digestion, immune function, cardiovascular function, fetal development and overall health.

↑ **Vitamin and Mineral Content:**
Vitamins – K, C, B9 (Folate), A, B6 (Pyridoxine), B1 (Thiamin), B2 (Riboflavin) & E
Minerals – Manganese, Potassium, Iron, Phosphorus, Magnesium and Copper

⊘ **Disease Prevention:** By increasing detoxification and reducing DNA damage, crucifers like Brussels sprouts reduce the symptoms or onset of many cancers more effectively than any other fruit or vegetable. Cancer examples: prostate, colon, bladder, breast and lung. The sulfur-containing phytonutrients slow or stop cell division of cancer cells and programmed cell death.

❦ **How to Grow:** Brussels sprouts take up extra space, but you can get varieties that last through fall and others that last through winter for a prolonged harvest. Choose site with full sun and well-drained soil. Soil pH needs to be 6.5 to 7; add lime to raise, if needed. Amend soil with highly fertile planting mix. Sow seeds in shallow drills 6 inches apart three to four months before the first expected frost. When they reach a few inches tall, plant them out centered in spaces 2-3 feet square depending on how large you want sprouts to be. Compress the well you plant into. Water initially and wait 1-2 weeks before repeating. Cover spaces between plants with compost, mulch or plastic to reduce weeds and need for watering. Keep watered through summer. In fall, pick off yellow leaves to avoid spreading disease. Harvest Brussels sprouts from the bottom up starting in early fall once they have hardened.

✗ **Insect Control:** Brussels sprouts are affected by a number of common garden pests, including cabbage butterflies, club, cabbage root maggot, cabbage moth, cabbage loopers and cabbage worms. Handpick and dispose of pests as they appear. Morning and evening are best times to remove. If infestation is uncontrollable manually, use insecticidal soap. Bt works in some instances. Sink shallow cups of beer in soil to induce slugs and snails to climb in and drown. Floating row covers protect against birds. If uncertain what to do, capture some pests and ask your local nursery for advice on best organic treatment.

✓ **Tips:** Best use of space may be to interplant another crop in the spaces between Brussels sprout plants. If you do, use little fertilizer as flooding Brussels sprouts with fertilizer softens them. If site gets windy, staking may be necessary to prevent toppling. Frost is not a problem and can even enhance taste, but if not insulated by snow, even the toughest sprouts will suffer with a hard freeze. You may need a season of trial and error to find the best planting time to get the healthiest yielding plants. Cook by steaming lightly to retain nutrients.

ooooo

� *BURDOCK* 🌣

✚ **Health Power:** Burdock has been used for centuries as an alternative herbal medicine. Diuretic (urine producing) properties help "flush" the body as it removes excess water. Some cancer patients say it enhances quality of life. Found in popular cancer remedies like Essiac and Hoxsey formula. May lower blood glucose levels, which helps prevent and manage diabetes. Useful in treating skin conditions (wounds, eczema, acne and psoriasis) by mixing into a cream-like lotion and applying directly to clean skin. Reduces throat pain and is found in some cold medicines. Detoxifies liver, kidneys, gallbladder and lymph system. Fiber stimulates digestive tract, helping relieve constipation. Side effects include dry mouth, slowed absorption of nutrients like iron, laxative action and slower heart rate. Not recommended if you take prescription drugs or are pregnant. (Can stimulate uterus.)

↑ **Vitamin and Mineral Content:**
Vitamins – B6 (Pyridoxine), B9 (Folate) and C
Minerals – Manganese, Magnesium, Potassium, Calcium, Copper and Iron

⊘ **Disease Prevention:** May help reduce symptoms or onset of diabetes, gout, ulcers, rheumatoid and osteoarthritis, acne, psoriasis and potentially many cancers.

❧ **How to Grow:** A great leafy vegetable native to Europe and Asia. Very efficient because both roots and shoot are edible. Hardy and able to grow in variety of climates (warm and humid to cool and dry). In cold winters (down to 0°F), plant loses leaves but regenerates them in spring. Sub-zero may compromise roots. Prefers well-drained, deep soil with light, sandy loam for deep rooting. Choose site with full sun. Needs soil pH close to 7 for best nutrient uptake. When preparing soil, avoid working in compost or manure, which may cause roots to fork out. Phosphorus helps spur root growth. Plant in site composted for previous crop and work in some ground rock phosphate or fish bone meal. When soil warms up (usually in spring), soak seeds for a half day to prepare for germination. Plant out directly about ¾ inch deep. Space or thin plants to 10 inches apart in rows 10 inches apart. Water regularly at first to keep surface moist. Seedlings pop up in about 2 weeks. A week after that, change watering regime to one deep watering weekly to promote downward root growth. (Roots go as deep as 2-3 feet.) When seedlings grow more than a few inches, mulch around plants to retain moisture and deter weeds. Harvest during any part of development. Expect roots to mature near end of summer or early autumn. Loosen soil around roots without damaging. Carefully wiggle roots out by pulling on tops. Harvest when mature, or they get too woody to eat.

✘ **Insect Control:** Common pests are nematodes. To prevent, plant French marigolds (*Tagetes patula*) or Mexican marigolds (*Tagetes minuta*). Work them into soil and let rot before planting burdock.

✓ **Tips:** Young roots are eaten raw similar to radish with a little salt. Older roots used more for cooking. Can be stir-fried, roasted, braised, pickled, added to soups, made into tea or used in a drink. Young leafy portions can be eaten as a green in salads and sandwiches.

ooooo

⚜ *CABBAGE* ⚜

✚ **Health Power:** Similar to Brussels sprouts, cruciferous vegetables like cabbage increase the production and action of enzymes that detoxify the body. Beyond antioxidant action that removes dangerous free radicals, crucifers make DNA produce more detoxification and anti-cancer enzymes. Enhance natural defenses by stimulating production of antioxidant compounds like glutathione. Supply sulfur compounds like sinigrin and sulforaphane that catalyze production of anti-carcinogens. Also affect the expression of cancer-related genes. Amino acid glutamine helps restore stomach lining after peptic ulcer. See Brussels Sprouts for more on the health power of crucifers.

↑ **Vitamin and Mineral Content:**
Vitamins – K, C, B6 (Pyridoxine), B1 (Thiamin), B2 (Riboflavin) and A
Minerals – Manganese, Calcium, Potassium and Magnesium

⊘ **Disease Prevention:** Reduces risk, symptoms and proliferation of cancer more than any other fruits or vegetables in prostate, colon, lung, stomach, breast, ovaries and bladder. Possibly occurs through increasing levels of isothiocyanate after eating crucifers. A potent anti-cancer molecule that binds to toxins inducing their removal, stimulates cancer cell death, prevents excess cellular dividing and promotes the healthy metabolism of hormones like estrogen.

🌱 **How to Grow:** Cabbages come in dense versions, with green, red and purple heads, and loose leaf versions including bok choy. Can be harvested all year long in a mild climate with moist winters. Three divisions among varieties based on harvest time: spring, summer and fall/winter. For spring cabbages, sow seeds in seed beds with shallow drills spaced 6 inches apart in mid- to late summer. Don't make the drills very long, as you only need 1.5 feet to produce 60-90 plants. Plant them out beginning early fall. Spring cabbages grow in moderate climates only. For summer cabbages, sow seeds in trays near the end of winter. These need to be transplanted indoors into a bigger container and kept under light or in a greenhouse. Or you may wait longer and sow them outdoors in the spring when air and ground temperatures rise. For autumn/winter cabbages, which include red cabbage, sow seeds in a bed with shallow drills in mid- to late spring with the same spacing as spring cabbages. For all varieties, transplant when seedlings have grown roughly 3 inches. Soften the seed bed with water the evening before. Fill a small dirt hole with water and soak the seedling roots until they are covered in muddy water. Plant each seedling in holes 6 inches deep and 18 inches apart in rows spaced out 18 inches as well. Keep weed-free and watered. Harvest when hearts feel solid. Cut at the base of stems. You can preserve some varieties in a cool shed hung upside down.

✘ **Insect Control:** See Brussels Sprouts for how to rid pests.

✓ **Tips:** Spring cabbages need a handful of fertilizer per plant in late winter to keep them growing. Cook lightly to retain more phytonutrients. Choose organic varieties, which have more phytonutrients that reduce cancer risk.

∞∞∞

✣ *CACTI* ✣

✚ **Health Power:** Nopales (pads of prickly pear cactus) are especially good for cardiovascular, colon and immune system health. Rich in vitamins A and C, both potent antioxidants that protect cells/tissues from free radical damage that leads to DNA mutations. Also preserve elasticity and integrity of blood cell walls and other epithelial tissues. Help reduce inflammations linked to arthritis or asthma. Rich in phytonutrients called flavonoids, also powerful antioxidants. Soluble and insoluble fibers aid digestion, lower blood glucose, cholesterol and triglycerides. Fiber, antioxidants and other phytonutrients work synergistically to combat oxidative stress, optimize immune function, maintain good systemic balance and help prevent adverse conditions.

⬆ **Vitamin and Mineral Content:**
Vitamins – A, C, K, B6 (Pyridoxine) and B2 (Riboflavin)
Minerals – Manganese, Calcium, Magnesium and Potassium

⊘ **Disease Prevention:** Reduces symptoms or risk of constipation, gastric ulcers, atherosclerosis, heart disease, diabetes, breast cancer and colon cancer.

❧ **How to Grow:** Several thousand species of cacti grow in the U.S., but only about 100 can grow outside arid regions of the Southwest. Prickly pears of the genus Opuntia are most common in northern areas, being hardy down to minus 40°F. Most cacti produce gorgeous flowers in spring; some even produce edible fruit or vegetables. *Opuntia ficus-indica* produces fig-shaped fruit (prickly pears) about 2 inches long, as sweet as peaches. Pads of this species, nopales, are edible. Others popular in China and Vietnam produce pitaya, also known as dragon fruit. Consult local nursery for which cultivar grows best in your area. Cacti require full sun (minimum 6 hours per day) and excellent drainage for optimum growth. Work in a generous amount of compost or planting mix rich in organic matter. Add coarse sand, gravel and some limestone. If soil naturally retains much water, create a raised bed. Plant in spring but plan for the function and mature size of cactus. Prickly pears spread about 2 feet, others more confined, some grow wider. Check with nursery before planting. Protect hands with gloves, or even magazine, newspaper or cardboard, from both visible spines and smaller, hooked spines called glochids. Post planting, put a layer of gravel around base to prevent rot. Little maintenance required. Apply liquid fertilizer or other micronutrient-rich mix each spring. When harvesting prickly pears from *Opuntia ficus-indica*, handle with care; tiny glochids hard to remove if wedged in skin. Can grow in containers indoors, but less than full potential with lack of sunlight.

✗ Insect Control: Tough, almost impenetrable, texture and sharp spines protect cacti from pests.

✓ Tips: Be careful while harvesting. Use gloves. Soaking prickly pears in scalding water for a few minutes makes peeling skin containing glochids much easier.

∞∞∞

❧ *CARROTS* ❧

✚ Health Power: Many health benefits. Great source of antioxidant compounds. Rank among highest carotenoid contents. Help regulate blood sugar levels and reduce insulin resistance, a common cause of diabetes. High vitamin A helps eyes adjust to changing brightness and promotes good night vision. Vitamin A reduces risk of emphysema from exposure to cigarette smoke.

↑ Vitamin and Mineral Content:
Vitamins – A, K, C, B6 (Pyridoxine), B1 (Thiamin), B3 (Niacin), B9 (Folate)
Minerals – Potassium, Manganese, Molybdenum, Phosphorus and Magnesium

⊘ Disease Prevention: One daily serving of carrots or squash cuts in half risk of heart disease among elderly. Beta-carotene from carrots converts to Vitamin A in liver; travels to eye where it helps produce chemicals needed for night vision. Beta-carotene has antioxidant properties that help prevent cataracts and macular degeneration. High levels of carotenoids with falcarinol defend against many cancers: postmenopausal breast, bladder, cervix, prostate, larynx, esophagus, colon and lung. Carotenoids in carrots may work only when grouped into biochemical team, since supplementation of only one carotenoid, beta-carotene, is not as effective.

❦ **How to Grow:** Easy to grow with quality soil. Varieties differ in maturation timing and size. Plant in less dense, finer soil. Need well-aged compost or mature organic matter to grow well. (Fresh manure or compost causes deformed root growth and atypical tastes.) Lacking light soil, grow in raised deep beds. Some smaller types will grow in shallower soil, but larger crop demands deep raised beds or deep sandy loam soil. To create a deep raised bed, dig a trench of desired width and one spade deep. Break up the bottom soil layer to create room for roots to explore. Mix in couple inches of well-aged, disease-free manure, compost or planting mix. Fill trench half way and add another couple inches. Finish by filling the trench with the remainder of the soil dug up. For good measure, throw over the top a few handfuls of planting mix containing alfalfa, fish bone or kelp meal. Needs pH near 6.5; add lime to raise. Sow seeds directly into permanent rows in late winter for warm climates and mid-spring in cooler areas. Place a pinch or about 5-6 seeds per inch of the row. Cover the row with a thin layer of topsoil (roughly ½ inch or slightly more in dry areas). Water softly, but keep seeds moist so they germinate and sprout in 1-3 weeks. When tops reach a few inches high, mulch around plants to help retain moisture. Ready for harvest when big enough to eat. Moisten soil to make it easier to pull out.

✗ **Insect Control:** Carrots usually problem free. Common pests include carrot fly, parsley worms and nematodes. Biggest threats are gophers, deer, woodchucks and rabbits. If these are large risk, erect large barriers or fences to block entry. Block gophers with underground fence or flood them out of their holes. Interplant with onions to repel carrot flies or cover rows with plastic lining. Crop rotation helps prevent nematode infestation. Plant marigolds year before to remove them from soil.

✓ **Tips:** Crowded carrots interfere with each other and grow deformed. When the sprouts are 2-3 inches high, thin the rows so plants are separated by 1inch. Repeat in several weeks to make them 4 inches apart. Carrots respond well to container planting if you want to grow just a few carrots and avoid effort of creating deeper bed of lighter soil.

∞∞∞

❧ CAULIFLOWER ❧

✦ **Health Power:** Like other crucifers, cauliflower contains glucosinolates (sulforaphane) and thiocyanates (isothiocyanate). Together, they increase the ability of liver cells to create compounds that remove harmful, sometimes cancer-causing, toxins. See Brussels Sprouts and Cabbage for more on the detoxification benefits of eating crucifers. Cauliflower itself also contains enzymes that assist in detoxification. Cauliflower also provides dietary fiber and the B vitamin folate. Fiber promotes healthy digestion and lower blood cholesterol levels. Pregnant women need folate to ensure the healthy development of their baby's nervous system.

↑ **Vitamin and Mineral Content:**
Vitamins – C, K, B6 (Pyridoxine), B5 (Pantothenic Acid), B2 (Riboflavin), B1 (Thiamin) and B3 (Niacin)
Minerals – Manganese, Potassium, Phosphorus and Magnesium

⊘ **Disease Prevention:** Eating cruciferous vegetables several times a week reduces the risk of many cancers, sometimes by up to 50 percent. Such cancers include lung, colon, breast, ovary, bladder, colorectal and prostate. Research has found the spice turmeric has a compound, curcumin, that, with the many isothiocyanates in crucifers, may retard or inhibit the growth of prostate cancer cells. Middle-aged men concerned about prostate enlargement may do well by regularly eating cauliflower with turmeric. Cauliflower may also protect from cardiovascular disease, arthritis, and indigestion.

❧ **How to Grow:** Cauliflowers are the most difficult crucifer/brassica to grow due to their sensitivity to nutrient deficiencies and club root disease. Try to grow these only if your land is free of club root. Like cabbage, cauliflower comes in three types: summer, fall and winter/spring. Choose a site with full sun. Amend the soil with plenty of organic matter from a planting mix, aged manure or compost. Cauliflower must have access to all the micronutrients for proper growth. Make the pH 6.5-7. Add lime to raise, if needed. For summer varieties, sow seeds in midwinter in a tray on a windowsill or in a greenhouse. Transplant into bigger seed trays when large enough to handle so they do not go hungry. Plant them out as soon as they reach 2 inches tall into spaces 18-22 inches square. Consider planting under cloches to protect from cold and pests. You can successively sow seeds on a windowsill in late winter and outdoors in shallow drills throughout spring for a continuous harvest. Autumn cauliflowers are the most popular. For them, sow seeds mid-spring in shallow drills separated by 5-7 inches. Plant out in early to mid-summer in holes as deep as they were, making sure to space them out about 24 inches square. For winter/spring varieties, sow seeds in mid- to late spring. Transplant into spaces 30 inches square when they reach 3 inches tall. Keep the area weed free. Cover soil around the plants with organic matter or plastic to retain moisture. Keep watered, as they wither quickly. Cut the curds as they develop into proper sizes. If too many of the summer types are ready at the same time, cut them and store in a cool shed. Remove stumps after harvesting and dispose or compost them. Leave the fall and winter/spring types to harvest when ready to eat to avoid their running to seed.

✗ Insect Control: Cauliflowers are bothered by a number of common pests. See Brussels Sprouts and Broccoli for common treatments. Your rapid response to infestation or disease is crucial with cauliflower to avoid compromising the crop by premature curding.

✓ Tips: Keep micronutrients available for cauliflower, as deficiencies cause deformities. Fertilizing with a nutrient-dense fertilizer (such as alfalfa, fish bone or kelp meal) halfway through growth may help avoid potential problems with soils bordering on deficient. For fall cauliflowers, compact the soil around the base to provide support. For winter/spring varieties, angle the plants away from the morning sun to prevent the middle curds from thawing out too quickly, which can ruin flavor and change the color. Keep the curds out of direct sunlight by bending over a large leaf to cover them. Also, spray stored cauliflowers with water to keep them happy.

∞∞∞

�֎ CELERY ✖

✚ Health Power: Excellent source of Vitamin C, antioxidant that fights free radicals and plaque build up in blood vessels. Phthalides linked with lowered blood pressure by helping arteries dilate. Lowers cholesterol. Diuretic helps get rid of excess fluids. Promotes overall health and optimizes function of immune and vascular systems.

↑ Vitamin and Mineral Content:
Vitamins – K, C, B6 (Pyridoxine), B1 (Thiamin), A and B2 (Riboflavin)
Minerals – Potassium, Folate, Molybdenum, Manganese, Calcium, Magnesium, Phosphorus and Iron

⊘ Disease Prevention: Celery contains many antioxidants including coumarins that decrease the build up of cancer precursors and promote white blood cell activity. Acetylenics also stop cancer cell growth.

❦ **How to Grow:** Two types of celery, self blanching and blanched. Prefer areas where growing seasons are long, moist and cool but not frosting. Choose site with minimum 6 hours daily sunlight. Requires soil that easily retains moisture; digging in organic matter is a must. Get started celery plants at nursery. If you begin from seed, start indoors 6-8 weeks before last frost. Celery likes soil pH near 6.5. Add lime to bring toward neutral. Harden off seedlings and transplant to garden when temperatures are consistently above 50°F. With blanching celery, dig a small trench for optimum growth. Before transplanting, dig a trench one spade deep and long enough to space celery plants 12 inches apart. Place a shallow layer of compost, manure and/ or plant mix in bottom. Cover organics with thin film of soil. Plant seedlings one foot apart and wrap stems with cardboard or a semi-resilient material. Keep soil saturated and feed animal manure liquid fertilizer or sprinkle another organic fertilizer on half-way through growing season. Mid-season and in one month intervals, fill trench with soil up to bottom of leaves. This is the blanching process. For self-blanching types, plant on flat ground in organic-rich soil. For both, keep soil moist and weed free.

✖ **Insect control:** Susceptible to slugs, celery fly and celery leaf. See Artichokes for anti-slug treatments. Celery fly causes leaves to turn pale green, then brown and shriveled. Remove affected leaves and destroy immediately. Celery leaf spots are brown spots on leaves and stems caused by fungus. Immune seeds available are treated with non-organic fungicide. For natural treatment, remove affected leaves and spray every two weeks with Bordeaux mixture until two weeks before harvest.

✓ **Tips:** Harvest self-blanching celery before the first frost. Use blanched types from first frost until well into winter. Use Golden-self blanching plants. If blanching yourself, do not let soil pack against the stems, which can cause rot.

∞∞∞∞

🙣 *CHAMOMILE* 🙣

✚ **Health Power:** Before modern medicine, herbal treatments were popular way to soothe ailments. Some of chamomile's powers discovered long ago still used effectively. Brewed tea from chamomile flowers is calming. Some say chamomile helps reduce nervousness, minor insomnia and aids digestion and upset stomachs. Essential oil from flowers gives more concentrated dose in a cup of tea. Oil obtained through steam distillation. Usually found at herb shops or some grocery stores. Blue color comes from the phytonutrient azulene, which has anti-inflammatory properties. Oil can be used to reduce skin conditions like rashes or eczema, help aid digestion and PMS symptoms. You may also enjoy the fragrance of dried flowers or soothe skin ailments (sunburn and others) by putting dried flowers in a permeable sack to soak in bath water.

↑ Vitamin and Mineral Content:
Vitamins – traces of B1 (Thiamin), B2 (Riboflavin), A and B9 (Folate)
Minerals – Manganese and traces of Copper, Iron, Magnesium, Potassium & Zinc

⊘ Disease Prevention: May help soothe symptoms of skin conditions eczema, psoriasis, sunburns and rashes. May also help with indigestion. Often used to help reduce infant crying (colic) from teething pain, anxiety and insomnia.

❦ How to Grow: Different varieties of chamomile available. Some perennial, others annual. Some used as ground cover or bordering. German variety is an annual used to make tea, as is the Roman perennial. Needs well-drained soil. Prefers site with partial shade, but can tolerate full sun. Can be grown in smaller areas, but may need to be kept in check later to keep from spreading. Growing in pots also an option. Work in compost or planting mix rich in organic matter/microbes into the soil of desired location. Start from seed or plant transplants from reputable nursery. In spring or mid-fall (in warmer climates), plant about 1.5 feet apart if growing for herb use or 8 inches apart for ground cover. Once they are a few inches tall, mulch around with fine fertile material that will not disrupt pH or block water absorption. Don't use pine bark or peat. Water just enough to keep soil moist. Trim off faded or dying flowers/leaves to promote new blooms. Chamomile peaks early through mid-summer with yellow and white flowers. Remove these to make tea. When frost comes, remove annuals and cut back perennials to just a few inches. To over winter perennials, insulate with a layer of mulch.

✘ Insect Control: No pest or disease problems if grown in open position with sun and wind, especially if a number of plants are grown.

✓ Tips: Chamomile thrives best in areas where summer temperatures stay below 100°F. Be careful using chamomile as an herbal remedy. If you are allergic to daisy or ragweed, you may have an allergic reaction to chamomile. Also has blood-thinning action. Discuss with your doctor if you take prescription blood thinner.

ooooo

❧ *CHERRIES* ❧

✚ Health Power: Red color of this tasty treat comes from the powerful antioxidants known as anthocyanins. Cherries packed with free radical destroyers; almost as many as blueberries. Help with pain of inflammatory conditions like arthritis and muscle soreness. Linked with heart benefits by reducing inflammation and total cholesterol, and lowering body fat and total weight. Low in fat, high in water content and helps boost metabolism. One of only a few foods with melatonin. (Produced in pineal gland and associated with sleep rhythms. Cherries may help you get to sleep.) The high potassium content also can help control blood pressure and maintain proper muscle and nerve cell functioning.

↑ **Vitamin and Mineral Content:**
Vitamins – A, C, B2 (Riboflavin), B6 (Pyridoxine), B9 (Folate) and K
Minerals – Iron, Copper, Manganese, Potassium and Magnesium

⊘ **Disease Prevention:** The flavonoids (anthocyanins and quercetin) as well as the phenolic acid amygdalin in cherries may help lower symptoms or onset of several conditions: heart disease, pain from rheumatoid arthritis and gout, diabetes and other connective tissue ailments. Some studies show a reduced risk for colon and breast cancer by controlling cell-damaging free radicals.

🌿 **How to Grow:** A tasty addition to the garden. Grow well in moderately cool temperatures but not constantly freezing. Many varieties self-pollinate. Must match the cultivar to your area. Consult trusted fruit tree supplier for one that grows well and matches your taste. Varieties are sweet, sour, dwarf and standard. Pick site with plenty of sunlight. Thrive in soil rich in nutrients and organic matter. Soil should be pH 6-8 with moisture retentive, well-drained loam. Prepare soil area of five square feet by adding generous amounts of organic matter and nutrient rich planting mix or well-aged compost. Rock dusts also good to work in, because they continue to release vital nutrients for years. One-year-old trees are best to start. Make sure to allow for space of branches and foliage, usually just over 20 feet in diameter for full-size tree. Dig the hole 6 inches to a foot wider and deeper than the ball of roots in the transplant. Loosen soil at bottom of hole by poking with pitchfork or similar tool. Cut off elongated roots with a clean tool, plant tree and firm in soil around roots. Water until air bubbles stop appearing. Prune tree/s back to around 2-3 feet by cutting slightly above connection to an adjacent branch. Decreasing demand for water and nutrients will buy time for roots to catch up with supply. Shape as desired. Most importantly, cut internal lateral branches close to the trunk to maintain room for air and sun. Other than that, leave them to grow or trim branches similar to peach trees to increase fruit size. Leave cherries on tree as long as you can, but pick before they split. Eat sweet cherries right away. Use tart ones to cook with, bottle or make into jam within a few days.

✗ **Insect Control:** Birds are main threat to cherries. Plan on losing about 30 percent of crop. If planting only one tree, consider planting a mulberry tree nearby to distract birds from cherries. They love mulberries. (If growing more than one tree, you will have more fruit than one family can think of consuming per season.) Sometimes aphids, winter moth or bacterial canker cause problems. Spray off aphids with a strong stream. Best way to get rid of winter moths: secure a grease band around the tree between fall and spring to stop females from crawling up to lay eggs. To rid bacterial canker, cut and dispose of all infected wood. Then spray copper fungicide three times with one month between applications.

✓ **Tips:** When planting in windy, more exposed locations, support tree with a stake until trunk and roots are strong enough.

∞∞∞

❧ *CHIVES* ❧

✚ **Health Power:** Provide only small amounts of vitamins, minerals and phytonutrients (from garnishing dishes with chives), but they add to the overall health of meals. High vitamin K, A and C content by weight. Vitamins A and C have antioxidant properties that help rid body of damaging free radicals. Vitamin K helps build bone and form blood clots. Some suggest they have antibiotic action, aid digestion, improve blood flow and stimulate appetite. Research still young on this member of the onion family, but more study may reveal potentially great benefits.

↑ **Vitamin and Mineral Content:**
Vitamins – K, A, C and B9 (Folate)
Minerals – Manganese

⊘ **Disease Prevention:** Much more research needed. Thus far, researchers say eating chives regularly may reduce risk of prostate cancer. Chives may be as beneficial as its cousins in the Allium family (onions, garlic, leeks, shallots and scallions).

❧ **How to Grow:** A great addition to the garden. Useful as ornamental piece along borders or inside garden. Nice flower blooms. Take well to containers, too. Hardy perennial herb tolerant of both sun and shade. Only soil preference is keep it moist. The pH can vary and chives will still thrive. Sow seeds in early spring spaced 12 inches apart. Or separate already-developed plants and replant 12 inches apart in early spring or fall. Keep them watered and watch them grow. Every three years or so, dig up the groups, divide in half, and replant in fresh soil. If you don't want to move, dig them up and plant temporarily in a pot or unused section of soil. Rework the original soil and amend with compost or planting mix. Then replant back in for another few years. Chives are stimulated to re-grow quickly when cut, so cut down to about half inch above ground as needed. Remove weeds as soon as noticed. Or lay down layer of mulch.

✗ Insect Control: No specific or common pests that damage them. If problem occurs, consult local nursery for treatment.

✓ Tips: Chives store well frozen, but not as well as dry herbs. Lose much of their flavor when stored. If they become woody, trim down to about an inch above ground.

ooooo

🏵 *CILANTRO* 🏵

✚ Health Power: Cilantro leaves and coriander seeds both packed with beneficial phytonutrients. Animal research shows promising health benefits for humans. Regularly eating coriander may reduce bad cholesterol levels (the LDL form), control blood sugar by stimulating insulin production in pancreatic cells and reduce cellular damage by free radicals. Coriander contributes fiber that promotes healthy digestion and nutrient extraction from foods. Coriander has antibiotic components. The volatile oil dodecenal kills Salmonella bacteria responsible for many food poisonings. Cilantro helps remove potentially toxic heavy metals that damage nerve functions. Many popular antioxidants help defend important cells from damage that could lead to reduced vision, higher cholesterol, weakened blood vessels and minor inflammation.

↑ Vitamin and Mineral Content:
Vitamins – traces
Minerals – Manganese, Iron and Magnesium

⊘ Disease Prevention: Cilantro in the regular diet may help reduce symptoms or even prevent heart disease, arthritis, Alzheimer's and anemia. Cilantro has also been a popular treatment to help defend against urinary tract infections.

❧ How to Grow: Cilantro is an annual plant with very aromatic leaves. Also known as the producer of coriander seeds, it grows easily in a container or on the plant bed in a garden. Grows best in sheltered, rich, moist and well-drained soil in full sun. If you get extreme heat, consider a site shaded part of the day. Difficult to transplant. If growing outdoors, plant seeds in spring after the last frost. Weeds tend to grow faster at first than your herb, so keep them weed free early on. Plant seeds half inch deep and spaced out about an inch. If growing in rows, keep rows 12-15 inches apart. Begin to harvest leaves when the plant is roughly 6 inches tall.

Harvest outside leaves first, and thin out the plant as you go to maintain good air circulation. For maximum leaf production, cut off the flower stalks when they develop, which forces more energy into leaf production. When the plant bolts to seed, collect seeds and use them as a spice or a way to get more cilantro later on. Cilantro loses its flavor quickly when it dries out, so keep it fresh in a cool area.

✘ **Insect Control:** Cilantro's pungent smell keeps most pests away. If any, aphids or white flies might attack. Aphids can be expelled with a strong stream of water, but cilantro is too weak to withstand it. Instead, destroy aphids, (which attack many plants) by planting French marigolds to attract their predators. Hoverflies and ladybugs eat aphids by the thousands. White flies are strongly attracted to the color yellow. Get rid of them by creating an old fashioned flytrap with yellow paper and a gooey substance to cover the paper. White flies will land on the paper and be stuck for good.

✓ **Tips:** Another way to experiment with the initial planting is to start a few indoors and transplant them outside after the last frost while also planting seeds directly outdoors. Get a continuous sowing of seeds going in the spring for continuous harvest, because cilantro runs to seed rather quickly after sprouting up.

∞∞∞

✤ *COLLARDS* ✤

✚ **Health Power:** Collard greens are nutritional rock stars loaded with beneficial phytonutrients, vitamins and minerals. Rich in antioxidants, B vitamins and important minerals. An excellent choice for heart health. Sulfurous phytonutrients (glucosinolates and cysteine sulfoxides) inhibit growth of many types of cancers. Some stimulate liver to produce detoxification enzymes that work synergistically to speed up removing free radicals and toxins. Vitamins and minerals promote cardiovascular, immune system, brain and overall health through direct interactions and antioxidant effects. Provide antioxidant vitamins A, C and E. Vitamin C protects water-soluble areas (inside and outside of cells). Vitamins A and E protect fatty molecules and structures, together protecting cell machinery (proteins, enzymes, cell membranes, DNA, mitochondria). Free radicals oxidize cholesterol, which converts to a form that sticks to blood vessel walls (initiating plaque build-up). Vitamin A and zinc help maintain healthy epithelial cells (skin, mucus membranes, gastrointestinal tract, vaginal epithelium), the first line of defense against infection. Folate and other B vitamins moderate homocysteine level in blood by converting to safe form. Potassium and magnesium help reduce elevated blood pressure. Manganese is enzyme cofactor (activator) and integral part of enzymes that make vitamin C useable. Also facilitates antioxidant superoxide dismutase, protecting mitochondria from free radical byproducts. Calcium, essential for healthy bone, also helps prevent menopausal bone loss, migraines, PMS symptoms and helps protect colon cells from carcinogens. Dietary fiber promotes smooth, healthy digestion, helps regulate blood sugar and lowers elevated cholesterol.

↑ Vitamin and Mineral Content:
Vitamins – K, A, C, E, B9 (Folate), B6 (Pyridoxine), B2 (Riboflavin), B3 (Niacin), B1 (Thiamin) and B5 (Pantothenic Acid)
Minerals – Manganese, Calcium, Potassium, Magnesium, Zinc and Iron

⊘ Disease Prevention: Collards may provide risk reduction or symptom relief for atherosclerosis, heart disease, osteoarthritis, macular degeneration, osteoporosis, diabetes, and cancers of lung, breast, ovary, prostate and colon.

❦ How to Grow: Very popular Southern vegetable, yet grow well in cooler regions, too. These crucifers are cold hardy, similar to kale and cabbage. See Kale for site, soil and maintenance needs. Spring usually best time for planting. Plant seeds ¼ inch deep a few weeks before last frost. When seedlings emerge, space them 1 foot apart in rows 3 feet apart. For fall harvest, plant seeds 2-2.5 months before the first frost. Collards slower to mature than kale (70-80 days). Keep soil moist. Collards like foliar feeding. Apply liquid fertilizer a few times during growth season and spread out evenly. Leaves ready to harvest when the plant is about 1 foot tall. Pick outer leaves first.

✗ Insect Control: See Cabbage and Kale for pest control methods.

✓ Tips: Flavor is better after cool weather, especially right after frost.

∞∞∞

❧ CORN ❧

✚ Health Power: More than just a source of starch and carbohydrates. Corn contributes to heart health, lung health, energy production, metabolism and memory. Yellow corn higher in carotene lutein than white corn, hence yellow color. Lutein great for eyes. B vitamin folate helps prevent birth defects and lowers homocysteine in blood, a molecule linked to cardiovascular problems. Phytonutrient beta-cryptoxanthin found in corn (also oranges and red bell peppers) may protect lungs from carcinogens. B vitamin pantothenic acid helps maintain energy by breaking down carbohydrates, fats and proteins. Thiamin helps provide energy and contributes to brain health by helping synthesize acetylcholine, a crucial neurotransmitter for memory and neural function in general. Fiber aids healthy digestion and lowers total cholesterol. Whole grain foods like corn and wheat are rich in antioxidant phenolics, which work in synergy to help deal with adversity and prevent many diseases.

↑ **Vitamin and Mineral Content:**
Vitamins – B1 (Thiamin), B9 (Folate), C and B5 (Pantothenic Acid)
Minerals – Phosphorus and Manganese

⊘ **Disease prevention:** Research incomplete on corn's antioxidant activity and general potential to prevent disease. Nutrients are linked with lower risks of heart disease, colon cancer, lung cancer, macular degeneration and Alzheimer's disease.

❦ **How to Grow:** Among oldest, most widespread foods. Grows in warm weather. Young corn very sensitive to frost and transplants. Start outdoors after soil warms up. To start earlier, use peat pots so roots are undisturbed when transplanting. Choose plot with full sun in area where they will not shade other crops that need sun. Amend soil well with aged compost or very fertile plant mix. Corn prefers slightly acidic pH. If below 5.5, add lime or dolomite to raise. Pollinated by wind, so plant in rectangles with rows close together. To ensure good pollination, plant 6 or more rows together in a group. Plant seeds outdoors (two in every one-inch deep hole) when temperature rises above 70°F. Space holes 8-12 inches. Cover holes with soil and compress a bit. Water thoroughly. Seeds will start showing after week one of watering. Keep weeds away, especially while plants are young. Cover surrounding area with mulch. Water regularly, especially on hot days. Corn is fully-grown and ready to harvest in about 3 months, when the top hairs turn brownish and kernels are plump.

✗ **Insect Control:** Corn grown in highly fertile soil usually has few problems. Most common pests are flea beetles, earworms, cutworms and corn borers. Flea beetles are most damaging to young crops by chewing many small holes in leaves. Apply parasitic nematodes to soil. In extreme cases, spray with insecticide like rotenone. Corn borers enter the stalk below the tassel. Look for sawdust-like material next to small holes. Squeeze stalk to kill pest. Earworms feed on ear tips when little hairs emerge from the tips forming tassels. Look for them then and dispose. Cutworms chew on plant base just under surface. Attract ground beetles to eat them by growing ground cover nearby. Dig up area surrounding plant and hand pick or use cutworm collars on transplants.

✓ **Tips:** Birds and raccoons can also be a problem during seed sowing and harvest. Aside from installing row covers, deter birds by getting rid of standing water, planting mulberry trees to distract them, removing trash and introducing an owl/ scarecrow. A barrier (like taping ears to the stalk), night lighting or electric fencing will deter raccoons.

∞∞

✂ CUCUMBER ✂

✚ Health Power: Cucumbers contain silica, a trace mineral, which we need for healthy connective tissue (bone, ligaments, tendons, cartilage and muscle). Silica also encourages healthy skin. Some use it topically for swelling under the eyes, dermatitis and soothing sunburn. Cucumbers are 95 percent water by weight, so eating is a good way to hydrate. Cucumber adds some fiber to the diet, aiding digestion. With vitamins A and C, cucumber helps the immune system and the liver disarm free radicals that cause cellular damage.

↑ Vitamin and Mineral Content:
Vitamins – C, A and B9 (Folate)
Minerals – Molybdenum, Potassium, Manganese and Magnesium

⊘ Disease Prevention: With lower nutrient concentrations, cucumbers are good, but not major, contributors. The magnesium, potassium and fiber may help reduce hypertension. The fiber and water helps avoid indigestion.

❦ How to Grow: Cucumbers grow best in a sunny spot with rich soil. Amend the site with lots of compost or planting mix to achieve a pH close to 6. Sow seeds twice in the year for two harvests. The first one is in small pots indoors in early spring. Place two seeds to a pot at least 3 inches in diameter. Thin down to the strongest seedling if crowding occurs. Keep in a sunny location with moist soil. They should be ready to plant in late spring. Place about 2 feet apart. Make another sowing outdoors about 2 feet apart. If still cold in your area, put cutoff plastic bottles over the sowings to protect from night cold. You can grow cucumbers on the ground or up along sticks. Making a thin tepee with strong sticks looks cool, and it also keeps cucumbers off the ground and reduces their risk for disease, rot or slug infestation. If you plant them in the ground, space them out a little more than 2 feet, as they will grow out like vines. To keep them attached to the sticks as they grow, regularly tie them to the sticks with thick string. When the seedlings are about a foot tall, mulch with some organic matter. Also, trim back the side shoots to encourage growth upward. Pinch the tops of cucumber plants when they reach the top of the tepee. Keep soil moist. Starting roughly half way through growing season, begin fertilizing every few weeks. To produce more cucumbers, harvest cucumbers when young and plant still contains blooms. Failing this, entire plant stops producing.

✗ **Insect Control:** Popular pests of the cucumber bush include slugs, aphids, and cucumber beetles. To deter slugs, embed a cup of beer in the soil. Slugs and snails fall in and drown. If the plant is big enough and aphids are infesting, spray them off with a strong stream of water. Otherwise, plant French marigolds to attract their predators (hover flies, ladybugs). Inspect all plants and handpick any cucumber beetles when you notice them. You can also wait until later in the season to plant when beetles are on the wane. If they are especially prevalent, you can place row covers over them or, as a last resort, spray with insecticide.

✓ **Tips:** Cucumbers are mostly water, so letting the plant dry out is not an option. During dry weather, water deep into the soil.

∞∞∞

❀ *DANDELION* ❀

✚ **Health Power:** Is the weed with the yellow flower in your backyard nutritious? Yes. Dandelion greens are a great source of many vitamins and a good source of many minerals. One serving has five times the recommended daily dose of vitamin K. Essential for bone health by increasing ratio of bone matrix development to bone breakdown, especially in the presence of calcium. Antidote for coumarin poisoning (rodent poison) since coumarins block liver production of vitamin K and cause internal bleeding. Greens loaded with antioxidant vitamins A and C, preventing buildup of harmful free radicals in water soluble areas of the body and promoting healthy cardiovascular function. Maintain elasticity in blood vessels and assist in blocking biochemical pathways that lead to plaque buildup. Potassium aids blood pressure by helping blood vessels relax. Enhance liver function, eyesight, immune system function and synthesis of connective tissue. Riboflavin and small amounts of other B vitamins assist in metabolism of carbohydrates, lipids and protein to provide energy or help develop body structure. Diuretic components cause kidneys to produce more urine, removing excess toxins, lowering high blood sugar and lowering blood pressure.

⬆ **Vitamin and Mineral Content:**
Vitamins – K, A, C, E and B (Riboflavin)
Minerals – Calcium, Iron, Manganese, Potassium, Magnesium and Copper

○ **Disease Prevention:** High content of vitamins and minerals may help delay or prevent heart disease, atherosclerosis, rheumatoid and osteoarthritis, osteoporosis and cell damage leading to many types of cancer.

❧ **How to Grow:** We know it as a common weed, but dandelions have an attractive flower. Very tolerant and grow in most soils. If growing to eat, increase nutrition by selecting sunny site, amend soil with compost or planting mix and check drainage. Sow seeds in spring; water during dry weather. Thin out to 6 inches or more between plants to reduce disease risk and provide room for leaf growth. Harvest leaves like other leafy lettuce before they flower and/or go to seed, which leads to bitter taste.

✗ **Insect Control:** No common pests for dandelions. Usually dandelion is the pest by growing as weed interfering with other plants. Strong taproot makes them hard to remove, which requires completely digging up roots without breaking off.

✓ **Tips:** When gone to seed, they spread rapidly and germinate. Alternative approach: grow in container to prevent spreading to undesired locations. Many highly nutritious juices and teas come from dandelion. Give them a try.

ooooo

❀ *DILL* ❀

✚ **Health Power:** The significant health benefits of dill come from unique phytonutrients, including monoterpenes (carvone, anethofuran, and limonene) and flavonoids (kaempferol and vicenin). Monoterpenes activate the antioxidant enzyme glutathione-S-transferase, which marks dangerous free radicals for destruction by other compounds. Dill's volatile oil has anti-bacterial properties. Like garlic and thyme, dill inhibits the growth of many common bacteria. Dill is also a great addition to dishes for its mineral and fiber content. A good source of calcium, dill contributes to bone maintenance. Its iron helps blood deliver oxygen to tissues. Fiber promotes smooth digestion and absorption of nutrients. Munching on dill seed has been used to stop hiccups. Making tea with dill is a popular cure for indigestion.

↑ **Vitamin and Mineral Content:**
Vitamins – traces
Minerals – Iron, Manganese and Calcium

⊘ **Disease Prevention:** In the small quantity dill is eaten, it does not significantly reduce disease risks. But added to dishes it helps prevent infection by pathogenic bacteria and bone loss (osteoporosis).

☙ **How to Grow:** Dill is an attractive, fast-growing annual herb native to the tropics. Many consider its taste a perfect complement to fish. The seeds are also used for flavoring pickles. The pleasant yellow flowers make a great plant for bordering. Dill plants prefer sunlight and well-drained soil. Plant in the spring. Amend the soil with compost or planting mix. Sow the seeds directly in the bed outdoors after the last frost when the soil begins to warm up. Thinly place the seeds in small rows spaced about 1 foot apart. Later thin the seedlings to 1 foot apart. If growing for the leaves, make successive sowings every month from mid-summer. Dill grows well in pots, too. Space them out 1 foot apart in pots. Avoid planting near their kin, fennel, as they may cross pollinate. Keep weed-free. Water enough to keep soil moist. Pick leaves fresh as needed. Or dry and collect leaves and seeds. If drying leaves, harvest the plant young before it flowers. Tie stems together in small bunches and hang upside down in a shady, well-ventilated area. If collecting seeds, cut just as seeds ripen, then hang upside down in small bunches in a dry, shady, well-ventilated area.

✘ **Insect Control:** No pest issues. Often used to attract beneficial insects in companion planting, including parasitic wasps and pollinating bees. Plant this herb near fruits and vegetables to help control pests and attract pollinators to get generous yields. If planted near tomatoes, dill strongly attracts hornworms, which are easier to spot and remove from dill.

✓ **Tips:** Difficult to grow from transplants. Another way to collect seeds: Remove the whole flower head when the seed pods turn brown, place them in a paper bag and shake carefully. Seeds will fall out, and you can separate them from other plant matter.

ﻌﻌﻌ

❧ *EGGPLANT* ❧

✚ **Health Power:** Eggplant has a nice mixture of vitamins, minerals and phytonutrients. Many of the phytonutrients, like phenolic compounds and flavonoids, are antioxidants. One flavonoid, nasunin, protects the membranes around each cell. Especially important because cell membranes control traffic in and out of each cell, contain receptors for messenger compounds that tell the cell what to do and are the protective barrier between inside and outside. Among phenolic compounds, chlorogenic acid is a potent antioxidant in highest concentrations.

With flavonoids, these compounds disarm free radicals in many locations to help stop oxidative cell damage (which could develop into cancer), help relax blood vessels, lower cholesterol and plaque buildup, help ward off microbes and viruses and reduce free-radical stress in joints, a primary part of arthritis development. Eggplant also has fiber, potassium and several B vitamins to help promote healthy metabolism, digestion and nerve/muscle function. All these benefits are low-cost, because eggplant is low in fat and sugar.

↑ **Vitamin and Mineral Content:**
Vitamins – B1 (Thiamin), B6 (Pyridoxine), B9 (Folate) and B3 (Niacin)
Minerals – Potassium, Manganese, Copper and Magnesium

⊘ **Disease Prevention:** Eggplant may help reduce risks for, or symptoms of, rheumatoid and osteoarthritis, heart disease, cancer cell development, type II diabetes and others.

🌱 **How to Grow:** Eggplants are native to the tropics and do not produce through cold winters. Grown as annuals in cooler climates and perennials in warmer ones. Can be found as seeds or bought as young plants. An earlier variety will produce longer. Choose a sheltered site with full sun and well-drained soil. Amend the soil with aged compost, manure or planting mix. Grow best in soil with pH 6.5. If you live in a cooler region, you may need to warm up the soil by covering with black plastic weeks in advance. In cool climates, sow seeds indoors on a windowsill or under fluorescent light in early to mid-spring. A week or two before planting out, harden them off by bringing outdoors for increasing periods. In late spring, plant out 2 feet apart in rows underneath plastic row covers. In warmer climates, row covers not needed. Eggplants get bulky for stems to hold, so tie main stem to a stake in multiple places to provide weight support and keep them off the ground. Water when needed and monitor regularly to see how they grow. If they do not branch out from the main stem when they are 10 inches high, pinch out the growth tip. Also, limit fruits to about 5 per plant to ensure all get loaded with nutrients and grow in a healthy way. Remove extra flowers after about 5 have fruited and begun to develop. Treat soil each week with nutrient-dense liquid fertilizer like compost tea, manure tea or liquid seaweed. Begin harvesting eggplants in late summer when they are fully mature and shining.

✗ **Insect Control:** Aphids, whitefly and red spider mite are common pests of eggplants. The spider mites thrive in dryness, so keep the plant moist by spraying regularly. Control aphids by planting French marigolds, which attract predators like hover flies and ladybugs that eat them by the thousands. White flies can be trapped in an old-style flytrap. They are attracted to the color yellow, so construct a trap by covering some yellow material with a sticky substance. Hang it near the plants at risk or under attack. Whiteflies fly into trap and get stuck in adhesive.

✓ **Tips:** Harvest before eggplants lose their shine or they will taste bitter.

ooooo

ENDIVE

✚ **Health Power:** Endive is particularly rich in vitamin K, which is essential for several proteins that make blood clot. (The name K comes from the German word koagulation.) If blood does not clot, wounds bleed out of control. Vitamin K plays an important role in bone formation. Many foods contain vitamin K, and a deficiency is rare. Endive is also a good source of vitamin A, folate and fiber. Vitamin A is a fat-soluble antioxidant that clears destructive free radicals and helps maintain healthy epithelial tissue around blood vessels and organs such as the liver and stomach. Folate protects blood vessel walls from early damage that can lead to stroke and heart attack. Folate converts the molecule homocysteine into harmless molecules used for other purposes. Folate also helps with cell growth and normal fetal development, making it essential during pregnancy. It also aids digestion by stimulating alkaline bile, which may help balance intestinal pH like a mild antacid.

↑ **Vitamin and Mineral Content:**
Vitamins – K, A, B9 (Folate), C and B5 (Pantothenic Acid)
Minerals – Manganese, Potassium and Iron

⃠ **Disease Prevention:** Endive may reduce the risk of anemia and cancer in the rectum, skin and bladder. It may also help ward off atherosclerosis or other cardiovascular disease. Due to its alkaline nature, endive can reduce minor symptoms of heartburn or acid indigestion.

❦ **How to Grow:** Endive is a salad vegetable great for late summer or early fall harvest (winter in warmer climates). Flavor is bitter like chicory and can be tough if not cared for properly. Choose a partly shaded site to prevent excess bitterness and running to seed too soon. Prefers rich medium loam soil that holds moisture well with a pH near 6.5. Work in highly fertile compost or planting mix a couple weeks before sowing. For a fall and/or winter harvest, sow in midsummer and/or late summer, respectively. Place seeds in shallow drills roughly 1 foot apart. Direct sowing is the best way to plant, since transplanting causes endive to run to seed quickly. Keep soil moist and weed as needed to keep beds free of competition. The most-recently-sown rows may need cloche covers in cooler climates to prevent cold damage. About 12 weeks after sowing, blanch the endive to create a more delicate flavor. Do this by placing flowerpots over them. Cover the pothole in the bottom to block sunlight. Leave as is for a few weeks. Ready to harvest when hearts are a light creamy color.

✗ **Insect Control:** Generally pest free. If you get an infestation of anything, ask your local nursery what might cause problems in your area.

✓ **Tips:** Toss mixed greens, sliced pear, candied walnuts, gorgonzola cheese and raspberry vinaigrette with endive for a tasty dinner appetizer.

∞∞∞∞

❧ *FENNEL* ❧

✚ **Health Power:** Fennel has promising phytonutrients with potent antioxidant activity, anti-inflammatory properties, and the ability to inhibit cancer cell development (according to early research). Most notable is phytonutrient anethole. In animal studies, anethole reduced inflammation and blocked the initiation of cancer cells through the inhibition of one or more biochemical pathways. Fennel is a great way to get vitamin C, potassium, folate and fiber. Vitamin C is a versatile antioxidant. It protects cells in water-soluble areas from free radical damage that can lead to arthritis and atherosclerosis. It may also be needed by the immune system for optimum function against harmful invaders. Fiber, folate and potassium together are great for the digestive tract and cardiovascular system. Fiber helps the intestines and lowers elevated levels of cholesterol and blood sugar. Folate prevents the buildup of homocysteine in the blood, a compound known to cause vessel damage in high concentrations. Fennel has potassium as well, which promotes healthy nerve and muscle functions and helps lower blood pressure.

↑ **Vitamin and Mineral Content:**
Vitamins – C, B9 (Folate) and B3 (Niacin)
Minerals – Potassium, Manganese, Molybdenum, Phosphorus, Calcium, Magnesium, Iron and Copper

⊘ **Disease Prevention:** Fennel may reduce symptoms or the onset of rheumatoid and osteoarthritis, cardiovascular disease, heart attack, stroke and colon cancer. High antioxidant activity (and the phytonutrient anethole) may reduce cell damage that causes many other types of cancer.

❦ **How to Grow:** You can grow fennel for its swollen base or leaves. It can reach a height of 5-6 feet tall. Varieties grown for stem bases are called Florence fennel. Both types need sunny site with well-drained, living soil holding the right micronutrients and microbes. The pH should be above 6.5. To gain these optimal growing conditions, work in some compost and planting mix. Fennel is a perennial that can be planted in either spring or fall. Sow regular fennel seeds or plant young seedlings roughly 2 feet apart. If planting Florence fennel, sow seeds only in spring in shallow drills 1.5 feet apart. Later thin the seedlings to 8-10 inches apart. Keep plants weed free. Water when soil begins to dry. If Florence fennel dries out, it runs to seed and compromises the crop. Trim regular fennel plants down as they grow to promote continuous growth of fresh young leaves. Let some shoots produce flowers and go to seed for a stock. Make sure not to plant fennel next to other spices like dill, coriander or caraway as they can cross pollinate each other. Every few years, lift fennel and replant somewhere else so the soil can reach its original balance again. Harvest the leaves as needed. To get seeds, hang the flowers upside down in a dry area with a cloth underneath to catch them when they fall.

✘ **Insect Control:** Most fennel is not affected by pests. Florence fennel can be bothered by slugs and celery fly. To rid the garden of slugs, embed a glass of beer in the soil. The slugs will be attracted, slither into the cup and drown. Celery flies are tough to notice until they cause leaves to turn pale and then brown. Remove these leaves and destroy them away from the garden.

✔ **Tips:** Many plants have trouble growing next to fennel, because its large taproot competes for nutrients. Best solution is to grow it at least 3 feet away from other plants.

∞∞∞∞

🌡 *FIGS* 🌡

✚ **Health Power:** Figs are a great source of potassium, which supports healthy nerve function and muscle contraction. A diet with many potassium-rich fruits and vegetables is linked to lower blood pressure compared to diets with little potassium. Figs have little calcium, but their potassium helps decrease the amount of calcium lost in urine, which makes figs a net supporter of bone health. The dietary fiber promotes healthy digestion, regulates cholesterol and blood sugar levels, and may support weight loss. Research on the benefits of fig leaves suggests phytonutrients within the leaves can help lower the amount of insulin needed by dependent diabetics. They may also reduce triglycerides in blood and inhibit the growth of some cancers. Watch for future discoveries of the health benefits linked to fig trees.

↑ Vitamin and Mineral Content:
Vitamins – trace amounts
Minerals – Potassium and Manganese

⊘ Disease Prevention: Figs are linked to a lower risk of post-menopausal breast cancer. They also support bone health, perhaps forestalling osteoporosis. Heart healthy, they may reduce complications of high blood pressure.

❧ How to Grow: Figs are a cool, tasty little specialty fruit to have growing in the back yard. They can be trained as fan trees, bush trees or left alone to do what they will. Bush trees will grow roughly 10 feet high, fan trees 15 feet. Let the tree shape itself with some minor pruning. Figs need a sunny site and soil that holds moisture well but has good drainage for the excess. The pH should be around 7 or just below. If your garden area is small and you don't want to risk casting shade over other plants, grow the figs along a south wall so it gets full sun. If growing more than one tree, plant trees 12-15 feet apart. Choose a tree well adapted to your climate. Self-fertilizing trees are easier to grow. The local nursery should have a young transplant geared for your environment. Dig a deep hole and amend it with aged compost, planting mix or well-aged manure. Plant the fig in and fill the hole with the amended soil. Water manually during first year and during dry spells. In winter, prune out old wood. Thin out branches in summer so fruit can ripen in sun. Also, cut away any sucker sprouts that come up from roots during growth. Replant these or give away. Figs are ready to harvest when skin changes color. Dark skinned ones turn dark purple; light skinned turn yellow. Eat straight off tree or store by drying or freezing.

✕ Insect Control: Figs rarely have serious pests. Sometimes birds, botrytis and canker can be a problem. If birds are a serious issue, the only sure way to protect the tree is to surround it with netting. You may also try planting a mulberry tree to divert them to what they love. Canker starts with eroding patches of bark that grow bigger. When you notice it, cut off the diseased patches or branches and dispose of them. Botrytis is gray mold that thrives in cold, moist conditions. To avoid Botrytis, make sure the tree has good air circulation, drainage and no excess water. Remove infected growth and destroy immediately.

✓ Tips: If fruit yield is your top priority, restrict root growth to encourage more energy into fruiting. Do this by digging a wider hole and putting sediment on the bottom. Then barricade the sides with bricks or metal sheets.

ooooo

❊ *GARLIC* ❊

✚ Health Power: Garlic, an antioxidant, slows plaque buildup (calcification) in coronary arteries. Studies show it stops calcium from binding with proteoheparan, (and then with LDL cholesterol) which begins the process. Slowing plaque buildup lowers the risk of later heart attack. Helps lower blood pressure and suppresses or removes oxidizing agents in blood stream and fat areas. Contains organosulphur compounds (ex. allicin and diallyl disulphide) that have antiviral and strong anti-bacterial activity, making garlic excellent for treating common colds. Compounds also help relax and enlarge blood vessels, which can help lower blood pressure and improve blood flow. These phytonutrients in garlic also show strong anti-carcinogen effects. Contains anti-inflammatory compounds that reduce painful swelling from conditions like arthritis. Vitamins, minerals and phytonutrients in garlic promote optimum general health.

↑ Vitamin and Mineral Content:
Vitamins – B6 (Pyridoxine), C and B1 (Thiamin)
Minerals – Manganese, Selenium, Calcium, Phosphorus and Copper

⊘ Disease Prevention: Reduces symptoms or risk of asthma, rheumatoid and os-teoarthritis, diabetes, heart disease and atherosclerosis. Reduces risk of, and impedes growth of, many cancers: oral, pharynx, esophageal, colorectal, laryngeal, breast, ovarian, prostate and kidney.

❦ How to Grow: One of the easier bulb vegetables to grow and a great addition to many dishes. Grow best in areas with ample sun. Prefers deep soils with lots of organic matter. Mix in generous amounts of aged manure, compost or other planting mix containing high concentration of organic matter. The pH needs to be at or above 6.5; add lime to raise, if needed. Garlic grows from individual cloves that make up the bulb. To plant, dig 1.5-2 inch holes spaced 4-6 inches apart. Place one big clove with point facing up in each hole. Lightly mulch around plants to provide frost protection and water retention. In the far North, do it near winter's end or the start of spring. Elsewhere, fall is a good time to plant. For nice growth, keep rows and area weed free. In windy location, prop up longer stems with something to prevent snapping. Dig up bulbs in summer, dry with sun exposure and store in a net or basket.

✗ Insect Control: Rather pest free. Avoid diseases by preventing bulbs from sitting in standing water. Occasional viruses, but the worst they do is cut down yield a bit.

✓ **Tips:** Weeds are biggest enemy; keep cleared. During spring, when leaves are emerging, encourage growth using an organic foliar spray. During the bulb-forming stage in early summer, prevent soil drying out.

ooooo

✿ *GINGER* ✿

✚ **Health Power:** Ginger has been used for years to soothe gastrointestinal discomfort, including motion sickness, cold sweats, dizziness and vomiting. Effects are also seen in pregnant women. Antioxidant compounds (gingerols) suppress free radicals and reduce inflammation, thereby relieving pain. They may help protect the lipids in cell membranes from becoming damaged, preventing the loss of the important, internally produced antioxidant glutathione. High antioxidant activity supports cardiovascular health. Compounds in ginger help perspiration, a good way to detoxify during colds and other illness. Sweat has antimicrobial properties, helping protect against skin-borne infections.

↑ **Vitamin and Mineral Content:**
Vitamins – B6 (Pyridoxine)
Minerals – Potassium, Magnesium, Copper and Manganese

⊘ **Disease Prevention:** Consuming ginger regularly reduces inflammation and pain of rheumatoid and osteoarthritis. Gingerols may also help prevent different cancers from forming. In animal studies, gingerols have inhibited the growth of rectal and ovarian cancer cell lines or induced apoptosis (cell suicide).

❧ **How to Grow:** Ginger only sprouts when at temperatures of 75-80°F. These plants like sun, but will grow indoors if exposed to some sun. Great for container growing and does fine outdoors in a warm climate. Buy a plump ginger root with many buds from a trusted quality market. Soak overnight in warm water. For container growing, use those at least 1 foot deep full of highly fertile soil. Plant ginger roots just under the surface (2 inches deep) evenly spaced, with buds facing upward. Keep plant indoors in warmest, sunniest spot until it emerges above soil. Afterward, seasonally move container indoors and outdoors to keep plant in 75°F air. Keep sheltered from higher winds. Keep soil moist, but let it dry a bit between waterings. In warmer climates, plant roots any time. Amend soil with plenty of well-aged compost or planting mix. Ginger needs nutrient-rich soil with great drainage. Choose warm, sunny, sheltered spot. Soak fresh ginger roots the same way and plant out in spring when temperatures exceed 75°F. Ginger roots take a year or less to reach 2.5-4 feet tall. Harvest newer, younger sprouts in front of originals. Some can be used, frozen and/or replanted.

✗ Insect Control: Relatively insect and disease free. Some varieties bothered by spider mites or aphids. Usually you can shower and handpick to remove. If infestation is heavy, rinse off plant and use insecticidal soap. Planting French marigolds attracts aphid predators. Recommended, especially if growing other green-leafed vegetables nearby.

✓ Tips: If the temperatures drop more than usual, cover them with either a row cover or plastic sheet to hold in some heat. The young stems are good for harvest at any point as they will hold a nice soft texture. Make sure the plant is indoors during cool weather (below 40 °F.) as it does not do well, and you will probably lose it if left outside then.

ooooo

❦ GLOBE ARTICHOKES ❦

✚ Health Power: Almost no food or drink has more antioxidants than artichoke. (Came in #4 out of 1,000-plus in 2006 study.) Beat out blueberries, red wine, dark chocolate and tea. With a nice balance of nutrients, they are ideal for general health. High potassium prevents kidney stones. Folic acid supports cardiovascular health and helps prevent folate-deficiency birth defects. Contains cynarin, which triggers production of bile and aids digestion. Contains phytonutrients that help stimulate regeneration of liver cells and improve gall bladder function, both improving detoxification and digestion. Great source of fiber, which promotes smooth digestion and helps regulate blood sugar and cholesterol. Low glycemic index and a good source of protein with no fat. High vitamin C defends body tissues from oxidative damage of free radicals.

↑ Vitamin and Mineral Content:
Vitamins – C, K and B9 (Folate)
Minerals – Magnesium, Potassium and Manganese

⊘ Disease Prevention: Contains many poly-phenol-type anti-oxidants shown to reduce risks of heart disease, cancer and birth defects. Help stimulate regeneration of liver cells, reduce blood cholesterol levels and improve digestion.

❧ How to Grow: A great addition to the garden and the dinner plate. Sensitive perennials needing moderate temperatures in winter. If winters freeze, you can treat them as annuals. Start with seeds indoors in winter or pick transplants in early spring from a quality local nursery. Avoid planting before final spring frost. Choose sunny, sheltered area of soil. Thoroughly mix in plenty of organic materials and/or fertilizer. If working with dense, heavier soils, try more organic matter to get good drainage. Plant roughly 18 inches apart. They grow up and sideways, spreading up to 5 feet by 5 feet in size. Deep beds give artichoke plants room for root growth, good drainage and high yields. Need a lot of water. Mulch the area with mature compost or manure, making sure to water on dry, hot days. In a colder climate, cut back plant in late fall and cover with a bushel basket or similar.

✗ **Insect Control:** Damaged by a variety of slugs, which are most active feeding at night on soft plant tissues. Several ways to remove. In the evening, physically pick them off plant or soil and drop in a jar. Or cut bottom off a plastic jug and place over seedlings. As plants grow larger, use a larger plastic bottle and cut off the top, too. A dishful of beer sunk in the soil attracts them. They fall in and drown. For problem aphids, plant marigolds nearby to attract predator bugs (ladybugs and hoverflies). You can also rub off or spray off. If severe, use an organic insecticidal soap.

✓ **Tips:** They like the soil just below neutral pH of 7. If pH is plus 7, add lime to bring down. When harvesting, expect 2-4 heads per plant. Cut off larger ones first, just before they open, to encourage smaller ones to grow to full size.

ooooo

🏵 *GRAPEFRUIT* 🏵

✚ **Health Power:** Excellent source of Vitamin C, giving more than 100 percent of RDA. Protects immune system cells that fight the common colds/ other illness. Antioxidant reducing free radicals associated with inflammation, high cholesterol and cardiovascular disease. Pink grapefruit among the highest in antioxidants. Studies of antioxidant lycopene suggest regular eating can dramatically lower risk of prostate cancer. Many other phytonutrients with great potential benefits. Compounds called limonoids trigger production of detoxifying liver enzymes. Bonus: Limonoids stay active in body up to 24 hours, making them more potent fighter of many toxins, many of which could be carcinogenic. Red and blond grapefruit contain soluble fiber, pectin, that reduces bad form of cholesterol (LDL) and triglycerides, providing cardiovascular benefits by preventing buildup in arteries. Regular eating of high-C foods (juices of grapefruit, apple and orange) lowers risk of forming calcium oxalate (kidney) stones.

↑ **Vitamin and Mineral Content:**
Vitamins – C, A and B5 (Pantothenic Acid)
Minerals – Potassium

⊘ **Disease Prevention:** Helps reduce severity of inflammatory conditions like asthma, osteoarthritis and rheumatoid arthritis. Grapefruit linked to lower risk of cancers of prostate, breast, mouth, skin, stomach, colon and lung. Flavonoid naringenin linked with anti-cancer properties, especially of the prostate, via its ability to repair DNA. (As we age, lifelong cell divisions increase the frequency of "duplication errors" [mutations] in DNA.) Naringenin may promote the health of DNA by preventing mutations. Note: Although studied individually, many phyto-nutrients or antioxidants give their benefits not from their solo action but the synergy of many acting in concert. Thus, prefer to get your nutrition from natural sources (fruits and vegetables) rather than from chemicals synthesized into single-variety supplements in pill form.

❧ **How to Grow:** Grapefruit flesh similar to orange but larger and with sharper flavor. Some cultivars are yellow fleshed with seeds and slightly more tart in taste. Others have pink flesh, no seeds and generally sweeter. All varieties are self-fertilizing. Except that grapefruits need a few more nutrients, they are grown with the same soil requirements, maintenance, harvesting and pruning as oranges. See Oranges for details.

✗ **Insect Control:** See Oranges, since these citrus cousins face the same pests.

✓ **Tips:** When planting, dig the bed deep when amending the soil with organic nutrients. For optimal health benefits, try eating a serving of grapefruit or similar fruit every day either as juice, part of a dish or raw.

∞∞∞

❦ GRAPES ❦

✚ **Health Power:** Recent extensive research suggests most beneficial attributes may lie in their phytonutrients rather than vitamins and minerals. Most notable phyto-nutrients may be polyphenols, which include flavonoids and phenolic acids. Flavonoids quercetin and resveratrol help prevent free radicals from oxidizing the bad type of cholesterol (LDL), turning it into a form that later leads to arterial damage and plaque buildup. They maintain normal blood vessel dilation and prevent blood clots that can cause strokes. Contain saponins, believed to reduce absorption of cholesterol and slow the biochemical pathways leading to inflammation.

Resveratrol and others play a large role in both of those health benefits and also prevent the secretion of the hormone angiotensin II, which can lead to stiffening of the heart. Contain pterostilbene, a promising compound for metabolizing fats, including cholesterol. Resveratrol, highly concentrated in red wine, is antibacterial and antifungal, making grapes a good fighter of food borne illness. Antioxidant action ditches free radicals and optimizes health of circulatory system, making grapes a great promoter of overall health. Nutrients available several ways: eating grapes fresh, drinking wine and juice or eating toast with grape jam.

↑ Vitamin and Mineral Content:
Vitamins – C, B1 (Thiamin) and B6 (Pyridoxine)
Minerals – Manganese and Potassium

⊘ Disease Prevention: Significantly reduces risk of heart disease and atherosclerosis. Research suggests consuming resveratrol may help protect DNA from damage leading to lung cancer or other damage leading to prostate, liver, colorectal and breast cancer. May also lower risk of Alzheimer's disease.

❧ How to Grow: Grapes prefer sunny site with great drainage. Produce fruit from second year forward. Self-fertile, so not essential to grow more than one variety. (Nice to have a few different flavors.) Many different cultivars make it possible to grow grapes almost everywhere. Certain locations (like the Deep South) suitable to grow grapes only for jelly, juice or wine. Ask experts what varieties and types work best in your area. Before planting, amend the soil around the planting area with plenty of organic matter and adjust the pH to around 6.0. Get year-old vines from nursery. Support with a wire or grow along a fence or over an arch in backyard. Nurseryman can tell you how to train them. Soak roots in a bucket of water with a handful of micronutrient rich fertilizer for a few hours before planting. Plant 5 feet apart in spring while still dormant before buds begin to swell. Once planted, cut each vine down to leave just two or three healthy looking buds. After planting and each spring, mulch underneath the area with well-aged compost or manure. If growing grapes to eat fresh, prune out any odd-shaped or diseased, and remove berries regularly in random spots in each cluster to allow others to grow larger. Harvest when stems turn brown and fruit is nice and sweet. Cut off clusters with pruning shears and store in cool, shady spot where they will last for about a month.

✗ Insect Control: Pests include birds, wasps, grape berry moths, Japanese beetles and red spider mite. Birds can be completely stopped only by covering with netting or some type of row cover. Birds also love mulberries. Plant a mulberry tree nearby to help distract them away from grapes. To control wasps, fill a container with a sweet liquid (like juice) and cover the container with a lid having a small hole. Wasps will crawl in and not find their way out. Grape berry moths lay eggs on the flowers; purplish larvae feed on buds and flowers. Hang pheromone traps to control. For Japanese beetles, shake them off in the morning and set out bait containers that trap them. Most nurseries have pheromone or other baited traps. To stop red spider mite, keep plants moist by regular spraying with water. If resilient, spray with organic insecticidal soap or oil.

✓ **Tips:** If the growth seems slow, apply a handful per vine of nutrient-rich fertilizer like kelp meal, fish bone meal, or alfalfa meal. One study found red wine contains about triple the valuable phytonutrients (like resveratrol) of white wine. Downside of regular wine drinking is the adverse affects of alcohol. Avoid this by drinking alcohol-free wine or 3 glasses of grape juice daily.

∞∞∞

❦ *GUAVA* ❦

✚ **Health Power:** Loaded with vitamin C (more than double the RDA per fruit) and beneficial phytonutrients. Vitamin C is a powerful antioxidant that prevents damage to many cells, organs and tissues such as eyes, blood vessels, heart and immune system. Full dose of vitamin C in one fruit assures water-soluble areas get protection from free radicals and that immune cells are active. High in lycopene, a powerful antioxidant known to reduce oxidative damage in cells. May also inhibit growth of some types of cancer cells. (Undergoing extensive research.) Fiber and potassium enable guava to lower blood pressure, blood glucose, plaque buildup in blood vessels, cholesterol and triglycerides while promoting smooth digestion. Some phytonutrients in guava have antibacterial and anti-fungal action that may help fight off common microbes (such as Staphylococcus, Shigella, Salmonella, Bacillus, E. coli, Clostridium, and Pseudomonas genera).

↑ **Vitamin and Mineral Content:**
Vitamins – C, A, B9 (Folate) and traces of others
Minerals – Potassium, Copper, Manganese and traces of others

⊘ **Disease Prevention:** Guava may help protect against asthma, rheumatoid and osteoarthritis, atherosclerosis, heart disease and cancers of prostate, lung, stomach, colon and many others. Can help reduce symptoms of gastroenteritis, recurring diarrhea and other digestive problems.

❧ **How to Grow:** Guava is a small, tropical native tree producing delectable green fruit with tender light-yellow or red/pink interior. Grow best in temperature range of 45-90°F. To produce fruit, mean temperature must remain above 60°F. for up to six months (depending on the cultivar). Mature trees can withstand an occasional light frost, but young trees die right away. Choose site with full sun where wind does not exceed 10-15 mph for long periods. Guavas tolerate soil types (except compacted) and pH range 5-8. For best fruit production, roots must penetrate well into soil. For full nutrient supply and good drainage, work in some fertile plant mix rich in organic matter several weeks before planting. If you have not planned ahead, hold off adding mix or fertilizer. If soil consistency is bad, mix in regular soil 1 to 1. Buy a resistant, healthy transplant from a reputable local nursery. If planting more than one tree, space minimum 7-10 feet apart. Dig a hole 3-4 times the diameter of the root ball and 3 times deeper. Position tree in the hole so that root ball lies just beneath soil surface. Fill hole and pat down to remove air pockets. Stake tree the first year so roots get nicely anchored. Use soft fabric to tie stake to tree so as not to damage trunk. Mulch over root zone, keeping 1 foot away from trunk. In first year, fertilize about 5 times (every couple months) with highly fertile, well-balanced mix with full range of macro and micronutrients. As tree grows larger, apply more fertilizer each time. Prune young tree during first year at around 1-2 feet high to promote branching. Also tip branches at 2-3 feet to promote more branching. Harvest just as fruit softens to the touch and is easily removed. Store harvested fruit in a cool place away from sun.

✗ Insect Control: Guava trees can be infested by a number of insects, diseases and nematodes. For most effective treatment, consult local county agricultural extension service or nearby nursery.

✓ Tips: For best flavor, let guavas ripen on the tree. Even in cooler temperatures, they do not store long when fully ripe. Or pick them when still a bit firm just before ripening. You can then store them up to five weeks in cool temperatures. To speed up the ripening process, put them in a paper bag with a banana or apple.

oooo

❀ *HORSERADISH* ❀

✚ Health Power: Horseradish contains glucosinolates (ex. isothiocyanate), potent phytonutrients promoting synthesis of compounds that fight cancer and suppress synthesis of compounds fueling cancer cell growth. Research suggests effects come not from isothiocyanate alone, but from synergistic action with other vegetables containing isothiocyanate. Also linked with increasing blood flow in infected areas and increasing liver's ability to detoxify. Many people use its antimicrobial properties as remedy for cold, flu and fever. Here's how: Blend or grind up tablespoon of fresh horseradish and add to boiling water. Steep for about 5 minutes. Drink this brew 2-3 times per day for fever relief. Can be an effective nasal decongestant by adding to food or eating straight. (Watch out for strong taste.) Excellent source of vitamin C and a little fiber. Small amounts of other vitamins and minerals.

↑ Vitamin and Mineral Content:
Vitamins – C and B9 (Folate)
Minerals – Potassium, Manganese and Magnesium

⊘ Disease Control: Horseradish may reduce the risk or onset of prostate cancer (and potentially many others from isothiocyanate action) and infections leading to coughs, colds, flu and urinary tract infections.

❦ How to Grow: Be careful. While this perennial root crop can be grown for a fantastic fish and meat sauce, it can proliferate beyond control. A crucifer like broccoli and cabbages, it prefers rich, water retentive soil. Digging deeply to loosen soil allows roots to grow thick and straight down several feet. In early spring, plant root pieces with the thinner end down and the thicker end 3-4 inches below surface. Space plants 1 foot apart and rows 4 feet apart. Horseradish spreads rapidly by its roots and fills void in no time. To harness its growth, dig up all roots each year and replant only a select few. Or let it grow in an area where space is plentiful and nothing is adjacent. Or grow in container or embed a pot/bucket in soil to block roots from spreading out. Not invasive. When horseradish gets established, it usually stays the same size. Once planted, water to keep soil moist. Hot summer days require more watering, but make sure to water well in late summer and early fall when they grow the most. Harvest a few young spring leaves to add to salads. Roots are ready to harvest in fall (October-November). Quite hardy. If not harvested, will sprout again in spring.

✗ Insect Control: Very resilient. No pest problems that threaten production or plant life.

✓ Tips: Can be companion planted next to potatoes to repel Colorado potato beetles.

∞∞∞

❧ KALE ❧

✚ Health Power: Kale is highly nutritious, with large variety of vitamins, minerals and phytonutrients. An ideal, all-in-one vegetable to add to your regular diet. Phytonutrients containing sulfur help activate detoxifying enzymes, which act synergistically to remove potentially toxic/carcinogenic chemicals. Other phyotchemicals in crucifers, like glucosinolates, metabolize to isothiocyanates, which inhibit development of many cancer cells. Great for vision. Carotenoids, like lutein and zeaxanthin, along with beta-carotene and vitamins A and C, protect from damaging free radicals and ultraviolet light. Antioxidant action of vitamins A and C help boost immune system, protect blood vessels, reduce inflammation and protect epithelial cells (skin and lining of internal organs). Vitamin K with calcium enhances bone-forming processes and helps prevent bone loss. Trace mineral manganese, along with the B vitamins, helps metabolize sugars, carbohydrates, proteins and lipids to produce energy. Eating leafy vegetables has been shown to extend cognitive function for years longer among elders. Excellent source of fiber, which promotes healthy digestion and regulates cholesterol and blood sugar levels.

↑ **Vitamin and Mineral Content:**
Vitamins – K, A, C, B6 (Pyridoxine), E, B2 (Riboflavin), B1 (Thiamin), B9 (Folate) and B3 (Niacin)
Minerals – Manganese, Copper, Calcium, Potassium, Iron, Magnesium and Phosphorus

⊘ **Disease Prevention:** May play significant role in reducing symptoms or onset of cancers in ovaries, breast, colon, prostate, lung and bladder, plus cataracts, rheumatoid and osteoarthritis and cardiovascular disease.

❦ **How to Grow:** A nutritious, hardy leaf vegetable that can grow in tough winters. Ask local nursery which varieties are best for your area. Choose semi-shady, moderately sheltered site. Soil pH should be near 6.8. Add lime, if needed. Amend soil by mixing in plenty of well-aged compost, manure or a planting mix rich in organic matter. Kale likes cooler weather but still grows in warmer climates during cooler months. In cooler areas, sow seeds outdoors in late spring for fall and winter harvesting. In warmer areas, sow seeds outdoors through early fall for late winter and spring harvests. Create shallow drills as long as desired, spacing each drill out by about 2.5 feet. Plant seeds half inch deep and 2 feet apart within rows. Cover with a thin layer of soil and water regularly. During growth, handpick or hoe out weeds out as they appear. Mulching helps deter weeds and holds in moisture. Harvest young and softer leaves from the center of the plant as needed, not all at once. Larger, tougher leaves are great for cooking.

✗ **Insect Control:** Kale generally less susceptible to pests than other crucifers. See Broccoli, Brussels Sprouts and Cauliflower for general pest control. Others include cabbage root maggot, cabbage butterfly and club root. Cabbage root maggots can be stopped by applying small plastic or foam ground covers that tightly wrap around the base of seedlings. Butterfly can be stopped by hand picking caterpillar and rubbing eggs off leaves. Club root is an incurable soil disease that can last 10 years. The only way around it is to transplant well-developed, resistant seedlings. This allows plants to have acceptable yield but stops club root infection.

✓ **Tips:** For continuous harvest, make successive sowings through start of growing seasons.

∞∞∞∞

🐚 *KIWI* 🐚

✚ **Health Power:** Kiwi fruit contain a solid mix of vitamins, minerals, and phytonutrients for a daily health boost. Research is still ongoing, but certain phytonutrients (probably carotenoids and flavonoids) in kiwi can decrease oxygen-related damage to DNA. Damage to DNA molecules can cause mutations that interfere with proteins and enzymes vital to all cellular functions. Studies show eating kiwis or other citrus fruits lowers the risk of respiratory problems. Highly concentrated source of natural vitamin C, the primary water-soluble antioxidant that neutralizes free radicals causing cellular damage, most notably in cardiovascular system, respiratory system, joints and immune cells. Fat-soluble antioxidant vitamin E gives some protection to fatty areas of the body. Good source of fiber, which reduces high blood sugar and cholesterol levels and helps remove toxins from the colon. The minerals in kiwi (magnesium, potassium and copper) support cardiovascular health. Some work individually, others synergistically, to reduce blood clotting, plaque buildup, triglyceride levels and blood pressure.

↑ **Vitamin and Mineral Content:**
Vitamins – C and E
Minerals – Potassium, Copper, Magnesium and Manganese

⊘ **Disease Prevention:** Kiwi may reduce symptoms related to or the onset of rheumatoid and osteoarthritis, asthma, macular degeneration, colon cancer (and potentially many others), atherosclerosis, cardiovascular disease and diabetic heart disease.

❦ **How to Grow:** Kiwis are a nice ornamental for the garden. Yields tasty treats with more than triple the vitamin C in oranges. Two main varieties, one hardy to as low as -40˚F.; the other down to 10˚F. Hardier variety has smooth skin and is the size of large grapes. Less hardy Chinese Kiwi are larger, fuzzy type we see more often at markets. Except for pruning, they need little maintenance and give high yield if trellised. If growing in colder region, main trunk of Chinese Kiwi needs winter protection. Except for a couple cultivars, most kiwis are not self-fertile. For non-self-fertilizing, plant 3-4 females per male. Most kiwis like full sun, but some prefer partial shade in warmer climates. They like well-drained soil at pH 6-6.5. To spread, kiwis need some help. Grow them along a sturdy trellis or strong fence. Work some compost or planting mix into soil to enrich with nutrients and organic matter and to create a nice loam. In spring, plant vines and trim back to 4 or 5 buds. When they grow a bit, choose one as main shoot/trunk. Secure it to trellis or fence so it grows upward. When it reaches the top, cut the tip to encourage growth of lateral branches. Every month in summer, prune new growth back to 4-5 buds for denser growth with large fruit clusters. Water enough to keep soil moist, taking care not to over water. At the beginning of each growing season, reapply a large amount of fertilizer rich in organic matter (aged compost, manure or planting mix). Kiwis need lots of nutrients. Vines give fruit 2-3 years after planting. For longer-lasting kiwis, pick off the vine in late summer right before they ripen. Let them ripen indoors. You can preserve some even longer in the refrigerator.

✘ Insect Control: Few pests or diseases plague the kiwi plant. If infestation is large, get advice from your local nursery or agricultural extension office.

✓ Tips: Remove soft, aged or damaged kiwis from fresh storage to prevent disease transmission or mass softening of fruit. Even the smallest damage can cause the release of ethylene, making other fruit ripen too quickly.

∞∞∞

🏵 *LAVENDER* 🏵

✚ Health Power: The soothing aroma in lavender plants alone is enough to calm the nerves after a tough day. Many say having the fragrance sprayed (or placed using the plant itself) on their pillow or in the bed linen gives headache relief and better sleep. Scientific studies support this phenomenon. Making it into a tea or extracting the oil can provide similar medicinal properties, such as reducing stress, anxiety, nervousness and nausea. Lavender's fragrance and soothing effects can be a great addition to body, bath and cleaning products. Lavender's essential oil has antibacterial and antifungal action. Lavender oil is great to have for applying to dressing of wounds and burns. Can be used for cooking to add a bit of flavor. Some create lavender sugar by leaving in a sugar container for a couple weeks. You can also grind it up and use it to bake or give flavor to anything you think needs it.

↑ Vitamin and Mineral Content: Non-sufficient data

⊘ **Disease Prevention:** Lavender is great for preventing microbial infections in wounds or burns. Its fragrance and oil extracts may also help treat insomnia, motion sickness and depression.

🌿 **How to Grow:** Lavender is an attractive fragrant perennial herb with purple flowers. About 30 species of this plant are known. The most popular for oil extraction is true (or English) lavender. They prefer site with full sun, superb soil drainage and excellent air circulation. The pH should be between 6.5-7.5. Amend soil with some all-purpose organic planting mix. Plant seedlings in spring when temperatures stay above freezing and soil is warming. Space them out about 20 inches. Water regularly in the beginning, but lightly. (Over watering quickly leads to root rot.) When fully mature, lavender plants are drought tolerant and need little water. Mulch annually to provide a little nutritional boost or insulate during winter. If attempting to grow in non-optimal conditions, plant in pots with holes in the bottom so you have option to take indoors during threatening weather. Lavender needs a couple of years before ready to harvest, even more if the goal is to extract oil (4-5 years). Harvest in morning hours when scent is the strongest.

✗ **Insect Control:** No common pest issues exist for lavenders.

✓ **Tips:** Using a bath bag filled with lavender, steep it in water for a soothing, muscle relaxing soak.

ᵒᵒᵒᵒᵒ

🐜 *LEEKS* 🐜

✚ **Health Power:** Leeks are in the Allium family and carry some of the same health benefits as garlic and onions. (See Garlic and Onion entries for the benefits of phytonutrients in this family.) Leeks differ from their family members in giving fewer nutrients per weight. Because they are less concentrated, you must eat more to get the same nutrition. Compared to garlic and onion, this is easy considering how mellow and sweet their taste is. In general, regular eating of veggies in the Allium family is linked with lower bad cholesterol concentrations and preventing or inhibiting the growth or spread of cancer. With a small dose of vitamin C, iron, folate and B6, leeks add a few antioxidants to get rid of dangerous free radicals, help activate hemoglobin molecules for oxygen transport, lower high levels of the compound homocysteine (damages blood vessels at high concentrations), and helps the body metabolize food to provide energy.

↑ Vitamin and Mineral Content:
Vitamins – C, B9 (Folate) and B6 (Pyridoxine)
Minerals – Manganese and Iron

⊘ **Disease Prevention:** With regular eating, leeks team up with other Allium veggies to help reduce the symptoms or prevent development of atherosclerosis, heart disease, prostate and colon cancer, ovarian cancer and many other cancers.

❦ **How to Grow:** Leeks are great to grow for a winter harvest. They need little attention and are hardy through all but the coldest winters when the soil gets too hard to dig. Choose a site with plenty of sunshine. Work in a generous dose of organic matter in the form of aged compost, manure or planting mix. They prefer a soil pH around 6.5. Add lime to raise, if needed. The pale color we are used to seeing near the bottom of leeks comes from the blanching process during cultivation. There are two ways to do this. First, you can multiple sow them in seed trays in mid-spring. Fill each cell with highly fertile soil (peat and planting mix). Make a small dip in each cell and place 6-7 seeds in each. Cover the seeds with a fine medium such as sand, cover with plastic, water well, and place on a windowsill, under a florescent light or in the greenhouse at or near 60°F. Once germinated, remove the plastic. When they reach 1-2 inches, they are ready to plant out (around early summer). Plant them about 10 inches apart in rows spaced 10 inches apart. Stagger the rows this way to prevent overcrowding. For an alternative technique that blanches each plant, sow seeds 6 inches apart outdoors in a shallow drill in mid-to-late spring. When they reach a couple inches tall, transplant them into pre-made dibber holes 6-8 inches deep. Place one plant per hole and space the holes out by 6 inches. Space rows out by 1 foot. Don't fill the hole with soil. Instead, water each hole a little after placing the leek to get some soil over the roots. As they grow, keep the area weed free by hoeing. Also, to keep the blanch going, push some soil up around the base throughout the growing season. Leeks are ready to harvest in mid-fall. They can be left in the ground until needed unless the weather will make the soil too hard to dig them up. In that case, dig them up early and store in a moist peat soil.

✗ **Insect Control:** Leeks are usually pest free. If you have problems, consult your local nursery.

✓ **Tips:** Companion plant leeks next to carrots and celery since they repel carrot fly. Do not plant next to beans, peas or parsley.

∞∞∞∞

�֎ *LEMON GRASS* ✖

✚ **Health Power:** Including lemon grass in your garden provides many benefits. Making tea with the stems helps digestion, promotes a calm night's sleep, reduces anxiety, eases headaches and even has antimicrobial abilities to fight some infections. It may help with respiratory problems and provide some calming effects as well. Adding lemongrass to the bath will help clear up oily skin. Lemon grass citronella oil is a natural, effective mosquito repellent. To get the oil directly from the plant, break off a stalk and peel off the outer leaves until you find a scallion-like stem at the base. Bend and rub with your palms until it turns juicy. Then rub thoroughly over exposed skin. Planting these plants around the patio will help deter mosquitoes. Lemon grass is able to repel fleas and ticks in the same way. If you are walking your dog through deep grasses, lemon grass can be a quick help for both of you. As a detoxifying agent, lemon grass has a diuretic effect (causing more urination) which helps flush out the kidney, liver, pancreas, bladder and digestive tract. Loaded with beneficial minerals, which can lower blood pressure, maintain healthy nerve/muscle function and act as co-factors for enzymes with many diverse functions.

↑ **Vitamin and Mineral Content:**
Vitamins – B9 (Folate) and B2 (Riboflavin)
Minerals – Manganese, Iron, Potassium, Magnesium, Zinc, Copper and Phosphorus

⊘ **Disease Prevention:** Lemon grass in your diet can only help, but we need more research before we can say it helps prevent disease. Very high manganese gives enzymes all over the body their co-factor and maintains the biochemical balance necessary for health. Good source of iron to help prevent anemia. Lowering blood pressure takes some stress off the cardiovascular system and may help prevent heart problems.

❦ **How to Grow:** Popular in Asian cuisine, lemon grass grows easily and has many uses from adding to fresh dishes to drying out to brew tea. Grows best in tropical regions, but also grows outdoors in warmer, temperate regions with a healthy dose of compost/planting mix and full sun. Alternatively, you can grow in slightly cooler climates in pots. Bring them indoors during the cool months and keep them in a sunny location. To grow lemon grass, pick up the greenest, healthiest looking plant with bulbs and roots still attached, if possible. Trim off the top couple of inches, get rid of any dead-looking growth and set the stalks down into a container of room temperature water in a sunny location (window sill). After the roots have matured a bit, take the started plant out of the water and set it down in fertile soil with the crown just below the surface. If you live in a climate where it gets cooler in the winters, plant in pots and place in a sunny, warm location of the patio or house. Lemon grass cannot survive freezing temperatures, so be swift to bring them indoors when temperatures drop. In warmer areas, plant outdoors in full sun. Water regularly to keep the soil damp, not soggy. Outdoor plants can reach 4-6 feet high and 6-8 feet wide, so allow them room to spread.

✗ **Insect Control:** Few problems with pests; none that threaten the life of the plant. In companion planting, some gardeners repel melon flies by planting and trimming lemon grass near their crop.

✓ **Tips:** Buy more than one stalk at the market to use as a backup if one or more plants do not sprout roots during initiation.

ooooo

🙐 *LEMONS & LIMES* 🙐

✚ **Health Power:** A great source of vitamin C and other phytonutrients, similar to other popular fruits and veggies. Vitamin C is the great immune booster and anti-oxidant that knocks out free radicals at the top of the inflammatory cascade. Helps reduce symptoms of inflammatory conditions like rheumatoid arthritis. Acting against free radicals, vitamin C can assist in cardiovascular health by preventing the oxidation of cholesterol, a step toward plaque buildup. Lemons and limes both have flavonoid compounds that act as antioxidants, too. Both help sterilize some foods by killing off bacteria. Citrus fruits also contain limonoids that fight a number of cancers and potentially lower cholesterol.

↑ **Vitamin and Mineral Content:**
Vitamins – C
Minerals – Many but none of significant daily value

⊘ **Disease Prevention:** Immune system health and cell protection (possibly against cancer) come from antioxidant concentration of lemons and limes. The citrus limonoids defend against cancers of the mouth, skin, lung, breast, stomach and colon. The flavonoids may prove to protect against many common disease-causing bacteria.

🌱 **How to Grow:** Naturally subtropical, all citrus fruits need protection from frost. An exception, the Meyer lemon can handle brief temperatures below freezing in a protected spot. Pick a protected site with plenty of sun. Prefer soil on the heavy side. Amend the site generously with aged compost, manure or highly fertile planting mix. Soil pH should be 6-6.5. Raise beds 1.5 feet above ground. Plant trees any time of the year, especially in the South, but spring and fall are usually best times. Plant tree so that grafting point is a few inches above soil level. Space multiple trees 15-20 feet apart to avoid competition for nutrients or sunlight. Best way to feed is by applying organic fruit tree fertilizers, kelp meal, fish bone meal, alfalfa meal, organic composts or compost tea. Keep tree well watered, especially in first few years. If tree becomes thick and bushy, remove a branch for better airflow and light absorption. Prune shoots that point inward or have dead/diseased spots. Cut fruit off tree when ripe and use or store. To store, place fruit in a container and surround with dry sand or dirt to preserve for several months. Tree produces fruit all year in moderate climates.

✘ **Insect Control:** See Oranges, which have identical pests as lemons/limes.

✓ **Tips:** Once all fruit is removed from a shoot, trim it back to 5 inches to encourage more fruit-bearing shoots.

ooooo

✺ *LETTUCE* ✺

✚ **Health Power:** Loaded with good stuff: Vitamins K, A, C, folate and manganese. Romaine especially supports cardiovascular health. Vitamins A and C help prevent arterial plaque buildup by eliminating free radicals that oxidize cholesterol and help keep arterial walls elastic. Fiber helps regulate cholesterol levels and promotes healthy digestion. Romaine lettuce's potassium may help reduce blood pressure and promote the proper firing of muscle and nerve cells. Folate helps prevent damage to blood vessel walls by lowering homocysteine concentration in blood. Folate also is essential for proper nerve development in fetuses. A few ounces of romaine lettuce give more than 100 percent RDA of vitamin K, which helps in making thicker bones. To help avoid lethargy, B vitamins and manganese in romaine help the body extract energy from food.

↑ **Vitamin and Mineral Content:**
Vitamins – K, A, C, B9 (Folate), B1 (Thiamin), B2 (Riboflavin), B3 (Niacin), and B6 (Pyridoxine)
Minerals – Manganese, Chromium, Potassium, Molybdenum, Iron, Phosphorus and Calcium

⊘ **Disease Prevention:** Romaine lettuce may reduce the risk or symptoms of cardiovascular disease, rheumatoid and osteoarthritis and macular degeneration. Provides general defense from many common cancers via synergistic effect of vitamins, minerals and phytonutrients acting as antioxidants, detoxifiers and possibly direct inhibitors of cancer cell growth.

❦ **How to Grow:** Great veggie to have in the garden for summer harvest. May grow all year round in moderate climates. Many lettuce varieties. Some mature quickly or slowly, are tolerant to heat; others that grow back after you cut them. Lettuce prefers a cooler spot. Choose a site with part shade if your garden gets warm. Soil pH should be near 6.5. Amend soil modestly with well-aged compost or planting mix; too much fresh treatment leads to rotting. Sow seeds in trays indoors around 65°F. under fluorescent lights or in greenhouse in late winter. After seedlings develop, prepare for transplanting outdoors by cooling temperature down to 50°F. In early spring, transplant seedlings 6 inches apart in rows 6 inches apart, underneath cloches if temperature is too cold. At the same time, sow a larger, later variety outdoors underneath the cloche. Continue to sow a new row of seeds in open ground every couple of weeks for successive harvesting, with the last sowing in midsummer. Keep soil moist by watering as needed. When heads look full and feel firm, pull plants and cut their roots.

✗ **Insect Control:** Cutworms, aphids, millipedes, and slugs are common lettuce pests. Cutworms live beneath soil and feed on the base of plants. If a plant falls due to its base being eaten, hoe around (without damaging roots) to expose worms to birds. Put cutworm collars on transplants if you have problems. Regulate aphids by planting French marigolds to attract hover flies and ladybugs, their natural predators. Millipedes are little black insects that live below the soil and feed on roots. They hide and breed under rocks or loose/fallen plant matter during daytime. Best way to control is keep garden area clean. Check under rocks and other hiding spots during the day. For slugs, embed a cup of beer in soil. They crawl into it and drown.

✓ **Tips:** If roots look infected, burn or dispose to prevent later return.

ooooo

❧❦ *LICORICE* ❧❦

✚ **Health Power:** The phytonutrients in licorice have been used for centuries as a natural remedy for many common ailments. Prepare as a tea, make lozenges or simply chew on the root. Stores carry it as an extract, powder or loose leaves. Many use it to help aid digestive problems, like indigestion, heartburn and irregularity; has mild laxative properties. May help produce energy and increase stamina. Most popular use is to relieve chest congestion, coughs or sore throats. Glycoside stimulates production of thin mucus in membranes of stomach and respiratory tract and helps clear out lungs and throat. Useful as a soothing skin ointment. Has antimicrobial properties (including antiviral and antibacterial). Inhibits the hepatitis virus. Some women use licorice root as a dietary supplement to relieve premenstrual syndrome and symptoms of menopause. Research suggests this effect comes from preventing spikes in estrogen levels. May also help decrease mood swings and hot flashes. Not to be used during pregnancy, because it is linked to increased risk of premature labor. Side effects of prolonged use include water retention and lower potassium levels. Use caution and consult physician if you have high blood pressure or heart disease.

↑ Vitamin and Mineral Content:
Vitamins – A, B1 (Thiamin), B2 (Riboflavin), B5 (Niacin), B6 (Pyridoxine), Folate & E
Minerals – Calcium, Iron, Magnesium, Manganese, Phosphorus, Potassium and Sodium

⊘ Disease Prevention: May relieve symptoms of ulcers, eczema, psoriasis, hepatitis C, bronchitis, sore throat, bronchial asthma and acid reflux.

❧ How to Grow: Native to Southern Europe, licorice grows as a perennial legume developing into a thin shrub with pretty lilac pea flowers. Prefers full sun and tolerates different soil types. Takes 3-4 years for roots to mature for harvest. Simple to grow but requires initial preparation. Scratch the surface of each seed with sandpaper or a file and soak in water for 24 hours. Fill 4-inch pots with soil/planting mix. Pack down firmly. Place each mini pot in a tray that can hold an inch or more of water. Fill tray with water and let soil saturate. Poke ¼-inch holes 1 inch apart in the center of each pot and place licorice seeds down one per hole. Fill holes with ¼ inch of soil. Place tray with pots where they will get 8-10 hours of filtered light and temperature between 60-70°F. Keep seedlings soil moist but not sopping. Transplant outdoors in spring. Clear site of weeds and work planting mix/aged compost into soil to achieve high fertility, water retention and good drainage. Prefers pH close to 6. Dig holes same depth as 4-inch pots and a bit wider. Plant seedlings 2.5-3 feet apart. Remove seedling along with its soil by turning the pot upside down and sliding it out. Place down in their holes and fill the hole with well amended fertile soil. Water deeply during the first year, keeping soil moist. After first year, water only in dry weather. Roots ready to harvest 3-4 years after planting.

✗ Insect Control: No real pests threaten healthy maturation.

✓ Tips: To extract the essential oils, chop and clean the roots. Soak the roots (if dried) overnight to plump them up. Place them in food processor or blender with equal amounts of water. Grind them down so root pieces are the size of sand particles. Pour water and root mixture into pot, cover (to retain volatile portions of oil), and simmer on low heat for an hour or more. Turn heat off, let cool, strain the roots out, place liquid in lightproof container, cover and refrigerate.

∞∞∞

❀ *LOQUAT* ❀

✚ **Health Power:** A great fruit low in saturated fat and sodium while high in a few vitamins, minerals and fiber. Good to eat while trying to lose weight. Vitamin A, a protective antioxidant, promotes eyesight, especially night vision. Also helps maintain healthy teeth, immune system, and skeletal and soft tissue (skin and membranes around organs). Fiber adds bulk to a meal, giving a full feeling faster that may help control weight. Promotes smooth digestion and lowers elevated cholesterol and blood sugar. B vitamins are necessary to encourage the breakdown (catabolism) and buildup (anabolism) of compounds in foods and vital nutrients needed for healthy function, respectively. Vitamin B6 helps immune system produce antibodies and break down proteins. Vitamin B12 helps form red blood cells and, with potassium, helps maintain healthy nerve function. Potassium also reduces elevated blood pressure and helps maintain proper functioning of muscle cells. Manganese is an important cofactor for enzymes involved with many functions like disarming free radicals, forming bone/cartilage, metabolism and wound healing.

↑ **Vitamin and Mineral Content:**
Vitamins – A, B6 (Pyridoxine) and B12 (Cobalamins)
Minerals – Manganese and Potassium

⊘ **Disease Prevention:** Loquats may help defend against infectious diseases while helping lower risk or symptoms of diabetes, heart disease, osteoporosis and cancers of the lung, skin, breast, liver, colon and prostate.

❦ **How to Grow:** Comes from an evergreen tree native to subtropics. Find a healthy transplant at a trusted local nursery. Choose a site with full sun and enough space away from buildings or other trees. Grows to average 20-30 feet. Spring is fruiting season. If spring frosts are a concern, plant in warmest part of garden. Tolerates many soil consistencies. Main requirement is good drainage. Dig a hole three times deeper than the root structure and triple the diameter of the tree. Work in plenty of aged compost or planting mix to the soil dug out. Fill the hole a bit and place the tree so that the top of the root crown matches ground level. Fill hole and pack down a bit. If your area has a low water table or is prone to flooding, plant tree higher in a raised mound. After planting, lay down a thick layer of mulch over the root zone, taking care to leave about a foot between base of trunk and mulch layer.

Water thoroughly after planting. Water every other day for first 4 weeks, unless it's raining. After a few years of growth, water tree only during longer dry periods and during fruiting. Fertilize every few months the first year and every 4-6 months every subsequent year. During fruiting season, remove half the loquats when they are pea size to increase fruit size and quality. Throughout the first couple years, prune shoots after harvest by tipping them when they reach 2-3 feet long. Prune older trees to restrain their growth. When pruning, aim to increase sun exposure and airflow to all foliage while promoting strong, healthy fruiting. When effectively pruned, loquat trees can be maintained around 10 feet.

✘ **Insect Control:** Main pests are birds and bees. If both are present at full force during fruiting season, preserve the fruit by bagging each cluster. Also try setting out hanging traps for bees and growing other trees, such as mulberry, to attract birds.

✔ **Tips:** Don't plant grass near the base of trunk. Lawn mowing and weed eating can damage and even kill the tree. If planting in a windy, exposed area, stake the tree the first few years.

∞∞∞∞

❦ *MANGO* ❦

✚ **Health Power:** Mangoes are a great source of powerful antioxidants such as beta-carotene, vitamin C, quercetin and astragalin. They combine to neutralize free radicals, which can damage cells in the form of DNA mutations that lead to uncontrolled cell division, i.e. cancer. The antioxidants zeaxanthin and lutein help stop age-related macular degeneration in the eye. Vitamin C helps the immune system and assists in preventing cataracts. The soluble fiber, pectin, lowers cholesterol, promotes healthy digestion and cardiovascular function. Pectin also helps reduce the risk of gastrointestinal cancer. The high iron content helps women recover after menstruation and assists during pregnancy. High potassium helps maintain healthy nerve signal transmission and muscle contraction. Contain proteolytic enzymes that help break down proteins and work with fiber for healthy digestion.

↑ **Vitamin and Mineral Content:**
Vitamins – A, C, B9 (Folate), B6 (Pyridoxine), B2 (Riboflavin), B1 (Thiamin), E & K
Minerals – Copper, Iron, Potassium, Phosphorus, Calcium, Magnesium and Selenium

⊘ **Disease Prevention:** The high iron content in mangoes can help prevent or reduce the symptoms of anemia. Vitamin C reduces inflammation and pain in rheumatoid arthritis, osteoarthritis and asthma. Antioxidants with vitamin E and selenium help ward off many cancers and heart disease.

🌱 **How to Grow:** Easy to grow this delectable fruit from the tropics, but are very sensitive to cold. Below 40°F they go dormant and die below 32°F. In an area like Florida, where it only frosts a few times a year, deal with it by manually protecting with a plastic cover. To start growth, buy the healthiest mango you can find and eat it, being careful not to disturb the husk inside. Wash off the husk and let the seed dry out for several days. Gently split open the husk with a butter knife and remove the seed inside. If it is starting to grow a root, keep it attached. Fill a small pot (6-8 inches) with fertile soil and a little planting mix. Moisten the soil and make a small pocket in the center of the pot. Place the seed with the rounded side just above the surface and cover all but the very tip of the seed with soil. Don't water for a couple days. Place the seed in a sunny, warm location. Cover the pot with a slightly perforated plastic to increase humidity and temperature. A greenhouse is ideal. Keep soil moist and wait for the seed to sprout. In a warmer area, transplant the seedling with the ball of potting soil in a bed of well draining fertile soil in a warm, sunny, protected area. You can also transplant to a bigger pot if you need to keep it inside for warmth during cooler months. Fertilize a few times during the first year (except in winter) and keep soil moist but not soggy. While the tree is young, keep the area around the trunk weed free. It takes 3-7 years for the tree to bear fruit. Fruit is ripe and ready when it gives a little to a squeeze.

✕ **Insect Control:** White flies, aphids, spider mites, scales and thrips are the main mango pests. Hang a yellow card covered in sticky grease to attract and trap white flies. Plant French marigolds to attract aphid predators. Scales are disc shaped insects that hold themselves tightly to leaves, eat them and secrete honeydew that kills leaves. Watch for scales and scrape them off as soon as you see them. Thrips are too small to see, but their dark droppings are visible. Leaves appear wilted or bleached. Introduce predatory mites as a biological control. If infestation is large, spray with insecticidal soap.

✓ **Tips:** When the main shoot reaches 3-4 feet long, trim it to encourage more side shoots to form. Prune any branches that over crowd the tree for optimal sunlight and air circulation. Sometimes you can find a transplant that is already a year old and closer to fruit bearing.

ooooo

❧ *MARJORAM* ❧

✚ **Health Power:** See Oregano for vitamin, mineral and fiber health benefits. Main difference between marjoram and oregano is in their essential oils, although the effects of the oils overlap. The chemical compounds in marjoram essential oil are primarily pinene, sabinene, camphor, borneol and origanol. The oil has anti-bacterial/viral properties. It also helps ease pain, calms the mood, promotes sleep, aids digestion and lowers blood pressure. Some use it as a diuretic or expectorant. Used to treat migraines, headaches, arthritis, asthma, respiratory infections, depression, anxiety, insomnia, constipation and stress.

⬆ **Vitamin and Mineral Content:**
Vitamins – K, A and C
Minerals – Iron, Manganese and Calcium

⊘ **Disease Prevention:** See oregano for disease prevention. Essential oil may help reduce the symptoms or development of arthritis, asthma, insomnia and many bacterial, viral or fungal infections.

❦ **How to Grow:** Wild and pot marjoram are both hardy perennials. The more flavorful sweet marjoram grows only as a semi-hardy annual in colder regions. Prefers a site with full sun. Relatively tolerant of soil types. Grows best with moisture-retaining, well-drained soil. Work in generous amount of compost or planting mix before planting in spring. Get young transplants from a nursery. Plant about 1 foot apart. If growing sweet marjoram as an annual in temperate zone, sow seeds indoors in early spring, plant outdoors after the last frost, spacing 8 inches apart. Water regularly and keep weeds away to prevent nutrient competition. Pinch main shoots often to encourage dense, bushy growth. Fresh leaves are ready to harvest from early summer until gone or winter returns. Marjoram dries or freezes well for winter use. Grows well in pots, too. Grow entire crop this way or a few to bring in for winter to have fresh leaves all year.

✗ **Insect Control:** No common pests that threaten its life.

✓ **Tips:** Divide and replant perennials every three years. Herbs are excellent added to many dishes.

∞∞∞∞

🍈 *MELONS* 🍈
(CANTALOUPE & HONEYDEW)

✚ Health Power: Cantaloupe is rich in vitamins A, C and beta-carotene. (More than 100 percent of RDA in one cup.) Vitamin A and beta-carotene essential to maintain healthy vision. Vitamin C protects circulatory and immune systems from cell-damaging free radicals and stimulates white blood cells to fight infection. (Honeydew has much less of the vitamins but similar amounts of the others.) Also contains folate, important in producing and maintaining new cells, especially during pregnancy or when healing a severe wound. Cantaloupe helps with energy by controlling metabolism of carbohydrates.

↑ Vitamin and Mineral Content:
Vitamins – A, B1 (Thiamine), B2 (Riboflavin), B3 (Niacin), B9 (Folate), B5 (Pantothenic Acid), B6 (Pyridoxine), C, E and K
Minerals – Potassium, Phosphorus, Magnesium, Calcium, Sodium, Iron, Selenium, Manganese, Copper and Zinc

⊘ Disease Prevention: Helps reduce risk of cataracts, heart disease, stroke, many cancers and promotes overall health with broad base of vitamins and minerals. Vitamin A may help prevent emphysema in smokers and those exposed to second-hand smoke.

❦ How to Grow: First cultivated in southwestern Asia and the Nile Delta. Melons grow best in hot, dry areas. Night temperatures should not go below 55°F. Melons need 3-4 months of warm weather. Do not plant until the soil has reached 65-75°F. Require full sun, complete drainage and air circulation to prevent fungal diseases. Mix in some broken-down compost to provide nutrients and improve soil structure. Avoid water build up on the surface, since melons rest on the ground during growth. A sprinkling of fish bone meal helps. Best soil pH ranges from 6.5-7. In 2.5 to 3 months they yield ripe fruit. If growing in a cooler area, start in a heated greenhouse until it gets warm enough outside. Create a small soil hill and plant two transplants per hill. If sowing seeds outdoors, plant 6-8 seeds in a 12-inch circle on each hill. Space hills 5 to 10 feet apart, depending on projected size. Mulch after onset of summer to prevent water stress if you live in very hot, dry area. Keep soil watered regularly but keep surface relatively dry. Females have swelling below the petal tube. As flowers begin to show, notice if females are aborting. Means lack of pollinating bees. If so, pick the male flower and pollinate the stigma of the female.

✗ Insect Control: Canteloupe and honeydue susceptible to spider mites. (In some areas the cucumber beetle, too.) Seaweed spray several times during growing season helps maintain robust plant growth. If the infestation is severe, use rotenone.

✓ **Tips:** Very prone to mildew. Grow on mounds or raised beds to prevent water build up. Cantaloupe is ripe when easy to detach from the vine. Another hint to ripeness is sweet smell and softness on each end of fruit.

ooooo

🌺 *MINT* 🌺
(PEPPERMINT)

✚ **Health Power:** Many varieties of mint, all with similar health benefits. Peppermint adds little in vitamins and minerals, but phytonutrients give excellent remedies. Peppermint oil has phytonutrients that help relax smooth muscles (the muscles lining internal organs and blood vessels), which help control symptoms of dyspepsia or indigestion. Also inhibits growth of many common harmful bacteria and fungi. Research suggests the phytonutrient perillyl alcohol can stop the growth of many types of cancers. Peppermint contains phytonutrient rosmarinic acid, an antioxidant. It also blocks some chemicals of inflammatory response. Eaten in high quantities, mint is a rich source of all nutrients below and has other health benefits through antioxidant, anti-inflammatory, and anti-cancer actions. Promotes bone health and overall wellness.

↑ **Vitamin and Mineral Content:**
Vitamins – A, C and B9 (Folate)
Minerals – Manganese, Calcium, Iron and Magnesium

⊘ **Disease Prevention:** Peppermint may reduce symptoms or onset of asthma, arthritis, and cancers of the pancreas, colon, skin, lung and breast.

🌱 **How to Grow:** Many different cultivars. Among most popular are spearmint, peppermint, apple mint, lime, chocolate, lemon and grapefruit mint. Challenge with mint is not getting it to grow but keeping it from taking over entire garden. Can make a fragrant ground cover. Hardy perennial grows in almost any soil and site condition, but prefers partial shade, rich moist soil and slightly acidic pH. Choose site with enough space to allow mint to spread without invading other garden plants. Take root cuttings in early fall. To prevent rapid mint invasion, plant mint in a container (bucket or tub) with the rim just above soil level. This keeps roots from traversing under the soil and sprouting in undesired areas. Or control spreading by planting in containers. Allow at least 2 feet between other herbs or plants. Little maintenance needed. Water during dry weather. Harvest regularly to keep under control.

✘ **Insect Control:** No common pests threaten mint. Some diseases, so keep soil moist.

✓ **Tips:** To have continuous winter supply, freeze in cubes or store in a box with compost.

ooooo

✻ *MUSTARD* ✻

✚ **Health Power:** Mustard greens are loaded with vitamin K, which increases bone formation and decreases its breakdown (osteoclastic processes). Especially helpful for postmenopausal women. Magnesium also an important cofactor for many enzymes, some involved with bone and cartilage building. (Others keep smooth muscles relaxed, which helps asthmatics.) With some calcium, mustard greens are good for bones. Great source of vitamin A and a good source of vitamin C. Besides being a protective antioxidant, vitamin A helps maintain healthy eyesight in low light, embryonic development and immune system function by helping develop and activate red and white blood cells. Vitamin A also helps increase blood vessel dilation and decrease blood vessel spasms. Antioxidant vitamin C protects water-soluble areas from cellular damage by free radicals. Also important in synthesis of collagen (part of blood vessels), ligaments, tendons and bone formation. (May also promote healthy immune system function, but more research is needed.) Together, antioxidant vitamins A, C and E help blood vessels relax and prevent plaque buildup. Folate is involved with DNA synthesis and protein catabolism. Folate also regulates homocysteine in the blood. (At excess levels, homocysteine is linked to hardening of blood vessels, which leads to heart disease.) Folate is also essential to proper fetal development. Mustard greens have many phytonutrients (e.g. glucosinolates) that get converted to isothiocyanates. These are being researched for their ability to inhibit cancer cell growth and stimulate production of detoxifying enzymes in the liver.

↑ **Vitamin and Mineral Content:**
Vitamins – K, A, C, E, B9 (Folate), B6 (Pyridoxine), B2 (Riboflavin), B1 (Thiamin) and B3 (Niacin)
Minerals – Manganese, Calcium, Potassium, Copper, Phosphorus, Iron and Magnesium

⊘ **Disease Prevention:** Mustard greens may help avoid cardiovascular disease, stroke, osteoporosis, rheumatoid and osteoarthritis, asthma, cataracts and cancers of the mouth, throat, vocal cords, esophagus, skin, lung, breast, liver, stomach, colon and prostate.

☘ **How to Grow:** Easy to grow and great in salads and sandwiches or as a garnish. Can grow indoors in winter and/or outdoors in spring and fall. Grows best in cool weather with full sun. Outdoors, grows best in sunny site with moist, highly fertile soil. Indoors, it does well in shallow pans or trays. For a winter sowing, place a bit of moist soil into a tray. Scatter the seeds thickly on it. Cover the seeds with a piece of paper (newspaper, magazine page, printer paper). When seeds germinate, remove paper and set in direct sunlight. When they begin to grow, put them in fertile soil. If sowing outdoors, sow in a container the same way or in the corner of a bed. Sow every couple of weeks to get continual harvest. Greens are ready for harvest in 10-20 days. Cut and enjoy, but remember to sow another tray.

✗ **Insect Control:** Mustard is largely trouble free, especially indoors. If you have a persistent infestation, consult local nursery or agriculture extension office.

✓ **Tips:** Mustard is a cool weather crop. Flowers want to develop during long, warm, summer days. Remove and compost them when hot weather arrives before flower stalks appear.

oooo

❀ *NECTARINES* ❀

✚ **Health Power:** Nectarines have high content of carotenoids and flavonoids, including phytonutrients lutein and lycopene, both supporters of healthy vision, heart health and the fight against carcinogens. Vitamins C and A also support immune system response to unwanted bacteria, viruses and fungi. Vitamins E and A help protect skin from UV or free radical damage and helps maintain elasticity in the inner lining of blood vessels. Nectarines give a good dose of dietary fiber, which works to promote healthy digestion and nutrient absorption from food and drink. Fiber helps balance cholesterol levels and prevents buildup of bad cholesterol. Very low in total calorie content, fat free and great source of natural sugars.

↑ **Vitamin and Mineral Content:**
Vitamins – C, A, B3 (Niacin) and E
Minerals – Potassium, Copper, Phosphorus and Manganese

⊘ **Disease Prevention:** Phytonutrients in nectarines help reduce risks of atherosclerosis, heart disease, macular degeneration and many cancers.

☘ **How to Grow:** See Peaches for growing guidelines. Cousin to the peach, nectarines are often called "beardless peach." During a break on a warm summer day, not much beats biting into a cool, juicy nectarine. Trees take 2-3 years to produce delectable fruit. Can be grown as a bush tree, fan tree or standard. Prefers sunny site with well-drained soil not overly nutrient rich. Note: If flowering occurs before pollinating insects arrive, you may need to hand pollinate from one flower to the next. Use soft-bristled paintbrush or similar device.

✕ **Insect Control:** See Peaches.

✓ **Tips:** Needs great drainage to get nutrients and grow disease free. If soil is thicker, in addition to amending with organic matter, sprinkle a layer of broken-down bricks or sediment into the bottom of hole to help create space for draining.

∞∞∞

🎇 OKRA 🎇

✚ **Health Power:** Okra is a powerful source of both soluble and insoluble fiber. The soluble fiber, in the forms of gums and pectins, lowers total cholesterol, mainly LDL (the bad form). It also helps regulate digestion, which moderates spikes in blood sugar levels. Soluble fiber puts less stress on insulin producing cells and could help prevent Type II diabetes. Insoluble fibers in okra help maintain intestinal health. They bind to wastes (some of which are toxic or contain cholesterol), absorb water and keep things flowing smoothly in the intestines. They also delay absorption of glucose and promote colon health by balancing pH levels. Okra's high quality fiber helps feed beneficial bacteria in the intestines, contributing to more efficient breakdown of food and nutrient absorption. Okra's vitamin K contributes to blood clotting and strong, healthy bones. Also low in calories, which makes it ideal for eating healthy while losing weight.

↑ **Vitamin and Mineral Content:**
Vitamins – C, A, B1 (Thiamin), B2 (Riboflavin), B9 (Folate), and B3 (Niacin)
Minerals – Calcium, Magnesium, Potassium, Manganese, Iron, Phosphorus, Zinc and Copper

⊘ **Disease Prevention:** Okra may help suppress or prevent the symptoms or onset of colon cancer, heart disease, diabetes, ulcers, and mouth and lung cancers. Vitamin C in okra is an antioxidant that helps ward off potential carcinogens and blocks cholesterol buildup. It is also anti-inflammatory and works to help prevent cataracts, atherosclerosis, asthma and arthritic conditions. Vitamin A, an antioxidant with other flavanoids, wards off carcinogens. They help the eyes, too, aiding night vision and slowing macular degeneration.

❦ **How to Grow:** Okra is an annual originating in the tropics. Popular in the South for thickening gumbos or stews. It grows as an upright bush that produces hibiscus-like flowers followed by five-sided pods used for eating. Okra wants full sun in moisture retaining soil with good drainage. It grows best outdoors in warmer temperatures, but you can start indoors and transplant in warm weather. Sow the seeds when temperature reaches the mid-60's. Soak for 24 hours and plant in highly fertile soil amended well with compost or planting mix. Place seeds ½ to ¾ inches deep and 3 inches apart. Thin out later to 2 feet apart. Keep about 3 feet between each row. Mulch when it is 4 inches tall to prevent weeds and hold moisture. Water okra well during dry times. Reapply organic fertilizer every month. Pods will appear 50-60 days after planting. Harvest when they are young and soft, no bigger than finger size, as they harden during maturation.

✘ **Insect Control:** Pests not a big problem for very resilient okra. Stinkbugs, corn earworms, flea beetles, aphids, or cabbage loopers may be a nuisance. Pick off stinkbugs or worms when you see them. Remove aphids with a strong spray of water or introduce predators such as lady beetles, lacewings or midges. If they do not work, use garlic spray, insecticidal soap or rotenone. For flea beetles, introduce parasitic nematodes or spray with rotenone. If attacks are severe, use rotenone for all as a last resort.

✔ **Tips:** Harvest daily to stimulate more pod growth and discard the firm pods that were missed or did not get harvested on time. Cook okra over low heat to maintain nutritional value.

∞∞∞∞∞

❧ *OLIVES* ❧

✚ **Health Power:** Olives are a great source of the fat-soluble antioxidant vitamin E, which helps protect fat-based areas of the body. They also have monounsaturated fats, which resist oxidative damage by free radicals much better than polyunsaturated fats. Olives also contain proactive phytonutrients including polyphenols and flavonoids, both having antioxidant and anti-inflammatory roles. They help protect cells from free radical damage that could lead to heart disease or colon cancer. The anti-inflammatory properties may also reduce pain or recovery time for "red and sore" conditions. Olives have iron and dietary fiber, too. The iron helps hemoglobin in the blood bind oxygen in the lungs for delivery to all tissues. Fiber promotes smooth digestion, helps lower excess cholesterol and regulates blood sugar levels.

↑ Vitamin and Mineral Content:
Vitamins – E
Minerals – Iron and Copper

⊘ Disease Prevention: Olives may help reduce the risk of developing heart disease, colon cancer, asthma, osteoarthritis and rheumatoid arthritis.

❧ How to Grow: Olives grow best in areas with cool winters and warm to hot summers. They come in two main types, African and European. The African ones are inedible, but you can use them to give the yard visual appeal. European olives provide edible fruit about six years after planting but continue to bear for many years. They are also self-fertile, so one is enough for olive production. An olive tree grows as a standard tree and needs minimal pruning. For soil, they need only good drainage. For best growth, work organic matter (compost or planting mix) into the soil. They can grow, though, in lumpy or stony soil and can be good filler for an area that cannot support many other plants. Trees can be purchased container grown as transplants. Best time of year to plant is in the fall before moist weather. With more than one tree, space them about 30 feet apart. The one nutrient olives need in quantity is nitrogen, so mulch over the roots of the tree every spring with well-aged compost, manure or planting mix. If growth seems stunted, treat the soil to nutrient-dense fertilizer like compost tea, feather or kelp meal. Throughout growth, prune off branches that cause overcrowding and block sunlight from the inner foliage. Harvest olives by hand in fall when they are green. Or leave them on a bit longer into the winter until they turn black.

✗ Insect Control: Grown organically, olive trees do not usually have pest problems. Some pests stay away from olive trees because of the "chemical quality" of olive oil. Some general garden pests may cause issues. Watch for any infestations. Remove larger bugs by hand and destroy them. If uncertain about a pest, collect a few or take photographs and visit the nursery for help on identification and treatment.

✓ Tips: Green olives are great for pickling. Black olives can also be pressed for olive oil.

ooooo

🦋 ONIONS 🦋

✚ Health Power: Onions have a dense collection of phytonutrients that give many health benefits. These include powerful sulfur-containing molecules like allyl propyl disulfide and a multitude of flavonoids including quercetin. Eating onions can help increase efficient processing of free-floating glucose in the body. Allyl propyl raises free-floating insulin in the blood by preventing it from becoming inactivated in the liver. Chromium also decreases blood sugar by making cells more responsive to insulin, resulting in cellular glucose uptake. Onions are also heart healthy by reducing the amount of cholesterol and homocysteine in the blood, both linked to heart problems. Quercetin is an antioxidant that benefits the colon by protecting against carcinogens. Another onion compound blocks osteoclasts (cells that break down bone), which is beneficial for elders whose bone production has slowed. Vitamin C, quercetin and isothiocyanates reduce joint swelling.

↑ Vitamin and Mineral Content:
Vitamins: C, B6 (Pyridoxine) and B9 (Folate)
Minerals – Chromium, Manganese, Molybdenum, Potassium, Phosphorus and Copper

⊘ **Disease Prevention:** Allyl propyl and chromium act to reduce demand for insulin, which can stave off or help manage diabetes. By lowering cholesterol, homocysteine levels and blood pressure, the vitamins (especially folate) and minerals reduce the risk of atherosclerosis, heart disease, stroke and heart attack. Eating onions regularly has also been linked with lower risk for a number of cancers: esophageal, oral cavity, pharynx, colorectal, laryngeal, breast, prostate, ovarian and kidney. The anti-inflammatory properties help deal with rheumatoid arthritis, osteoarthritis and asthma.

❦ **How to Grow:** Onions are great to have in the kitchen. They are versatile, store well, come in many different flavors and cook easily. Choose a site full of sunshine. Work in plenty of organic matter in the form of aged compost, manure or planting mix. Best pH is roughly 6.5; add lime to raise if needed. To save space and a few dollars, sow multiple onion seeds together. They grow next to each other and push each other over slightly to make room as they enlarge. Sow 6-7 seeds together. If you want to start early, they germinate well indoors in trays on the windowsill or under a fluorescent light. Indoors, you need to gradually accustom them to being outside before transplanting. Otherwise, sow them similarly in shallow drills roughly 1 foot apart just after spring begins. Thin seedlings to a couple inches apart. Sow the Japanese varieties toward the end of summer in the same way. Fertilize this variety in the spring to encourage the rest of growth. With onions, you must keep beds weed free to minimize nutrient and sunlight competition. Water during dry weather but not overmuch. When tops turn brown, pull or dig up bulbs and let them dry in the sun for a couple days. If weather is unpredictable, put them in shelter to dry out. Once they are dry, remove their tops, and store them in a perforated sack or net in a well-ventilated, warm, shaded place to cure and avoid rot.

✕ Insect Control: Pests are not generally a problem with onions, especially the Allium species. Common pests include onion maggots, onion eelworm and onion flies. Attacking from early to mid-summer, the onion fly can be controlled by hoeing around each plant to expose the maggots to birds. Or put sand around the base of each plant to deter female egg laying. Alternatively, multiple sowing avoids the need to thin out the plants, which prevents releasing the attractive smell to female onion flies. Onion eelworms get inside the bulbs. The only way to get rid of them is to dig up the affected plants and replace for a couple years with something that is not a host (broccoli, lettuce, cabbage or another crucifer). If the risk of infestation is high in your location, interplant onions among other plants to give pests a smaller target to attack. A number of the Allium species ward off pests like aphids, beetles and carrot flies from other garden plants like carrots, lettuce and parsnips.

✓ Tips: For a continual harvest, grow a main crop variety and a Japanese crop that harvests first. To avoid sun burning while waiting for onions to dry on a hot day, cover one plant's bulb with another's shoots.

∞∞∞

🍊 *ORANGES & TANGERINES* 🍊

✚ Health Power: Besides high vitamin C, oranges contain flavanoids under the sub-category flavanones. The flavanone herperidin, in animal studies, has shown it can lower blood pressure, cholesterol and inflammation. This flavanone and others are found mostly in the peel and pulp of the orange rather than the juice. Thus, you can be less meticulous about removing all the peel before eating. Vitamin C is vital in protecting cells in the immune system and disarming aqueous free radicals that cause cell damage (potentially carcinogenic DNA mutations). Compounds known as limonoids remain active for extended periods. Along with folate, potassium, fiber and many phytonutrients, citrus fruits are antioxidant, anti-allergenic, anti-carcinogenic and anti-inflammatory. They also help lower blood pressure, promote proper digestion and prevent kidney stones.

↑ Vitamin and Mineral Content:
Vitamins – C, Folate, B1 (Thiamin) and A
Minerals – Potassium and Calcium

⊘ **Disease Prevention:** Oranges help reduce the potential for a multitude of cancers: lung, colon, esophageal, mouth, pharynx, larynx and stomach. Antioxidants in vitamin C reduce effects of inflammatory conditions like asthma, osteoarthritis and rheumatoid arthritis. Phytonutrients, vitamins and minerals help reduce the risk of ulcers and atherosclerosis.

❦ **How to Grow:** Oranges grow best in climates moderately warm year-round. Extended frost deforms or kills fruit. In cool climates, oranges must be grown in a greenhouse. Orange trees are bushy. Two types of oranges, sweet and sour. Sweet oranges are common for eating and comprise most of what is in the produce section of a grocery store. Best time for planting is spring or fall. They need as much sun as possible with as little wind as possible. This may require planting close to a fence corner, house corner or building a wind barrier. Soil should be slightly acidic; pH just above 6.0, and consist of a sandier loam with great drainage. Planting orange trees decreases soil drainage. If soil is denser, raise planting area by about 18 inches. Baby orange trees can be found at any nursery in a habitable climate. Before planting, amend the area with plenty of organic material. Plant the tree so the point at which branches converge is 4-5 inches off the ground. With multiple trees, space them about 25 feet apart to avoid nutrient competition or light deprivation. Throughout the first couple years, make sure roots get plenty of water. Be careful not to add too much chemical fertilizer, which can damage roots. Add a few fistfuls of planting mix heavy in fish bone, feather, kelp and other meals once in the spring and summer over the soil where roots are growing. During growth, if tree becomes too thick in certain areas, thin out by removing branches. Harvest when oranges have deep color. Twist off gently so as not to break off the fruit-bearing shoot. Fruits can hang ripened for up to six months. Immediately after harvesting, trim the same shoot (not branch) to roughly 5 inches to encourage more fruit-bearing shoots.

✗ **Insect Control:** Popular outdoor pests include gall wasps. Indoor pests are aphids, scale insects and/or red spider mite. Gall wasps lay their eggs into new shoot growth in spring. Once hatched, larvae embed themselves in shoots, causing unnatural looking swellings (galls) to show up. The only way to control these creatures is to cut out galls when they appear and destroy them. Aphids prefer dry weather. They can be warded off via biological controls such as introducing ladybugs or by growing a plant like marigolds to attract them. Insecticidal soap controls a large infestation. Red spider mites, like aphids, thrive in drier temperatures. Attacks can be prevented by frequently spraying with water. If they attack heavily, a controlled spraying of rotenone gets rid of them.

✓ **Tips:** Without fertilizer containing trace elements such as zinc, orange trees develop little leaf. This causes mottling of leaves and possibly deformed fruit. Avoid this by applying well-aged compost, manure or fertilizer with seaweed meal.

ᴓᴓᴓᴓ

✿ OREGANO ✿

✚ **Health Power:** Contains the potent volatile oils thymol and carvacrol, known to have antibacterial action stronger than some prescriptions. Thymol and rosmarinic acid are effective antioxidants, helping to eliminate cell-damaging free radicals. Oregano is also a great source of some minerals and vitamins, especially vitamin K. This often-overlooked vitamin may help promote heart health by helping to keep calcium from forming plaque in arteries. It also promotes bone health and blood clotting.

↑ **Vitamin and Mineral Content:**
Vitamins – K, A and C
Minerals – Manganese, Iron and Calcium

⊘ **Disease Prevention:** The high fiber in oregano makes it a good way to reduce cholesterol, defend against colon cancer and promote healthy digestion by absorbing good nutrients and eliminating toxins. Also, omega-3 fatty acids are polyunsaturated fats that also help create the healthier HDL form of cholesterol. It may help prevent high blood pressure associated with heart disease. Oregano's essential oil helps prevent many bacterial, viral and fungal infections. It also helps digestion and calms the nerves.

❧ **How to Grow:** Many species of oregano, some not suitable for cooking. Watch out for *O. vulgare*, which has a purple flower. It is tasteless and sometimes mistakenly sold for cooking. The most aromatic and common one for cooking is *O. heracleoticum* or, confusingly, *O. vulgare* subsp. *hirtum*. These produce white flowers rising a foot above the leaves. Oregano is a perennial that grows best with full sunlight in well-drained soil. The low-cost way is to start from seed or get healthy labeled transplants from a good local nursery. After the last frost, loosen the soil up with garden spade. If the soil is shallow or needs some amending to help drainage, create a raised bed by mixing in some fine gravel, grit or sand. Plant the transplants outdoors 14-18 inches apart. If starting from seed, plant these 6 inches apart about 1/2 inch deep. If planting more than one row, space them out 18 inches. When seeds sprout up, thin out the plants to one foot apart. Keep the soil moist for the first couple months. After that, it tolerates dry weather and only needs water when soil dries out. As the plant grows, trim back straying stems and pinch off flower buds to encourage optimal growth and desired shape. When the plant reaches 5-6 inches tall and/or has more than a dozen leaves, harvest as needed for cooking. When the season ends, cut the plants all the way down and mulch around them before winter to insulate roots from freezing temperatures. If you have too many leaves to use, dry them in a cool, dark place, chop up and store in an airtight container.

✘ Insect Control: Oregano deters some common garden pests and can be planted methodically to help protect other plants. Since we eat the leaves, if pests become a problem, avoid using chemical pesticides or sprays. Although unlikely, sometimes aphids or thirps will attack. If the problem is not serious, let the pests do a little damage rather than introduce chemicals. If needed, try an organic treatment such as insecticidal soap.

✓ Tips: Avoid using fertilizer to promote stronger flavor in the leaves. Oregano seeds can be sown in containers and transplanted 12 inches apart after the last frost or just left to grow spaced out in containers. When harvesting, cut the leaves off in the morning just after dew recedes. They have the most flavor and aroma before the sun causes oils to move into the shoots. Replace the plant after 2-4 years when it starts to become woody. Eat fresh oregano as much as possible to get all the beneficial oils. Oregano is a great source of omega-3 fatty acids.

∞∞∞

❀ *PARSLEY* ❀

✚ Health Power: In addition to great plate décor, parsley has excellent potential health benefits. It contains volatile oils such as limonene, myristicin and eugenol and beneficial flavonoids like apiin, apigenin and luteolin. The volatile oils act as anti-carcinogens (in animal studies) and may act similarly in humans. Myristicin activates an enzyme that attaches glutathione to highly reactive molecules (some are carcinogens) neutralizing them. The flavonoids have antioxidant properties and help neutralize oxygen-containing free radicals, preventing them from damaging cellular components (membranes, DNA, enzymes, etc.). Parsley is a great source of vitamins K, C and A. Vitamin K helps maintain a healthy bone matrix and may help prevent some cancers. Vitamin C is an antioxidant protecting cells from damage in water-soluble areas all over the body. Both vitamins C and A strengthen the immune system. Folic acid renders homocysteine in the blood harmless, protecting blood vessel walls from damage.

↑ **Vitamin and Mineral Content:**
Vitamins – K, C and A
Minerals – Iron and others in trace amounts

⊘ **Disease Prevention:** Reduces risk and helps stop cell growth in lung cancer. Research suggests vitamin K helps resist liver and prostate cancer. Eating foods rich in vitamins C and A, like parsley, lowers the risk of atherosclerosis, colon cancer, diabetes and asthma. Arthritis sufferers may also gain relief by the anti-inflammatory actions of vitamins C and A. Folic acid is important for proper cellular division in both the colon and cervix, reducing the risk of those cancers. Folic acid's effect on homocysteine helps prevent cardiovascular diseases.

❦ **How to Grow:** Whether used as a topping or worked into a sauce, parsley puts a finishing touch on dishes. There are two main types: flat and curly leafed. Flat leafed is the pungent Italian parsley. Curly leafed is used for cooking and garnishing plates. Both are biennials and grow about 14 inches. Plant out in the spring or start them indoors, which might be better, since the seeds take a month to germinate. In either case, soak them in warm water for a few hours or over night before planting. Space seeds out about 6 inches. They grow in well-enriched fertile soil in both pots and the ground. They prefer a bit of shade. For a harvest every year, plant new parsley every spring. They are frost hardy and come back to life the second year to flower if the winter is not too harsh. If you cut off the flower stalks, they will not die in the second year. Conversely, if they flower and go to seed, they can sow themselves and need little effort to reproduce. Those able to sow themselves are healthier and taste better. Harvest the leaves as needed from the outer leaves in. Taking inner leaves first prematurely sends the parsley to seed.

✗ **Insect Control:** Generally, no pest problems with parsley. Herbs attract pollinating insects, like bees, for other plants and beneficial predatory insects to control other pests.

✓ **Tips:** Parsley does not keep long. Either freeze it or dry it in an oven to preserve for later use. If you want to grow it during winter, sow seeds in a pot during midsummer and bring them in just before the weather cools down. To save seeds, harvest the stems as the seeds ripen and hang them upside down over a cloth in a ventilated shed.

ooooo

✿ *PARSNIPS* ✿

✚ Health Power: Benefits are similar to potatoes. The main difference: parsnips have more fiber and folate but less vitamin C per weight. (Still a great source, with half the RDA of C in one parsnip.) With more dietary fiber, parsnips better support digestion. They help everything flow smoothly, get rid of excess cholesterol and regulate blood sugar. Folate is known to lower homocysteine in the blood, preventing plaque buildup that harms blood vessel structure. Pregnant women need folate to promote healthy fetal nerve development. Also a good source of vitamin K, which helps develop a dense bone matrix. Parsnips have some B vitamins that help boost fat, protein and carbohydrate metabolism to provide energy.

↑ Vitamin and Mineral Content:
Vitamins – C, K, B9 (Folate), E, B1 (Thiamin), B5 (Pantothenic Acid) and B6 (Pyridoxine)
Minerals – Manganese, Potassium, Magnesium, Phosphorus and Copper

⊘ Disease Prevention: Vitamin B6 and folate help reduce homocysteine levels, helping to prevent heart attacks and strokes. Vitamin B6 also fights cancer by attaching signals to molecules that lead to turning on tumor suppressive genes. This type of signaling, methylation, also signals to destroy toxic, potentially carcinogenic, chemicals. The fiber in parsnips helps prevent colon cancer and the onset of diabetes. The fiber may also reduce the risk or onset of heart disease, stroke and heart attack.

❧ How to Grow: Parsnips grow in many different soil types. For best results, choose a sunny, sheltered site with deep soil. The pH should be around 6.5; add lime to raise, if needed. In cooler climates, sow seeds as soon as the soil starts to warm and is workable (early to mid-spring). In warmer climates that do not freeze, sow seeds in the fall. Loosen the soil to 2 feet down. Remove any large solid chunks like rocks. Amend the soil with a few inches of compost or equivalent planting mix. Soak seeds in warm water for several hours to promote germination. Create shallow drills 1 foot apart and sow seeds 1 inch deep 6 inches apart. Do not let soil dry out while waiting for germination. Mulch lightly around the base of the plants once they are a few inches tall. Hoe to keep rows weed free, making sure not to damage roots. Water deeply once a week to supply the whole root and avoid rot from sitting water. If soil dries out, water again to keep it moist and prevent cracking of roots. Parsnips take 3-4 months to mature. They are usually ready in late fall to early winter. Use a garden fork to loosen soil around plants before pulling. Lift roots after first frost. Enjoy or store for winter use.

✗ **Insect Control:** Common pests for parsnips are carrot root flies. They are also susceptible to canker. The larva of the female fly burrows into the root, leaving tunnels and brown marks. To prevent females from laying eggs at root base, put a plastic barrier around parsnips, carrots or celery supported by posts. This keeps females from approaching the base of the plant. Parsnips have canker if they show red-brown marks on the top of the roots, which leads to rot. To prevent, do not over water or over fertilize. Use balanced practices to develop a healthy plant. Also, look for resistant cultivars.

✓ **Tips:** To store parsnips, gently place undamaged ones in a container and fill in gaps with moist peat, sawdust or sand. Put the container in a cool, frost-free area.

∞∞∞∞

❧ PEACHES ❧

✚ **Health Power:** Peaches are an excellent source of vitamins A and C. Vitamin A is an antioxidant that stabilizes free radicals associated with cancer and other diseases. It also aids proper vision in low light. Vitamin C is famous for its many benefits: healing cuts and abrasions, building connective tissue for muscles and bones, protecting immune system, preventing bruising and helping build new red blood cells. Peaches also contain other vitamins and minerals, including fiber, that aid in proper digestion and help enhance skin color.

↑ **Vitamin and Mineral Content:**
Vitamins – A, B1 (Thiamin), B2 (Riboflavin), B6 (Pyridoxine), C, B3 (Niacin), B9 (Folate), B5 (Pantothenic Acid), C, E and K
Minerals – Potassium, Phosphorus, Magnesium, Calcium, Iron, Selenium, Manganese, Copper and Zinc

⊘ **Disease Prevention:** The anti-oxidant glutathione, with vitamins A and C, correlates with preventing cancer cell development. Eating peaches reduces the risk of heart and cardiovascular disease.

❧ **How to Grow:** A gorgeous addition to the backyard, peaches work miracles in summer. They grow throughout the U.S. but do best in warm summers. They thrive in healthy, well-drained soil. Pick a transplant from your nursery and put it in a fairly sunny spot. Amend the soil with plenty of compost or organic planting mix. Plant the tree deep. The first few years set the stage for the tree's shape and size. Stake the tree after it grows taller than a foot to help it grow straight up. In spring, when growth buds appear, cut the central growth down to two feet above the ground right above the bud. Remove all the lower shoots except for the top 3-4. Later, remove any shoots under those top 3-4 branches. Before fruit bearing age, mulch widely around the trunk with compost or organic planting mix twice a year, once in March and again in May. After that, one application a year is good unless you see signs of deficiency. Keep soil moist. Water thoroughly if the soil might dry out. If soil stays too dry too long, fruiting suffers. When peaches are about cherry size, remove some, leaving 1-3 peaches per stem. If clusters form on branches, remove all but one to avoid stunting growth. When they are the size of golf balls, check the branches again and remove enough to ensure branches withstand the weight. They are ready to pick when skin softens to the touch.

✘ **Insect Control:** The most serious pests are peach tree borers. Aphids and spider mites are also common. Borers enter on the lower trunk and leave sticky sawdust around their entry. Prevent by keeping the lower trunk uncovered. Kill them by sticking something in the hole such as the end of a wire coat hanger. Or cut out damaged areas until you see healthy wood. Treat with a 1:1 mix of lime-sulfur and latex paint. Aphids are a common garden pest. Control aphids by companion planting marigolds to attract their predators (hover flies or ladybugs). You can also wipe or spray off with a strong stream of water. If infestation is too great, spray an organic insecticidal soap. Red spider mites are barely visible, but their webs are easy to see. They succeed in dry conditions, so keep plant regularly sprayed with water. For a bad infestation, spray with an organic pesticide like rotenone.

✓ **Tips:** The more peaches on a tree, the smaller they are. After a few growing seasons, you can determine the size that yields the best fruit to your taste. Quickly remove any shoots emerging from the roots. Also, completely remove any infested peaches or branches damaged during the previous year. This restores vigor to branches and fruit growing. Many vitamins are in the skin, so eat peaches whole.

ooooo

❦ *PEARS* ❦

✚ **Health Power:** Pears give a solid defense against damaging free radicals and are a great source of dietary fiber. Vitamin C and copper help keep highly reactive free radicals from causing oxidative damage to cells all over the body. Vitamin C is water-soluble and defends almost the entire body except areas of fat. It stops free radicals from oxidizing cholesterol into a sticky form that leads to plaque buildup in blood vessels. It also protects white blood cells while they fight off infection and reactivates antioxidant vitamin E. Because vitamin E is fat soluble, by activating it vitamin C helps disarm free radicals in both water-soluble areas and fat-soluble areas. Dietary fiber in pears acts to reduce cholesterol, regulate blood sugar levels and support good digestion.

↑ **Vitamin and Mineral Content:**
Vitamins – C and K
Minerals – Copper and Potassium

⊘ **Disease Prevention:** Reduced risk of colon cancer, postmenopausal breast cancer, heart disease and macular degeneration.

❦ **How to Grow:** Make sure your pear tree suits your climate. They flower early. If frosts extend well into spring, choose a late-flowering variety. Except for flowering, they are winter hardy. Most cultivars need cross pollination to fruit properly. Plant at least two trees that flower at the same time to get fruit to set. Tree height depends on the cultivar you choose. You can find self-pollinating dwarf trees with three cultivars grafted to one rootstock. This is a good option if space is limited. Best time to plant is early spring. Choose a sunny, sheltered spot with deeper soil. Prepare the soil by amending all around planting area with well-aged compost or planting mix rich in organic matter. Be careful not to over fertilize with nitrogen. This may stimulate too much new growth vulnerable to the deadly fire blight disease. Test the soil to be sure pH is 6-6.5. If not, nutrient deficiencies can cause deformities. Dig a hole wide enough and deep enough to set the bare rooted tree so the existing soil line on the trunk matches up with ground level and roots are unobstructed. A small mound of soil in the center of the hole may help support the tree. Fill the hole with the amended soil and pack it down lightly. Mulch around stem with a thick layer of well-aged manure or compost to ensure nutrient availability. Keep the soil moist by thorough watering. No need to water every day, but make sure to water long enough to reach the root level. (Watering just the surface encourages roots to grow upward.) You can thin out clusters or leave them alone, depending on how big you want fruits to be. If you want large fruit, thin the center fruit in each cluster near mid-summer. With several clusters on a branch, the weight can make a branch break or severely warp. Avoid this by thinning clusters on these branches to one fruit per cluster. Prune thick branches that block sunlight from reaching the foliage. Each spring, spread a thin layer of organic fertilizer and mulch over the roots. Pears take 2 or more years to bear fruit. Harvest fruit when it easily detaches with a slight tug. Store in cool temperatures. Bring up to room temperature before eating to soften and sweeten them up.

✗ **Insect Control:** Pear tree pests are aphids, wooly aphids, winter moth, coddling moth, sawfly and wasps. Fire blight is the most common disease. Remove aphids with a strong water stream. Also, draw their predators (hoverflies and ladybugs) by planting French marigolds nearby. Wooly aphids are more difficult to remove.

They form colonies on branches and cover themselves with a white waxy substance. Scrape off as soon as you see them. Or spray with rotenone after petals fall. If that does not work, cut them out. You can stop female winter moth caterpillars from breeding on the lower trunk by securing a sticky ring around the tree to catch them as they crawl up to lay eggs. Coddling moths lay eggs that hatch into fruit maggots. Deter them with a pheromone trap hung from a branch. (Find at your local nursery.) Sawfly quickly eat leaves off. Spray with an insecticide when you see caterpillars on leaves. If wasps are a problem, make a trap by putting sweet liquid in a container covered with a thin layer that has a hole in it. Hang this from the tree. Wasps will enter the container and be trapped. For fire blight, find out if your area is susceptible and buy a resistant cultivar. Otherwise, don't prune too much as new soft growth is most susceptible.

✓ **Tips:** When fruit stops growing and starts changing color, stop watering to keep the tree free of diseases. Pear trees grow tall but can be easier to harvest if shaped correctly.

∞∞∞

✿ *PEAS* ✿

✚ **Health Power:** Green peas promote overall health with seven vitamins, eight minerals and other phytonutrients. Vitamin K, crucial for bone health, is most abundant in peas. Some of it converts to vitamin K2 and is part of bone mineralization. Deficiency in K2 hinders mineralization and makes osteoporosis more likely. Incompletely researched, folate and vitamin B6 may contribute to bone health by blocking the buildup of homocysteine, a molecule that interrupts proper bone matrix formation. Vitamin K and folate also help the cardiovascular system. Vitamin K is essential for blood clotting, while folate and vitamin B6 lower homocysteine, which may reduce damage to arterial walls and reduce the risk of cardiovascular disease. Green peas also contain B vitamins that help break down carbohydrates, fats and proteins for energy. Iron is crucial for blood cell formation and oxygen delivery to muscles. Vitamins C and A protect many types of cells in the eye, liver, immune system, adrenal glands, connective tissue and the circulatory system.

↑ **Vitamin and Mineral Content:**
Vitamins – K, C, B1 (Thiamin), B9 (Folate), A, B6 (Pyridoxine), B3 (Niacin) and B2 (Riboflavin)
Minerals – Manganese, Phosphorus, Magnesium, Copper, Iron, Zinc and Potassium

⊘ **Disease Prevention:** Green peas are linked with reducing cell damage that causes osteoporosis, lymphoma, leukemia, and cancers of the lung, colon, cervix, breast, prostate and ovary. Eating green peas regularly with other nutrient-rich fruits and veggies promotes overall health and helps prevent many adverse health conditions.

❦ **How to Grow:** Peas are one of the oldest cultivated vegetables. Eating them fresh, right after picking, makes a big difference in flavor. Peas do not need much done to the soil for healthy growth. They produce their own nitrogen and need very little fertilizer. Peas are frost hardy, but do not deal well with heat. They slow down when temperatures go above 70°F and stop growing above 75°F. Early varieties will do well in sandier loam that warms up quickly. Later varieties may benefit from heavier soil to keep them cool. Pick a sunny spot for early varieties and part shade for later varieties. Make sure soil is well drained. Sow seeds outdoors in early spring and also in fall for mild climates. Make successive sowings to get a continuous yield. Seeds should be planted in drills 2 inches deep and roughly 2 inches apart. If planting a vine type, plant in double rows spaced 6-8 inches apart with roughly 3 feet between each double row. Support each plant with a stick roughly 4-5 feet long. Keep soil moist, but make sure not to over water. Harvest (2-3 weeks after blossoming) as close to cooking as possible.

✗ **Insect Control:** Common pea pests are birds, pea moths, mice, pea and bean weevils and aphids. To deter birds, install netting around the crop. (If you don't mind, sacrifice a little bit of the yield.) Pea moths lay larvae (maggots) on plants during flowering. If attack is severe, dust with rotenone. Use this as a last resort, as rotenone kills beneficial insects. See your local nursery for pheromone traps. Mice are not usually a big problem, but cats are great to have around if they are. Pea and bean weevils are not a problem unless they attack seedlings. Dust sparingly with rotenone. Spray aphids with strong stream of water or plant marigolds to attract ladybugs.

✓ **Tips:** Mulching between rows with well-aged compost or manure helps hold moisture, deter weeds and nourish the plant, especially if soil is depleted. Pea vines are very sensitive, so handpick weeds if needed.

∞∞∞

⚜ *PEPPERS* ⚜

✚ **Health Power:** All peppers are a great source of vitamins A and C, which eliminate cell-damaging free radicals. Vitamin A also counters the effects of cigarette smoke, which may help prevent lung conditions such as emphysema. Bell peppers have the B vitamins folate and pyridoxine. Both decrease homocysteine in the blood, blocking the start of a process linked with higher cholesterol and risk of heart attack or stroke. Fiber in bell peppers helps maintain healthy heart function by lowering harmful cholesterol. Bell peppers also have a carotenoid lycopene and beta-cryptoxanthin, all linked to lower risk of many cancers when eaten regularly.

↑ **Vitamin and Mineral Content:**
Vitamins – C, A, B6 (Pyridoxine), K, B9 (Folate), B1 (Thiamin) and E
Minerals – Molybdenum, Manganese, Potassium and Copper

⊘ **Disease Prevention:** The antioxidant properties of vitamins C and A suppress or prevent the symptoms of atherosclerosis, heart disease, vascular damage, both osteoarthritis and rheumatoid arthritis, emphysema, macular degeneration and the airway swelling of asthma. Regularly eating bell peppers may reduce the risk of cancers of the bladder, prostate, pancreas, lung and cervix.

❦ **How to Grow:** Peppers are easier to grow than eggplant in cooler climates, but are not frost hardy and do best in warmer areas. They have two main subdivisions, sweet (bell) and spicy (chili). Hundreds of varieties to choose from. The best for your area depends on climate and soil conditions. All peppers prefer warmer climates with lengthy summers. Some are specially bred to handle cooler climates with a cover. Choose a spot with full sunlight. The soil pH needs to be just above 6. In cooler areas, warm up the soil a couple of weeks before sowing by covering the plot with plastic. If starting from seed, sow in a greenhouse or under a fluorescent light. Get them ready for planting outside by gradually exposing them to outside air, starting with just daytime, until they are fully exposed day and night. You need a cold frame to do this, which is a shallow box outdoors with an air-tight framed glass/plastic lid that can be lifted up to expose plants. Or you can get acclimatized transplants from a trusted local nursery. Amend the soil with nutrient-rich planting mix, aged compost or manure. In warm climates with no late spring frosts, plant outdoors 2 feet apart. In cooler climates, cover plants with a frost-proof perforated plastic, called a cloche. Pinch the growing end when the plants reach roughly 6 inches and attach them to a skinny rod for support. Tie side shoots for when they grow out to help support the weight of peppers. Water as regularly as it takes to keep the soil moist as they grow. Apply a liquid fertilizer rich in micronutrients every other week. Harvest the peppers after they plump up. Red and green peppers are of the same variety. You can pick them when they are green or wait a little for them to turn red. With others, harvest when plump and hold a nice deep color. Hot peppers can be refrigerated, frozen or dried in the sun to store for winter usage.

✘ **Insect Control:** Most damaging are aphids, spider mites, slugs and the white fly. See Artichokes for slug and aphid control. See Strawberries for red spider mite control. The white fly sucks the sap off many plants. Like other flies, they are attracted to the color yellow. To get rid of them, hang a thick piece of yellow paper or plastic with a thin coating of grease, or use old-style flypaper. Make sure to prevent it from attaching to the plants.

✓ **Tips:** If you are de-seeding many hot peppers to save seeds or to cook, protect your hands with gloves and make sure not to touch your eyes until after thorough washing. Capsaicin is the powerful molecule that causes the burning sensation of pepper. It is insoluble in water and stays bound to the tongue no matter how much water is used to wash it down. Milk and cheese can break capsaicin's bond with tongue receptors if it gets too hot. These varieties will grow in cooler climates: Bell (sweet) pepper: Corona, Canape, Golden Summit, Sweet Banana, Yolo Wonder, Perma Green and Merrimack Wonder. Chile (hot) pepper: Hungarian Wax (hot banana peppers) and Czechoslovakian Black. For warmer climates: Bell (sweet) peppers: Cubanelle, Pimento, Aconcagua and World Beater. Chile (hot) pepper: Cayenne, Anaheim, Jalapeno, Pablano, Serrano, Black Cuban, Holiday Cheer and the very hot Chiltepin.

∞∞∞∞

🌸 *PERSIMMONS* 🌸

✚ **Health Power:** Persimmons are an excellent source of vitamins A and C, dietary fiber and manganese. Vitamins A and C help strengthen the immune system, maintain healthy vision and defend the body against harmful free radicals. Some notable antioxidant properties help reduce inflammation, prevent plaque buildup in blood vessels and maintain the elasticity of the inner lining of organs that have epithelial cells. Their excellent fiber promotes digestive efficiency and helps prevent the buildup of bad (LDL) cholesterol. They are also noted for their tannins, proanthocyanidins and other phytonutrients including beta-carotene, lycopene, lutein, zeaxanthin, cryptoxanthin, catechins, gallocatechins, betulinic acid and shibuol. All act as protective antioxidants throughout the body. Shibuol is a double-edged sword, however, because it can cause globs to form in the digestive tract. For this reason, wait for persimmons to ripen, and do not eat astringent varieties on an empty stomach. The tannin concentration of shibuol is very low in soft, ripened persimmons. Eating them with food in the stomach mixes them in, and they react less with stomach acids. Proanthocyanidins in the skin are linked to helping metabolic processes within cells, preventing unnecessary blood clots from forming, protecting blood vessel cells from hardening and lowering blood pressure. The nutrient content and value of a persimmon depends on which cultivar you choose and how healthy it develops. For its high antioxidant content, this is a promising fruit for overall health.

↑ Vitamin and Mineral Content:
Vitamins - A, C, B6 (Pyridoxine) and E
Minerals - Manganese

⊘ Disease Prevention: In addition to protective vitamins, the phytonutrients work in slightly separate ways, which may contribute to an overall lower risk for many cancers, macular degeneration, hypertension, cardiovascular disease and diabetes. Also, cigarette smoke can deplete the body of vitamin A. Persimmons are a great source of vitamin A and may help prevent or forestall emphysema.

❦ How to Grow: American persimmon trees, growing about 40 feet high, produce smaller fruits than Asian varieties and can tolerate brief periods of temperatures down to –20°F. Asian persimmons grow larger fruit on shorter trees (about 30 feet high) but can tolerate temperatures only down to 0°F. Get a cultivar from a trusted local nursery that can guide you on a particular variety suited for your area. They are self-fertile, but bear more fruit if you grow more than one tree. Both varieties prefer a lot of sun. Early spring is great for planting. Before planting, prepare the soil by digging a big hole and amending the dug up soil as well as some of the surrounding soil with fertile organic matter, such as compost or planting mix. Adding compost tea or manure tea is smart when planting fruit trees. Plant bare root trees in a hole big enough so that the roots are free and the soil line on the trunk matches the ground level. Fill in the hole with the amended soil and pack down. The compost mulch provides plenty of nutrients for healthy growth. A small application of fertilizer once a year helps. Give Asian persimmons a little shelter by planting near a house or other trees. You may need to stake in a windy area. Space them about 20 feet apart if you plan to grow more than one. Persimmons need little pruning. If you want to control the size, prune every spring before buds form. Since persimmons produce fruit on new wood, pruning back old wood encourages new growth and leads to more fruit. When trimming, train the tree to grow around a central leading shoot that grows roughly straight up. Trim down desired shoots to the outward growing branch they grew from. Persimmons usually ripen for harvest in early to mid-autumn. Clip off the fruit when it's still firm. Let the astringent varieties soften fully before eating.

✗ Insect Control: Persimmons are pest free and tolerant in the home garden. Check with the nursery to see if your area has pests to watch for. Sometimes citrus mealy bug, borers, Psylla and scale can be a problem. Growing a tree in healthy, highly fertile soil is the best way to defend against most pests and diseases. Psylla are invisible to the eye but excrete a visible honeydew that enables a black mold to grow on the foliage. If you notice these symptoms and find the insects on inspection with a lens, or if the leaves at the top of the tree begin to turn black, spray with an insecticidal soap that has rotenone or other recommended treatment. Mealy bugs look like little white furs and live underneath leaves or stems. If noticed, spray with an insecticidal soap. Borers will enter into the lower trunk or injured limbs. If you see gooey sawdust next to a small hole, probe up into the hole to kill the borer. If the hole is on the lower trunk, close it off with paraffin or putty. If on an injured limb, remove the limb and seal off with the same material. If scale appears, spray with a copper fungicide and dispose of the leaves after they fall.

✓ **Tips:** Persimmons produce many root suckers. Remove them on sight. Mulching over the root area helps deter them. Never eat unripe, astringent persimmons. They have chemicals inside that can lead to stones and intestinal disruption. Also, choose a young persimmon tree with a relatively small taproot, which transplants better. Ask the nursery about the persimmon's astringency.

∞∞∞

❦ *PISTACHIO NUT* ❦

✚ **Health Power:** Pistachios are packed with great overall nutrition including phytosterols, polyphenols, other antioxidants (some carotenoids), vitamins, minerals and fiber. They are one of the best nuts to get all of these nutrients, especially since they are low-fat. What they do have is "good fat," the unsaturated fats (mono- and polyunsaturated). The nutrients in pistachios make them a heart-smart snack. They are rich in the amino acid arginine, which in moderate concentrations can help relax blood vessels. The vitamins B6, B12 and folate reduce elevated levels of homocysteine, known to damage blood vessels when too high. The nut's potassium helps bring down high blood pressure and maintain proper muscle and nerve function (especially valuable for the heart). The antioxidants protect water-soluble and fat-soluble areas of the body, especially in preventing the oxidation of cholesterol. When oxidized, cholesterol becomes "sticky" and more easily adheres to artery walls, leading to plaque buildup. Antioxidants also protect against oxidative damage to DNA. Since DNA is used continuously to create new proteins, we need to protect it against "corruption" leading to mutation and loss of proper function. Fiber provides many key benefits. It promotes smooth digestion, helps expel potentially toxic substances faster and regulates blood sugar and cholesterol levels. Fiber also gives a quick, long-lasting satisfied feeling that leads to eating less often. Pistachios are a rich source of phytosterols, known to decrease the absorption of cholesterol by 30-40 percent and lower serum cholesterol in the blood.

Pistachios may promote visual health from their high carotenoid content. They are also a great source of minerals that serve as cofactors for activating enzymes.

↑ Vitamin and Mineral Content:
Vitamins – B6 (Pyridoxine), B1 (Thiamin), K, B9 (Folate), E, B2 (Riboflavin), B3 (Niacin) and B5 (Pantothenic Acid)
Minerals – Copper, Manganese, Phosphorus, Magnesium, Potassium and Iron

⊘ Disease Prevention: Eating pistachios regularly may help reduce the symptoms and risk of atherosclerosis, cardiovascular disease, macular degeneration, constipation, diabetes, colon cancer and possibly many other cancers.

❦ How to Grow: Pistachios love a dry warm climate like that by the Mediterranean Sea. They grow to 20-25 feet. In nature, pistachio trees have the male and female flower on separate trees, but for home gardens, nurseries have grafted female trees with male branches such that only one tree is necessary to produce nuts. If planting more than one tree, space them 20 feet or more apart. Pistachio trees take a number of years before they begin to bear heavily. After the fifth year, they bear a little. It takes another 10 years to reach full maturity and full productivity. Time to plant is in the spring. Buy a grafted cultivar adapted to your area from a local nursery. In general, they grow best in areas with cool winters and long, hot summers. They are thoroughly drought resistant. Pistachios need a site with full sun and deep soil with excellent drainage. Work in a modest amount of all-around planting mix rich in organic matter and nutrients. Taking care not to disturb the grafting point, dig a wide hole and set the tree down inside so that when filled in the soil will just cover the root crown. Water deeply more frequently when they are young. Once established, water only occasionally. The fruits are a dark red color and grow in clusters like grapes on the branches. During harvest time, the fruit husk surrounding the shell will loosen and release the nuts. Lay a sheet underneath the tree to catch them as they fall.

✗ Insect Control: Pistachios are safe from pests. Consult with a nursery, and pick a cultivar that resists common infections in your area.

✓ Tips: You may have to shake the tree to release the ripe nuts. Let them to dry for 1-2 days. They store well for months in a sealed container in a dark, cool spot.

∞∞∞∞

❦ PLUMS ❦

✚ **Health Power:** Plums are known for a unique group of phytonutrient phenols called neochlorogenic and chlorogenic acid. These phenols help prevent oxidative damage to fats all over the body. They also disarm the free radical superoxide, which is highly reactive and can cause major damage to cells all over the body. Plums increase the absorption of iron, the mineral needed to form hemoglobin, which transports oxygen to every cell. Plums offer a nice dose of dietary fiber to promote healthy digestion. They are also a good source of vitamins A and B2, which contribute to vision, blood vessel health and metabolism of lipids, carbohydrates and sugars for energy.

↑ **Vitamin and Mineral Content:**
Vitamins – C, A, B2 (Riboflavin)
Minerals – Potassium and others in trace amounts

⊘ **Disease Prevention:** Eating fruits and vegetables high in vitamins C and A has been linked to lower risk of atherosclerosis, heart disease, stroke, asthma, colon cancer, osteoarthritis and rheumatoid arthritis.

❦ **How to Grow:** Plums come in many different sizes, shapes, colors and flavors. There's a type right for everyone. Some trees grow nearly 20 feet tall. You can also find dwarfs growing as small as 6 feet. You can let them be, with minimal pruning, or train them to grow as fans or pyramids. You can decide on the tree shape, how much fruit to harvest and how much area to devote to it. Plums like deep, heavier loam soils that have good drainage and a pH near 6.5. Plant plum trees in spring. Dig a deep hole and amend the soil with plenty of organic matter (compost, planting mix or a combination of nutrient rich organic matter with fertilizer). Drive a support down into the hole. When placing the tree into the hole, line up the soil line on the tree with the ground surface. Fill in the hole with the amended soil, pack it down and mulch around the trunk with a thick layer to conserve moisture and deter grass and weeds. Attach the support with a tree collar that will not erode the tree, making it prey to silver leaf disease. With standard cultivars, leave at least 20 feet between trees. With dwarf varieties, 12 feet is enough. Keep the soil moist but not water logged. It takes 3-4 years after planting to bear fruit. Each spring, reapply planting mix to the soil and mulch over the area of root growth with well -aged compost to provide all the macro- and micronutrients needed. Thin small fruits to about 2 inches apart and 4 inches between large ones. During growing season, prune off extra thick growth that blocks sunlight from the interior so fruits can properly ripen. Over winter, prune off old wood to stimulate new growth. Harvest plums for cooking just before they soften. Or pick them off as they soften.

✘ **Insect Control:** Pests attacking plums are plum sawfly, wasps, red spider mite, aphids and birds. Deter aphids with a strong stream of water or by planting French marigolds to attract their predators, ladybugs and hoverflies. See Apricots for spider mites, sawflies and birds. If wasps become a problem, put something sweet in a jar (beer, juice, cider) and cover it with a film. Put a small hole in the cover and hang it from the tree. Wasps will be attracted, crawl inside the jar and get trapped.

✓ **Tips:** When watering, do it long enough for water to penetrate to the root level. Otherwise the roots will try to grow toward the surface for hydration. Also, never prune plums during the winter, as the wounds will remain open and susceptible to silver leaf.

∞∞∞

✂ *POMEGRANATE* ✂

✚ **Health Power:** Pomegranates have many vital vitamins and minerals. They also contain polyphenols, tannins, anthocyanins and ellagic acid, all highly beneficial phytonutrients that lower the risk of many diseases. All act as antioxidants, helping disarm damaging free radicals as they form. Most valuable, these phytonutrients might inhibit the initiation/growth of cancer cells. They also help the immune system with antibacterial, anti-viral and anti-inflammatory properties. Pomegranates also help thin the blood, increasing blood flow, oxygen delivery to tissues and exchange of compounds to and from organs. Thinning blood and donating antioxidants prevents cholesterol from being converted into a sticky form that begins the process of plaque buildup. The polyphenols and folate help protect and maintain elasticity in the blood vessels, which lightens the pumping load on the heart. Pomegranates are one of the richest sources of dietary fiber among fruits, promoting smooth digestion, regulating blood sugar and lowering high cholesterol. Research shows that pomegranates contain a phytonutrient capable of blocking an enzyme that breaks down cartilage in humans and other animals.

↑ **Vitamin and Mineral Content:**
Vitamins – K, C, B9 (Folate), B1 (Thiamin), B5 (Pantothenic Acid), B3 (Riboflavin) and E
Minerals – Copper, Potassium, Manganese, Phosphorus, Magnesium and Zinc

⊘ **Disease Prevention:** Pomegranate is a promising fruit to eat for reducing the risk of heart disease, atherosclerosis, rheumatoid and osteoarthritis and cancers of the breast, lung, prostate and colon.

❧ **How to Grow:** Native to the Middle East, these specialty fruits add beauty to the landscape with their glossy green leaves and glowing giant red-orange flowers. They are well adapted to many climates, but need a hot, dry summer for fruits to ripen. Plant them in deep soil with great drainage in a sunny site sheltered from strong winds. They will naturally develop into a bush or a small tree up to 15 feet tall and 10 feet wide. They can also be pruned as a hedge to conform to the shape of the yard or to look pretty. Planting from both seed and cuttings are the most popular methods. If you already have a pomegranate tree, cut off one of the suckers and transplant it as a cutting. Sow seeds after the first frost in the spring and/or plant cuttings in warmer weather (late spring to summer). You can get pomegranate cuttings 1-2 feet long in February or March. Work in compost or planting mix rich in organic matter and nutrients. Plant them so that 2/3 of the cutting is covered in soil. When the plant is young, water more often (every two days) to stimulate growth and help it get established. Once growth accelerates, and the tree sets a solid root foundation (about 2 months), give one deep watering every couple of weeks. Fertilize twice a year (once in early spring and fall) to help the plant grow strong, hardy and insect resistant. If you plant from cuttings, the tree should bear after 3 years. You may get a few in the season before. Harvest when they are the correct ripe color for the variety you are growing (ranging from purple and red to pink).

✘ **Insect Control:** Pomegranates usually are unaffected by pests or diseases that threaten yields in the home garden. Aphids are the most common but rarely leave damage behind unless the infestation is large and resilient. Monitor your plants. If aphids come, spray them off with a strong stream of water. Or plant French marigolds to attract their predators (ladybugs and hover flies) which eat aphids by the thousands. If something else comes up, photograph the pest and see your local nursery or agricultural extension office.

✓ **Tips:** Check with the nursery to see which cultivar is best suited to grow in your area. Remember, they need a hot, dry summer for fruit to ripen. Watch for shoots growing up from the base of the trunk. These are suckers and should be pruned and discarded or replanted

ꝏꝏꝏ

🜲 *POTATOES* 🜲

✚ **Health Power:** Potatoes are wrongly maligned as a high-carbohydrate starch with little or no nutritional value. Not so. The "problem" with potatoes is how they are often prepared (deep fried in oil) and/or what people put on them (high-fat dairy products and/or bacon bits). Potatoes have many different vitamins and phytonutrients. A crucial one is Vitamin B6, which helps build new cells and assists proper signaling in the brain. B6 also helps give us energy by breaking down carbohydrates during exercise. It also has fiber that helps lower cholesterol and supports digestion.

↑ Vitamin and Mineral Content:
Vitamins – B6 (Pyridoxine) and C
Minerals – Potassium, Copper and Manganese

⊘ Disease Prevention: Vitamin B6 helps control homocysteine, which helps prevent heart attacks or strokes by keeping vessel walls flexible and free of plaque. It also fights cancer development by attaching signals to molecules that turn on tumor suppressor genes. This type of signaling is called methylation and also serves as a signal to destroy toxic chemicals. The fiber in potatoes helps prevent indigestion and colon cancer.

❦ How to Grow: One of the cheapest, easiest foods to find at your local market. But most places offer only a few choices. Grow them yourself and choose among many different kinds. You can also enjoy a fresher, more flavorful 'tater.' With so many varieties, choose a few different types to find those that grow and taste best to you. If you buy seeds, get those certified disease-free. You can also create them yourself by saving the strongest, healthiest ones from a shop or your garden. When making potato seeds, place potatoes with the eye face-up adjacent to each other in a container in a cool room with plenty of air and light. After 4-5 weeks, they will be bright green and sprout. Discard the thinner, smaller sprouts (risk of disease) and keep the bigger, bushier ones. If they have more than one sprout, cut them into a few pieces before planting. Choose a sunny, warm, sheltered area. Amend the soil well with nitrogen-rich planting mix and/or compost. The soil needs to drain well or the tubers will rot. Cover the dedicated area with polypropylene to protect youngsters from weeds and frost. Cut slits in plastic and plant them a couple weeks before the last frost with sprouts facing up about 8 to 10 inches deep, a foot apart. Rows should be 2-3 feet apart. If shoots come up before frosting ends, work a bit of soil over them. When shoots grow about 10 inches above soil, work a fistful of high nitrogen plant mix like bone meal or seaweed meal along each meter of each row. Then pull soil almost to the tips of each shoot. Do this again later if the above ground growth is not very close to each other within the rows. For smaller, sweeter tubers, harvest only as they flower by cutting foliage and digging them up from the side with a garden fork. Store clean, blemish-free ones and use others right away. If you want larger mature potatoes, wait until the stems of the vines start to die back before harvest. Potatoes are also great for growing in large pots. Use the same method except start with the pot half full and add amended soil as the stem grows.

✘ **Insect Control:** Potatoes are affected by slugs, wireworms, cyst nematodes, leaf hoppers and many other diseases. Remove slugs by hand on moist evenings or mornings. Beer traps work as well. Start the growing season as early as possible to get the tubers well developed before pests arrive. As a general method, apply organic insecticide/fungicidal soap to prevent many pests and the development of common diseases like early blight, late blight, scab, dry rot and silver scurf. Powdering the roots with sulfur before planting also helps prevent bacterial rots.

✓ **Tips:** Eat the skin! Most of the vitamins and minerals are in the tissue just below the surface. To prevent rot, dig a slightly deeper trench and line it with a little mulch first. Do not let tubers see sunlight or they will develop a toxic alkaloid. Monitor the foliage closely for signs of pests or diseases, and apply proper treatment right away.

🧩 PUMPKIN 🧩

✚ **Health Power:** We most often see the seeds of large pumpkins around Halloween in late October, but they are full of important nutrients all year round. Ongoing research suggests pumpkin seeds help in maintaining prostate health. (Components in the oil prevent the enlargement caused by over-stimulation from the male hormones testosterone and dihydrotestosterone.) Pumpkin seeds also contain carotenoids and omega-3 fatty acids, which have antioxidant action and are beneficial fats compared to saturated fats. Pumpkin seeds also have magnesium and zinc, two minerals important for calcium uptake and bone building, among other benefits. The seeds are being investigated as potent anti-inflammatory agents. Animal studies show they reduce inflammation without the undesired side effects of fat damage in joint linings. Perhaps most exciting about eating pumpkin seeds: They are rich in phytosterols, molecules thought to lower cholesterol and boost the immune system. More research is needed to be conclusive, but they may also help lower the risk of some cancers.

⬆ **Vitamin and Mineral Content:**
Vitamins – K
Minerals – Manganese, Magnesium, Phosphorus, Iron, Copper and Zinc

⊘ **Disease Prevention:** Regularly eating pumpkin seeds may reduce the symptoms or onset of osteoporosis, rheumatoid and osteoarthritis, anemia and other conditions (depending on the results of current research).

❧ **How to Grow:** See Winter Squash for how to grow. These round orange fruits, closely related to winter squash, are common for pies, seeds and Halloween décor.

✗ **Insect Control:** See Summer/Winter Squash for how to manage pests.

✓ **Tips:** Pumpkins can grow large. Make sure you allow enough space for your chosen variety. Pumpkins grow on one main vine with secondary vines coming off. Tertiary vines grow off the secondary vines, and the pattern continues unless controlled. The most popular pruning method is the "Christmas tree" method. Prune the main vine when it reaches 10 feet past the last fruit you want. Prune tertiary vines when they begin to grow from buds on secondary vines, and pinch off secondary vines when they reach about 10 feet. This promotes fruit growth while limiting plant growth. Pinch off any new growth from the pruned sections. Cover vines with soil to promote secondary root growth. Rotate pumpkins once in a while to maintain symmetry, but be careful not to damage the vine.

∞∞∞

❧ *QUINCE* ❧

✚ **Health Power:** Quince is a great source of vitamin C and a good source of fiber, potassium and iron. Due to the high pectin content, it is rarely eaten raw. Rather, it is popular for making special jams and, since it holds shape well, is popular for baking, stewing or poaching as a dessert. Rich in fiber, quince aids digestion and lowers elevated blood sugar and cholesterol. Vitamin C helps protect cells (including blood vessel and immune cells) from oxidative damage by free radicals. This makes the immune and circulatory systems function more efficiently and helps maintain the body's biochemical balance. Some studies suggest the phytonutrients (phenolics) in quince have anti-viral properties.

↑ **Vitamin and Mineral Content:**
Vitamins – C
Minerals – Copper, Potassium and Iron

⊘ **Disease Prevention:** Quince may help treat or lower the risk of heart disease, arthritis, constipation, dysentery and gastric ulcers.

❧ **How to Grow:** Cousin to the pear, quince needs a moderate climate much like peaches to set fruit. Depending on variety, size will range from a large shrub to a small tree. They produce large, beautiful flowers in spring. Flowering a bit later than pears, the risk of frost damage is lower. Quinces take roughly 4 years for a light harvest. After 8 years, the harvest reaches full potential and can be quite large. You can find them in the local nursery in bare rooted form or propagated by cuttings of suckers from other quince plants. They are self-fertile; only one is needed for fruit production. They prefer a sunny site and heavier soil with a pH of 6-6.5 on a slight slope for good drainage. Work in a modest amount of plant mix to the site. Plant the tree and scatter a couple handfuls per square meter of planting mix over the root zone. Mulch over where roots will grow, keeping mulch at least 1 foot from the trunk. Water more frequently at first to get established. When watering, keep going until water reaches deep into the soil. This prevents roots from wanting to grow upward and protects them from drying out. Each spring reapply a couple handfuls of plant mix to encourage growth. Quinces are ripe when they are full yellow color and begin to smell sweet. Harvest and use immediately or store in a cool dry place.

✗ **Insect Control:** Common pests for quince include aphids, wooly aphids, winter moth, coddling moth, sawfly and wasps. Remove aphids with a strong spray of water or by companion planting French marigolds, which attracts hoverflies and ladybugs that prey on aphids. Wooly aphids are more difficult. They are hard to treat with sprays, because they cover themselves in a white waxy layer. As soon as you see these layers, scrape them off. If that fails, spray with a strong stream of rotenone after flowers have fallen. As a last resort, cut them out. Cover excess bare wood. Female winter moths have no wings and crawl up the tree to lay eggs in fall and spring. The best way to stop them is to tie a sticky band around the lower trunk during egg laying seasons. Coddling moths lay their eggs directly on the fruit, which give rise to tiny grubs that burrow directly into the fruit. Use a pheromone trap to control. Sawfly do damage as small brown caterpillars. As soon as you see them, spray with an insecticide like Bt, pyrethrum, or quassia. Wasps can be deterred by hanging a jar full of a sweet liquid (cider, stale beer, fruit juice) with a perforated top just big enough for the wasp to crawl in. Before taking these precautionary steps, ask the nursery which pests are most threatening in your area.

✓ **Tips:** Throughout growth, cut out the old wood and thin the long branches to encourage lateral growth. Remove the suckers that pop up from the base.

ooooo

✿ *RADICCHIO* ✿

✚ **Health Power:** The most significant nutrient in radicchio is vitamin K followed by phytonutrients like anthocyanins. Often overlooked, vitamin K plays an important biochemical role in blood clotting and bone matrix building. It is needed for the activation of many proteins in the clotting process. The overall biochemical processes require more research, but thus far vitamin K appears to help encourage the formation of bone matrix (osteoblastic processes), while discouraging the breakdown of bone (osteoclastic processes). Responsible for the deep red color, anthocyanins are promising phytonutrients that have anti-inflammatory properties and inhibit the growth of pre-malignant cancer cells, induce apoptosis (programmed cell death) in cancer cells, inhibit angiogenesis (the growth of new blood vessels that feed tumors) and reduce cancer-causing DNA damage.

↑ Vitamin and Mineral Content:
Vitamins – K, B9 (Folate), C and E
Minerals – Copper, Manganese and Potassium

⊘ **Disease Prevention:** Early research suggests radicchio may help reduce the risk of osteoporosis, hemophilia and many types of cancers.

❦ **How to Grow:** With its white-veined, deep red-purple leaves, radicchio is a great fall/winter veggie to add to a salad. Best time for planting is in late spring to early summer or late summer to early fall, depending on regional weather averages. The color and flavor of leaves develops in the transition to cooler temperatures. It may take a trial run to decide which one you like better. Radicchio prefers a sunny site with highly fertile moisture-retentive soil at a pH of 6.5. Amend the soil with a generous amount of aged compost or planting mix. Sowing seeds too early may cause the plants to run to seed. Start in late spring. Sow the seeds densely ¼ inch deep in shallow drills spaced about 1 foot apart. Later, thin the seedlings out to 9-10 inches apart. Keep the beds weed free and the soil moist, not soggy. If you let it dry out, they might become bitter. Right after first frost, remove outer leaves, leaving the curled interior leaves. Frost sweetens the leaf. Continue to keep the bed weed free and the soil moist. The colors should darken, and a head should begin to plump as weather cools. When the head gets plump and firm, they are ready for cutting.

✕ **Insect Control:** Radicchio is insect resistant but may be bothered by slugs and snails. To trap them, embed a cup of beer into the soil so that the rim is flush with the soil. Snails and slugs are attracted to the beer, slide in, get stuck and drown. For other problems, ask your local nursery what might affect radicchio in your area.

✓ **Tips:** When watering, soak the soil, not the foliage. This prevents any type of rotting.

∞∞∞

� RADISHES ✲

✚ Health Power: Like some other popular fruits and vegetables, radishes offer a substantial dose of vitamin C. Much research has been done on vitamin C's effects on the immune system, but whether it plays a significant role is disputed. Vitamin C is an effective antioxidant molecule that works in the water-soluble portions of the body to disarm free radicals. Vitamin C helps reduce oxidative stress on blood vessels in the cardiovascular system (leading to plaque buildup) and lung cells. The anti-oxidants also deter free radicals from damaging plasma membranes and DNA, which may help prevent cancer-causing mutations. Vitamin C also works with an antioxidant compound, glutathione peroxidase, to help restore the activity of vitamin E (a fat-soluble vitamin). Vitamin C is an important part of collagen formation involved with healthy bone, skin and connective tissues. Radishes have phytonutrients that help aid digestion (by encouraging bile flow) and stimulate the liver to produce detoxifying enzymes that remove harmful chemicals in the blood. Radishes, both red and daikon, have the phytonutrient myrosinase, which acts as an enzyme to break down other phytonutrients in radishes (glucosinolates) to isothiocyanates. Ongoing research with isothiocyanates suggest these compounds may have strong anti-cancer properties.

↑ Vitamin and Mineral Content:
Vitamins – C, B9 (Folate), B6 (Pyridoxine) and B2 (Riboflavin)
Minerals – Potassium and Manganese

⊘ Disease Prevention: Regular eating of radishes may help reduce the symptoms or development of atherosclerosis, cardiovascular disease, cataracts, kidney stones and many types of cancers.

❦ How to Grow: Radishes are a fast-maturing root to grow between slower-maturing vegetables. Highly tolerant of soil types but need cool weather to grow correctly. Like most veggies, radishes grow quickest in soil that has been worked with organic matter like aged compost or planting mix. Loosen up the soil to a depth of at least 1 foot to allow unhindered growth. Plant at the start of spring. Sow the seeds in rows 6 inches apart. Place seeds close together, roughly 1 inch apart. Thinning usually is not an issue. For a continual harvest, sow seeds weekly until weather begins to warm. You can begin sowing in mid- to late summer as the weather begins to cool for a fall harvest. Radishes are low maintenance. Most important is to water when the soil starts to dry and keep the area weed free. Mulching helps retain water and deter weeds. Harvest as soon as roots are mature. If they sit too long, they crack and get tough. Discard any that look diseased or damaged so they do not pass it on to other roots.

✘ **Insect Control:** Cabbage maggots, flea beetles and carrot fly may affect root growth. If you suspect cabbage maggots, deter them by making floating row covers or make slits in a piece of foam carpet pad or tar paper, securing it around the base of each plant. This prevents maggots from burrowing down to the roots. You know you have flea beetles if they jump in the air like fleas as you bring your hand a few inches over them. To control, take a piece of cardboard or wood and coat one side with a sticky substance. Hover the board a few inches over the radishes and watch the beetles jump up and get stuck. The female carrot fly lays her eggs at the base of root plants. The larvae burrow into the roots. To prevent it, surround the bed with plastic screen.

✓ **Tips:** Radish greens have up to 6 times the vitamin C of radishes themselves. Daikons are an Asian white radish grown the same way as red radishes with similar nutrient content and health benefits. Try both to see which you prefer.

ooooo

❧ *RASPBERRIES* ❧

✚ **Health Power:** Red raspberries are delicious and contain powerful phytonutrients that have antioxidant, antimicrobial and anti-carcinogenic properties. Aside from vitamins C and E, the tannin ellagic acids and a collection of flavonoids are the antioxidants in raspberries, (which outdo kiwis, strawberries and tomatoes). These compounds help protect critical cells and organs from damage caused by free radicals. They also have antimicrobial properties that help suppress certain bacterial colonies (and others like fungi). Research studies suggest some of the phytonutrients in raspberries inhibit initiation of, or halt the growth of, certain cancer cells. Both vitamin K and manganese help build bone matrix and are an excellent source of fiber. Raspberries have a fair amount of sugars, but the fiber and B vitamins slow the absorption of sugars and help break them down faster. Fiber plays a large role in a healthy digestive tract and helps regulate cholesterol levels. Raspberries also provide some folate, which reduces damage in blood vessel walls and supports fetal nerve development.

⬆ **Vitamin and Mineral Content:**
Vitamins – C, K, B9 (Folate), E and small amounts of B complex
Minerals – Manganese, Magnesium, Copper, Iron and Potassium

⊘ **Disease Prevention:** Cardiovascular disease, atherosclerosis, osteoporosis, arthritis, macular degeneration and many cancers (especially colon cancer).

❦ **How to Grow:** These delectable berries are simple to grow in moderate climates and do really well under organic methods. They take up a lot of room, but produce a plethora of berries. They are self-fertile and require only one variety to fruit. You can usually find healthy, disease resistant cultivars from a local nursery. They grow best in a sunny site in deep, thoroughly worked, moisture-retentive soil. The pH should be 6 or just under. (A pH above 7 causes iron deficiency in raspberries. Bring down the pH well before planting.) Plant in fall to early winter. With bare rooted plants, dig a trench a spade deep and 2 feet wide. Loosen the bottom and amend it with a few inches of well-aged compost, manure or planting mix. Place the canes down into the soil. Amend the soil you dug up as you did on the bottom while filling up the hole. Cut the canes to within 6 inches of the ground to encourage root growth. Separate plants by 3 feet and rows by at least 6 feet. For many varieties, create a post and wire support for the canes to grow along. Embed 6-8 posts in the ground. Connect the posts with wire, one 2 feet above the ground, one in the middle and one on top. As the canes grow, fasten them to the wires as they develop, maintaining a few inches between each cane. In late winter, mulch around the canes with compost or other organic matter. This prevents an iron deficiency. Before the fruit turns red, cover the canes with netting to prevent bird damage. Berries are ripe when the taste is right. To cook with, harvest some just before full ripening. Leave the central core of the fruit on the canes. If you cannot eat them all, store by freezing or canning. For ever-bearing varieties, fruit bears a small crop on the tips of first-year canes each fall and a larger crop on second-year canes. After you harvest all the fruit, cut all the canes that fruited to ground level. Space new canes 3-5 inches apart on the support and remove excess canes.

✘ **Insect Control:** Most common pests are birds, aphids and raspberry beetles. Netting deters birds. Planting French marigolds reduces aphids by attracting their predators, ladybugs and hover flies. Raspberry beetle larvae feed on ripe fruit and fall into soil to form pupae. If you see deformed fruit, hoe the soil to bring pupae to the surface for birds to eat. If infestation is severe, spray with insecticide like rotenone when the first fruits turn pink.

✓ **Tips:** Yellowing between veins on the leaves shows an iron deficiency. Quickly apply some foliar spray and spread a couple handfuls of nutrient rich fertilizer over the roots.

ooooo

❧ *RHUBARB* ❧

✚ **Health Power:** Rhubarb is a great source of dietary fiber and helps resolve indigestion issues with its gentle laxative properties. It may also help lower cholesterol and blood pressure. The potassium supports proper nerve functioning and muscle contraction, including the heart. Vitamin C gives rhubarb antioxidant, anti-inflammatory and antiallergenic properties. Vitamin K with calcium adds to bone formation and helps prevent bone breakdown. Rhubarb is low in carbohydrates, saturated fat, sodium and cholesterol. It increases metabolic rate, which is excellent for eating while trying to lose weight. Rhubarb has antibacterial and antifungal properties that may help prevent infections. If applied topically, rhubarb prevents staph infection.

↑ **Vitamin and Mineral Content:**
Vitamins – K and C
Minerals – Calcium, Potassium, Manganese and Magnesium

⊘ **Disease Prevention:** Cholesterol lowering properties support a healthy cardiovascular system free of diseases like atherosclerosis. Vitamin C is an antioxidant that eliminates water-soluble free radicals, many of which may later contribute to cancer. C also protects blood vessels by helping prevent the formation of arterial plaque via its interactions with the bad form of cholesterol (LDL). Vitamin C promotes heart health by stopping potentially fatal plaque-induced clots from causing a heart attack or a stroke. With vitamin K, calcium and manganese, regularly eating rhubarb may help prevent osteoporosis.

❦ **How to Grow:** Rhubarb is an interesting food because it produces fruit, but we eat only the stems. It is an easy, long-lived perennial plant and very cold hardy. Harvest it toward the end of winter through the middle of summer. Prepare the soil by shifting the pH to 7 if not already there. Amend the area with a generous amount of aged compost, manure or highly fertile planting mix. Generally, gardeners do not need more than a few plants. If you want to grow many, plant individuals 2 feet apart in rows 3 feet apart. Depending on time of year, you may find root crowns or potted plants. In spring, or in pots before spring, plant root crowns in soil and cover with a thin layer. Keep the soil moist but never waterlogged. Weed the bed as needed. Let the plants continue to grow through the first year without harvesting. In the second season, harvest the larger stems first as needed, making sure not to take all the stems from one plant. Stems are ripe when they change from green to purplish red. After harvesting each year in the spring, apply another layer of compost or planting mix to promote healthy rejuvenation of reserves once more.

✗ **Insect Control:** Common attacking insects include aphids. They are also susceptible to viruses. To deter aphids, companion plant marigolds. They attract both ladybugs and hover flies, which lay their larvae on colonies of aphids for food. They consume thousands this way. Or rinse off the aphids with a strong stream of water that does not damage the host plant. To avoid viruses, get the plant or seeds at a trustworthy nursery. Make sure there is good air circulation and do not waterlog the soil. Keep plants out of low, shady areas. Dispose of infected sections of plants immediately. If all else fails, spray with a copper- or sulfur-based treatment found at nurseries.

✓ **Tips:** Enjoy the flowers in the summer time, but do not let the plants run to seed, as this greatly reduces the following harvest. Note: Never eat the leaves of rhubarb, as they contain very harmful toxins, especially if you eat significant amounts.

∞∞∞

❀ *ROSEMARY* ❀

✚ **Health Power:** Rosemary adds wonderful flavor and aroma to potatoes, pork, lamb and chicken. It also adds helpful substance to a meal by exciting the immune system. It increases circulation (especially to the brain) and improves digestion. It has anti-inflammatory agents that might moderate the severity of asthma attacks or other conditions. The essential oil of rosemary, obtained by steeping in boiling water or steam distillation of all parts of the plant, may help improve memory and support healthy adrenal and lymphatic functions. Some people say its role in aromatherapy is unmatched. Some students use it at exam times to help with memory, mental stimulation and calming the nerves. It has also been noted to relieve headaches, soothe sore muscles, clear out nasal passages and help treat skin conditions like eczema, acne and rashes. Users derive these benefits by adding a bit to topical oils/creams, rubbing a few drops on directly or adding to bath water. A couple of drops have been added to shampoos and conditioners to help condition hair. The oil also has some antiseptic properties and is used to treat respiratory allergies, sore throat and flu.

↑ **Vitamin and Mineral Content:**
Vitamins – traces
Minerals – Iron and Calcium

⊘ **Disease Prevention:** Given the amount of rosemary included in meals, it is not likely to have a large role in preventing disease. It does add some healthy nutrition to a meal, and the essential oil may prove to be effective in our overall natural health.

❦ **How to Grow:** Rosemary is an attractive, fuzzy little herb that grows up to 3 feet tall and produces fragrant blue flowers. Great for borders and a generally good plant to have in the garden, as it attracts beneficial insects for pollination and predation. Rosemary does best in a sunny site with soil that has good drainage and plenty of organic matter worked in. It also grows well in containers. Grow them as you like; hedges spaced 1.5 feet apart or individuals 2-3 feet apart. Trim the bushes after flowering, as they will spread along the ground more. If they do, time to re-place them. Rosemary is an evergreen. It supplies fresh greens all year round unless temperatures get too cold (as in cold northern climates). To conserve trimmings you cannot eat, dry in a shady, well-ventilated shed. Then put them in airtight jars.

✕ **Insect Control:** Virtually no pests threaten rosemary. Use its fragrance to ad-vantage. It repels moths and, in many cases, can attract pollinating insects like bees.

✓ **Tips:** Growing rosemary in a container, put pebbles on the bottom for good drainage. Repot container-grown rosemary each year to help the roots spread equally with the plant above ground. Fertilize again each spring.

∞∞∞∞

❧ *RUTABAGA (SWEDES)* ❧

✚ **Health Power:** Rutabaga is a great source of vitamin C, folate, fiber, potassium and manganese. See Radishes for the many benefits associated with the antioxi-dant vitamin C. Folate and vitamin B6 help protect blood vessel walls by con-verting homocysteine into an inert compound. This keeps homocysteine from reaching high levels where it damages blood vessel walls. Folate is also important for pregnant women to support healthy fetal nerve development. Fiber facilitates smooth digestion and slows down the absorption of sugar and cholesterol, helping to reduce and regulate elevated levels of both. Potassium assists in the proper func-tioning of muscle and nerve fibers. It can also replace some sodium in the blood and bring down elevated blood pressure. Magnesium is an important cofactor for enzymes involved in detoxification, most notably superoxide dismutase. We need this antioxidant constantly to reduce oxygen free radicals that result from normal respiration in cell mitochondria. If left unchecked, oxygen free radicals can dam-age cell membranes, mutate DNA and denature proteins. We need magnesium for bone growth and maintenance.

↑ **Vitamin and Mineral Content:**
Vitamins – C, B1 (Thiamin), B6 (Pyridoxine), B9 (Folate) and B3 (Niacin)
Minerals – Potassium, Manganese, Magnesium, Phosphorus, Calcium and Iron

⊘ **Disease Prevention:** Regularly eating rutabaga may help reduce the symptoms or onset of atherosclerosis, heart disease, osteoporosis, diabetes, constipation, diverticulitis and colorectal cancer.

❦ **How to Grow:** Swedes, another name for rutabaga, are a member of the cabbage family and one of the easiest veggies to grow. Several varieties to choose from, some of which resist club root and mildew. Choose a resistant cultivar if those problems occur in your area. Swedes also need well-drained soil and a pH above 6.5 to minimize club root. Add lime if necessary. Work some planting mix into soil. Sow the seeds thinly in shallow drills from late spring to early summer. This will help prevent mildew. Space the rows 1 foot apart. Later, thin seedlings to leave the dominant ones 1.5 feet apart. Keep the area weed free. Water when necessary, but do not over water. Mulch overtop with organic matter like aged compost or manure. Harvest after the first frost in fall, remove tops and store in a shady, cool, dry place. Destroy any appearing damaged or diseased.

✘ **Insect Control:** Rutabagas are susceptible to flea beetles, which are fun to remove, because they jump when approached. Attach a sticky layer (honey or grease) to one side of a small piece of cardboard and run it a couple inches above the seedlings. Watch the flea beetles jump and get stuck. For other pest problems, consult a trusted local nursery for identification and treatment.

✓ **Tips:** They store longer in a container covered lightly with moist peat. If buying in a store, choose heavy, firm rutabagas with smooth, undamaged or unwrinkled skin.

ooooo

❀ *SAGE* ❀

✚ **Health Power:** The benefits of sage lie in its potent phytonutrients and volatile oils. Cousin to rosemary, sage is another source of rosmarinic acid. The acid is easily absorbed in the intestines and is known for its antioxidant properties. Sage is also a great source of flavonoids and two of the most powerful antioxidants, superoxide dismutase (SOD) and peroxidase. SOD and peroxidase convert strong oxygen free radicals into non-toxic forms. These antioxidant compounds give sage a unique ability to help neutralize toxic forms of oxygen formed during cellular respiration. This in turn prevents oxygen-related damage to cell membranes, vital enzymes and DNA. Some studies suggest sage helps improve cognitive function and memory by preventing the degradation of acetylcholine, a vital neurotransmitter. Sage is also known for antiperspirant, antiseptic, calming and digestive properties. Some commercial antiperspirants contain extracts from sage. Rubbing crushed sage leaves over an open cut or wound can help prevent infection. Regularly eating sage also helps smooth digestion and may help reduce blood sugar levels. In addition to adding sage to your food, you can also prepare a tea with it, which gives a more concentrated dose of the phytonutrients and essential oils.

↑ Vitamin and Mineral Content:
Vitamins – traces
Minerals – traces

⊘ Disease Prevention: Regular incorporation of sage in the diet may help reduce the symptoms or the onset of rheumatoid and osteoarthritis, asthma, atherosclerosis, Alzheimer's disease, diabetes and other diseases caused by oxidative damage to cells/organs.

❧ How to Grow: Easy on the eyes and aromatic, sage always serves as a pleasing component of borders. In addition to their colorful, velvety flowers and relaxing aroma, many cultivars add depth to a culinary creation. Sage is a hardy shrub, tolerant of many types of soil pH. Its main site requirements are full sun and good drainage. Amend the soil with plenty of organic matter, especially if it's naturally dense and compacted. Perhaps add some coarse sand to heavier soil. Spring is the time to plant. You can sow from seed, but starting with sage plants in containers or purchasing them bare rooted is easier. Plant both container and bare rooted styles in the ground about 2 feet apart. As they grow, pinch the shoots out to prevent them from getting too lanky. If a couple shoots do get this way, they may be used to layer with (see Tips). Keep the area surrounding them weed free to alleviate nutrient competition. Leaves can be harvested all summer long as needed. Do it before flowering. After that, the flavor is compromised.

✕ Insect Control: Sage has no common pests that threaten its life.

✓ Tips: Propagate sage by layering or taking soft wood cuttings. To layer, put an object on top of some of the shoots so they are stuck against the soil. After new roots form, sever the shoot that connects the two plants. You can leave the new plant alone or pot it up and plant it out again in spring. For soft wood cuttings, select a newly grown, healthy shoot about 4-5 inches long. Cut the 4-inch section in half below the leaf joint. Remove the rest of the leaves and plant the end of the cutting in a tray with highly fertile soil. Perhaps dip the cuttings in a fungicide solution and rooting hormone before planting.

oooooo

❦ *SCALLIONS* ❦

✛ Health Power: These young onions have beneficial phytonutrients like flavonoids and sulfur compounds that work together to lower cholesterol, promote heart health, and suppress inflammation. The flavonoid quercetin may bring a number of benefits, including the antioxidant effect in protecting colon cells. Quercetin, along with vitamin C, strengthens the immune system and works against harmful bacteria and viruses that cause common colds or worse. Vitamin C also has antioxidant and anti-inflammatory properties that help deal with arthritis and protect the cardiovascular system from cellular damage and plaque buildup. Vitamin K supports healthy bone development by helping support bone laying components and reducing bone break down by osteoclasts. Also lowers blood pressure. Scallions are a good source of dietary fiber, helping promote healthy digestion and preventing diarrhea. Folate promotes heart health and is critical for healthy fetal nervous system development. Scallions also encourage sweating and urination. In combination with those and the fact that scallions are low in saturated fat, sodium and cholesterol, they are an ideal food to include in a weight loss diet.

↑ Vitamin and Mineral Content:
Vitamins – K, C, A and B9 (Folate)
Minerals – Potassium, Iron, Manganese, Calcium, Magnesium, Phosphorus and Copper

⊘ Disease Prevention: Eating vegetables in the Allium family, like garlic, onions, and scallions, may reduce the risk of esophageal, stomach, colon, prostate and possibly breast cancer. Regularly eating reduces pain associated with arthritis and symptoms of asthma.

❧ How to Grow: Scallions (also known as green, spring or salad onions) are a type of onion pulled before they have the chance to develop a full root bulb. The most popular and widely used varieties are perennial versions, *Allium fistulosum* and *Allium cepa*. They produce high quality scallions in large quantity. They can be grown from seeds or transplants. Plant seeds thickly about one-half inch deep in well-amended fertile soil. If you want to start during cold winter conditions, sow the seeds indoors until nighttime temperatures rise above freezing. You then need to gradually wean them outdoors when the weather warms up a little. Otherwise, plant the seeds or seedlings outdoors a few weeks before the last frost. Keep rows more than 2 feet apart and slowly thin seedlings out to 6 inches. Once the soil warms up, mulch around and between the plants to deter weeds, retain moisture and buffer the soil so it changes temperatures more slowly. Weed as needed. Be careful not to damage the bulbs. Dry conditions cause bulbs to split. Monitor the moisture level in the soil. Harvest when the shoots are a deep green color and before base begins to swell, usually around mid-summer to fall. The tips should be crisp yet forgiving. You can store in a plastic bag in the refrigerator for about a week. They hold on to their flavor surprisingly well when frozen.

✘ **Insect Control:** Scallions are generally disease and insect free. They help deter pests like Japanese beetles, carrot flies and aphids from other garden plants. Interplanting is a great way to keep them disease and pest free while helping others. As a preventative, work a good amount of humus into the soil to create good drainage and prevent any potential bacterial or fungal infections. Removing weeds also prevents pests like thrips from persisting over winters. If you have a large, uncontrollable infestation, an insecticidal soap works well in small quantities.

✓ **Tips:** Mix in radish plants among the onions to deflect root maggots away from the onions.

∞∞∞∞

🕸 *SHALLOTS* 🕸

✚ **Health Power:** See Onions, which have similar vitamins, minerals and phytonutrients.

↑ **Vitamin and Mineral Content:**
Vitamins – C, B6 (Pyridoxine), B9 (Folate), B1 (Thiamin) and B2 (Riboflavin)
Minerals – Manganese, Potassium, Phosphorus, Magnesium and Calcium

⊘ **Disease Prevention:** See Onions

❦ **How to Grow:** Shallots are a smaller version of the main crop onion with a mild flavor. Harvest them earlier than main crops, too. Shallots need a site with full sunshine and soil full of organic matter. Work in a generous amount of aged compost or planting mix. The pH should be above 6.5; add lime to raise if needed. Shallots are most easily grown from sets (last year's bulbs). Try to choose a variety that stores well for the following year's crop. Remove any dead growth from the top of the bulb and plant in drills in spring. Place each bulb 6 inches apart. Barely cover the tip of the bulb with soil. Don't pack the soil down around the bulb, as this will make them pop themselves out when they start to grow roots. They grow best in looser soil that allows for their bulbs to expand and roots to grow without much resistance. Space the rows out by 1 foot and stagger them so sets do not grow right next to each other. Weed as necessary and water during dry weather. Early in summer, loosen the soil around the bulbs to help them ripen up. They are ready for harvest when the foliage dies off. Lift them out, brush the bulbs clean and store. Ideally, put them on a net for optimal airflow, but storing them in perforated sacks in a cool, dry, frost-free place works, too.

✗ Insect Control: Shallots usually grow trouble free. If you cannot control an infestation by hand, and it threatens the welfare of the crop, consult a local nursery or agricultural extension office.

✓ Tips: In warmer climates, plant shallots in the fall and take them through winter. Exposure to cool temperatures makes a larger, more flavorful shallot. If your soil is at all dense and drainage is an issue, plant shallots in raised ridges.

∞∞∞

❧ *SPINACH* ☙

✚ Health Power: Spinach is remarkable in the myriad of vitamins, minerals , and phytonutrients it gives in one serving. It contains an important carotenoid and a collection of flavonoids that, in addition to vitamins A and C, act as important antioxidants ridding the body of dangerous free radicals. This prevents plaque build up in artery walls by preventing cholesterol from being oxidized. In the end, this helps protect against serious heart problems. Folate and magnesium in spinach also add to heart health by decreasing plaque build up, arterial wall damage (folate) and blood pressure (magnesium and potassium). Because some nutrients are water soluble and others fat soluble, spinach helps resist the growth of various cancerous cells beyond the first day after its consumption. Moreover, nutrients like calcium and Vitamin K add to creating and maintaining healthy bones. The list keeps going with properties that help reduce inflammation in conditions like osteoarthritis, osteoporosis and rheumatoid arthritis. Eating many green leafy vegetables slows down the decline of mental functioning associated with age. Spinach is also an excellent source of iron for helping hemoglobin in blood deliver oxygen to tissues, and lutein that helps maintain eye health. This super food is a great addition to a meal and an ideal way to promote optimal health. Its effects may be profound.

↑ Vitamin and Mineral Content:
Vitamins – K, A, C, B9 (Folate), B2 (Riboflavin), B6 (Pyridoxine), E, B1 (Thiamin) and, B3 (Niacin)
Minerals – Manganese, Folate, Magnesium, Iron, Calcium, Potassium, Copper, Phosphorus, Zinc and Selenium

⊘ **Disease Prevention:** Spinach may help reduce risks in of heart disease, anemia, arthritis, and cancers of the stomach, colon, prostate, breast, ovaries and potentially many more.

❦ **How to Grow:** Spinach is a garden must. It's packed with great nutrition and easy to grow. Seeds are commonly found in most local nurseries and are more successful than transplants. Plant and harvest spinach in both spring and fall. True spinach is best for cooler climates, but if you want to plant during the summer in a southern, warmer climate, New Zealand spinach copes well with summer heat. If growing in cooler weather, choose a site with lots of sun. In warmer weather, choose a site with plenty of shade. If it gets too warm, spinach will go to seed and reduce yields. The soil needs to be at a pH near 7. Add lime if it's too low. Soil also must be light, fertile and able to hold water well. Adding organic matter in the form of fully aged compost, manure or planting mix works well. Sow each seed in rows roughly half inch deep, spacing seeds a couple inches apart. Space out rows 9-12 inches apart. Spring sowing should begin 6-8 weeks before the last frost. Summer sowing should start in mid-August for cooler climates, later for warmer ones. Thin the sprouts to 6 inches apart to avoid over crowding and premature seeding. Keep the soil moist and free of weeds. Mulching around the plants after they have grown a bit may help retain moisture and deter weeds. The leaves or whole plants should be ready to pick 7-10 weeks after initial sowing.

✗ **Insect Control:** Spinach grows in cooler weather and naturally escapes the wrath of many pests. If any, insects that may cause problems are spotted cucumber beetles, leaf miner larvae, aphids, and cabbage loopers. Remove the beetles by hand and dispose of them right away. The larvae of leaf miners embed in the leaves and cause light brown blotches. Remove any leaves showing signs of this infection to stop it from proliferating. This holds true for aphids as well. Remove them or spray with a strong stream of water. Planting French marigolds attracts ladybugs, a natural predator of aphids. If the infestation is too large with beetles, aphids, or loopers, spray with an organic treatment such as insecticidal soap/oil.

✓ **Tips:** If you want a continual harvest, try consecutively sowing seeds through spring or early fall. If you're looking to get as much iron from spinach as possible, cooking in iron pans or skillets increases its availability. Make sure to harvest the whole plant at the first hint of bolting to stop the plant from putting all its energy into forming seeds, rendering its the leaves tougher and inedible. Lastly, apply a micronutrient rich fertilizer half way through growth. A planting mix containing soluble seaweed extract or fish bone meal will provide sustenance and steady growth.

∞∞∞∞

🦑 *SQUASH (SUMMER)* 🦑

✚ Health Power: Summer squash adds similar nutrients as winter squash but in smaller amounts. See Squash (Winter) for health benefits.

↑ Vitamin and Mineral Content:
Vitamins – C, A, B9 (Folate), K, B6 (Pyridoxine), B1 (Thiamin), B3 (Niacin) and B2 (Riboflavin)
Minerals – Manganese, Magnesium, Potassium, Copper, Phosphorus, Calcium, Zinc and Iron

⊘ Disease Prevention: See Squash (Winter)

🌱 How to Grow: Common Summer Squash (zucchini, crookneck and straight neck squash and scallop squash). Thrives in warmer weather. Take about 2 months to ripen. All prefer rich soil in full sun with plenty of organic matter and great drainage. Dig in a generous amount of well-aged compost, manure or planting mix. The pH should be near 6. In mid-spring, sow seeds indoors in 3-inch pots, two seeds to a pot. Sow on a windowsill, under fluorescent light or on a sun porch. Keep soil moist. Thin out seedlings if needed to provide room for the strongest seedling. Plant bush types in late spring 3 feet apart in rows 5 feet apart. Plant vining cultivars 3 feet apart in rows 8 feet apart. Sow directly outdoors in mid- to late spring when soil temperatures rise to a minimum of 65°F. Create small hills 3 feet apart, with amended soil. Sow seeds 6 per hill. Keep them watered, and thin out to the two best seedlings per hill. Mulch around the seedlings with straw, hay or leaves when the vines are longer and stronger. Fertilize every few weeks, especially after fruits set, with a nutrient-rich fertilizer like compost tea, manure tea or liquid seaweed extract. Summer squash should be nice and plump by late summer. If the ground is always moist at this time, raise them off the ground on bricks or blocks. Harvest summer squash before it matures, and it will continue to set buds. Take care to harvest during a dry time, using a sharp knife you wash between each cut to prevent spreading disease. Cure by letting them dry in the sun until the stems wither. Store in a cool, shaded area.

✗ Insect Control: Slugs, aphids, vine borers and squash bugs are common pests for squash. Embed a cup of beer in the soil. Slugs and snails are attracted to the cup, crawl in and drown. Plant French marigolds to attract predators of aphids (hover flies and ladybugs) who eat them by the thousands. Or spray aphids off the leaves with a firm stream of water. Avoid this on smaller seedlings. Vine borers are about 1 inch long, look like caterpillars and eat their way into the base of plants leaving behind a sticky sawdust substance. Watch for this sawdust, and cut into stems to remove them or insert Bt (*Bacillus thuringiensis*) into the stem. Dig dirt up to the stem wound so it can again lay down roots. Watch for the orange and black wasp-like moth in late June when it lays its eggs at the base. They are tiny and reddish orange. If you find them, destroy them and dust or spray with an organic insecticide. Marigolds also help deter squash bugs. They are ¾ inches long and gray brown. They lay their red-brown eggs on the underside of leaves. Handpick them and scan for eggs. Dispose of the pest and eggs when you see them.

✓ **Tips:** To avoid disease, water soil not foliage. Keep beds weed free. To ensure fertilization, use a paintbrush to transfer pollen from the male stamen to the female pistil.

∞∞∞

✖ *SQUASH (WINTER)* ✖

✚ **Health Power:** Research is limited, though some phytonutrients found in winter squash have been linked with anti-cancer properties in studies of other plants. Winter squash is a good source of all the vitamins and minerals listed. More nutrient-dense than its cousin, the summer squash. Most notable in one serving of winter squash are vitamins A (more than 100 percent RDA) and C (more than 30 percent RDA). These vitamins team up for many functions. They support the immune response of white blood cells toward pathogens. They act as antioxidants in water soluble areas of the body, protecting cells from free radical damage. Some major antioxidant actions help prevent the buildup of plaque in blood vessels, reduce inflammation and help prevent damage to cells in the eye. Winter squash gives potassium, key to maintaining normal blood pressure, nerve cell transmission and muscle contraction. High fiber content supports digestion, removes excess cholesterol and helps regulate blood sugar. Pregnant women need the B vitamin folate for normal fetal neural development. Also contributes to heart health by preventing homocysteine, an amino acid that in high concentrations causes blood vessel stiffening. With other B vitamins, squash helps make energy through the metabolism of lipids, carbohydrates and proteins.

↑ **Vitamin and Mineral Content:**
Vitamins – A, C, B9 (Folate), B1 (Thiamin), B6 (Pyridoxine), B3 (Niacin) and B5 (Pantothenic acid)
Minerals – Potassium, Manganese, Copper, Iron and Magnesium

⊘ **Disease Prevention:** May reduce risk and symptoms of benign prostate hypertrophy (BPH), atherosclerosis, diabetic heart disease, heart attack, stroke, colon cancer (potentially others), asthma, osteoarthritis and rheumatoid arthritis.

❦ **How to Grow:** Common Winter Squash (butternut, acorn, delicious Hubbard, banana, buttercup and spaghetti squash). Thrives in warmer weather. Winter vining cultivars may grow 10-20 feet long and require generous space. Winter squash takes 3-4 months to mature. Prefers rich soil in full sun with plenty of organic matter and great drainage. Dig in a generous amount of well-aged compost, manure or planting mix. The pH should be near 6. In mid-spring, sow seeds indoors in 3-inch pots, two seeds to a pot. Sow on a windowsill, under fluorescent light or on a sun porch. Keep soil moist. Thin out seedlings if needed to provide room for the strongest seedling. Plant bush types in late spring 3 feet apart in rows 5 feet apart. Plant vining cultivars 3 feet apart in rows 8 feet apart. Sow directly outdoors in mid to late spring when soil temperatures rise to a minimum of 65°F. Create small hills 6 feet apart with amended soil. Sow seeds 6 per hill. Keep them watered, and thin out to the two best seedlings per hill. Mulch around the seedlings with straw, hay or leaves when the vines are longer and stronger. Fertilize every few weeks, especially after fruits set, with a nutrient-rich fertilizer like compost tea, manure tea or liquid seaweed extract. If the ground is always moist at this time, raise them off the ground on bricks or blocks. Harvest only when it is fully mature, as the taste depends on it. Do this just before the first expected frost, and they will store longer. Harvest during a dry time, using a sharp knife you wash between each cut to prevent spreading disease. Cure by letting dry in the sun until the stems wither. Store in a cool, shaded area to extend storage time.

✘ **Insect Control:** See Squash (Summer) for common pests and their control methods.

✓ **Tips:** To avoid disease, water soil not foliage. Keep beds weed free. To ensure fertilization, use a paintbrush to transfer pollen from the male stamen to the female pistil.

ooooo

🕸 *STRAWBERRIES* 🕸

✚ **Health Power:** Loaded with Vitamin C. (A single berry can have up to 20 percent of the RDA.) This antioxidant combined with ellagic acid and anthocyanin helps heal wounds faster, strengthens the immune system and helps delay age-related memory loss. The folate in one serving helps reduce neural tube birth defects and damage to arteries. The fiber helps prevent constipation.

↑ **Vitamin and Mineral Content:**
Vitamins – C, Folate, B2 (Riboflavin), B5 (Pantothenic Acid), B6 (Pyridoxine) & K

Minerals – Manganese, Iodine, Potassium, Magnesium and Copper

⊘ **Disease Prevention:** Strawberries are anti-inflammatory, helping prevent rheumatoid and osteoarthritis and asthma. The diverse content of minerals and phytonutrients in strawberries may also greatly reduce the risk of atherosclerosis, heart disease, macular degeneration and many cancers. Acts like aspirin and ibuprofen but without the negative side effects.

❧ **How to Grow:** A great addition to the garden. Easy on the eyes and taste buds with great health benefits. Four different types of strawberries bear fruit at different times: June bearers, Ever-bearers, Day-Neutrals and Alpine. June bearers yield all fruit within a month, depending on climate variation. Ever-bearers offer a good amount at the beginning of summer, scattered in the middle and a small spread in late summer. Day-Neutrals bear fruit throughout the season between frostings. They are sensitive to extremes and require babysitting. Buy at your local nursery, but ensure they are certified disease-free. Strawberries do well in both pots and garden rows. They like a soil pH just below neutral (7). They also need good drainage and moisture-retentive soil. Pick a site with plenty of sun and good airflow. If drainage is poor, you can increase it by tilling and raising your bed. Work in a couple handfuls of planting mix per square yard or a few inches of compost. Plant them 2 feet apart in rows separated by 1.5 feet. You can also lay down polypropylene and plant them in slits. This warms the soil and protects from weeds, but is not a requirement. Dig holes deep enough that the soil will come up to where the leaves begin on the shoots. In the bottom of the hole, form a small cone and set the plant over it, arranging the roots around it. Fill in with the amended soil. If you trim back most of the runners sent out during the growing season, the plant will dedicate more energy to growing large fruits. Water them thoroughly with about one inch of water a week (more in warmer climates). Avoid water logging, as strawberries can mildew. Harvest berries when they are a nice red. Freeze if necessary.

✘ **Insect Control:** Pests include birds, slugs, snails, aphids and red spider mite. Stop slugs and snails with a beer trap implanted in soil. A scarecrow might work for some birds but not many. Only row covers effectively stop birds. Stop aphids by planting marigolds to attract their predators (ladybugs and hover flies). Spider mites, most active on dry days, cause leaves to mottle yellow and fall off. Spray regularly with water. If the attack is bad, use rotenone as a last resort.

✓ **Tips:** Weeding is a must to produce healthy strawberries. Lay down a layer of straw mulch around plants during growing season to separate the strawberries from soil and help keep them weed free. Harvest ripe berries as soon as they are ready. Immediately discard any that are malformed or mildewing. Rotate crops every three seasons to maintain healthy soil and good yields. Create new plants for the next season by collecting runners in pots. Choose disease-resistant cultivars adapted to your temperatures and day length. To avoid mildew and viruses, do not over water, and keep air circulating well.

ooooo

❀ *SUNFLOWER* ❀

✚ **Health Power:** Providing nearly 100 percent of the vitamin E RDA in ¼ cup, sunflower seeds are an excellent source of the main fat-soluble antioxidant. It helps reduce oxidative damage that can cause plaque build up in the arteries, thickening of arteries and joint inflammation. Of the nuts and seeds, sunflower seeds have one of the highest concentrations of phytosterols, phytonutrients with similar structures to cholesterol and linked to lowering their levels in the blood. Some research evidence shows if we eat a moderate amount of these cholesterol substitutes, they have high potential to reduce the damaging effects of cholesterol. Sunflower seeds are a concentrated source of the intermediary mineral magnesium, which is important for biochemical processes in energy production, the synthesis of essential compounds (proteins, enzymes, DNA, lipids, the antioxidant glutathione), cellular communication (proper muscle, nerve function) and bone matrix formation. A deficiency in magnesium may contribute to higher blood pressure, migraine headaches, muscle spasms/cramps, soreness and fatigue. Selenium is a trace mineral in these seeds that is a cofactor/activator for many enzymes and proteins that help the body maintain healthy DNA, prevent proliferation of cancer cells (by inhibiting growth and inducing apoptosis), and helping detoxify the body by marking dangerous compounds for destruction.

↑ **Vitamin and Mineral Content:**
Vitamins – E, B1 (Thiamin), B5 (Pantothenic Acid) and B9 (Folate)
Minerals – Manganese, Magnesium, Copper, Tryptophan, Selenium and Phosphorus

⊘ **Disease Prevention:** Regularly eating unsalted sunflower seeds may reduce the symptoms or onset of asthma, hypertension, rheumatoid and osteoarthritis, osteoporosis, hot flashes, diabetes, atherosclerosis, cardiovascular disease and many cancers.

❧ **How to Grow:** A great way to brighten up both the garden and daily nutrition. Grow sunflower for its visual appeal and its seeds, sprouts and greens. All are highly nutritious. Sunflowers are easy to grow and tolerant of soil types. Choose a sunny site next to vegetables or in the flower garden where they will not shade other plants needing sun. For optimum growth and a beautiful flower, work in some compost or planting mix to increase soil fertility. The time to plant is spring after the last frost. Sow seeds directly into the bed where they will grow. Place them ½ inch deep and 1 foot apart. They sprout soon afterward as the seeds germinate in roughly 3-5 days. Water regularly when they are young and keep the bed weed free. After they reach 1 foot tall, mulch around the base to help retain moisture and deter weeds. The heads grow to the size of a dinner plate in some cultivars. Keep the soil moist during flowering to promote productivity. They are ready to harvest when they dip over. Cut them 2 feet below the flower and hang upside down in a dry, sheltered area for a few days with a cloth underneath to catch any seeds that fall. Then rub off the seeds and store for any occasion.

✗ **Insect Control:** Sunflowers are generally pest free and attract beneficial insects to the garden that can help control other pests. Protect the seeds from birds by covering the flowers with mesh, pantyhose or hole-punched plastic bags.

✓ **Tips:** Save a couple heads with their stalks to hang up to use as bird feeders. This may help keep the birds from other plants in the garden and provide them with good sustenance.

∞∞∞

❧ *SWEET POTATOES* ❧

✚ **Health Power:** A great source of vitamin A (in the form of beta-carotene) and vitamin C. Sweet potatoes have antioxidant properties that help remove damaging free radicals that affect the cardiovascular system, eyes and digestive tract. They also slow the biochemical reactions that cause inflammation, which helps with a number of painful conditions. Vitamin B6 reduces homocysteine levels in the blood. (High homocysteine levels are correlated with increased vascular and heart conditions.) B6 also supports nervous system function by helping nerve cells communicate and helping to synthesize neurotransmitters. Vitamin B6 helps relieve bloating and acne during premenstrual stress. Potassium good for maintaining normal blood pressure. Fiber and B vitamins promote smooth digestion and efficient metabolism of nutrients from food.

↑ **Vitamin and Mineral Content:**
Vitamins – A, C, B6 (Pyridoxine), B5 (Pantothenic Acid), B3 (Niacin), B1 (Thiamin) and B2 (Riboflavin)
Minerals – Manganese, Potassium, Copper, Magnesium, Phosphorus and Iron

⊘ **Disease Prevention:** The antioxidants in sweet potatoes help treat or prevent atherosclerosis, colon cancer and diabetic heart disease. Their anti-inflammatory properties help reduce the severity of arthritis and asthma. The vitamin B6 in sweet potatoes helps defend against heart attack and stroke. High levels of vitamins A and C help protect eyes against cataracts and macular degeneration. Vitamin A deficiency is linked with cigarette smoke, raising the risk of emphysema for those exposed to it. Vitamin A in sweet potatoes can help counter the effects of inhaling smoke.

❧ **How to Grow:** These tubers grow only in warm, sunny climates. Sweet potatoes prefer loose, sandier soil, but will grow in heavier soils if amended with plenty of organic matter for good drainage. Work in a bit of compost or planting mix to create raised ridges or beds about 8 inches high. Buy plants from a nursery. Plant a few weeks after the last frost in rows or beds, spacing plants 1.5 feet apart in rows 3.5 feet apart. You can also plant single plants in hills 3 feet apart. Water regularly after planting, but reduce watering near the end of growing season (end of summer) so potatoes do not crack. During growing season, gently lift vines and shift them around so they do not lay down roots in unplanned spots. Keep the area weed free. In a cold climate, cover the rows with black polythene and plant through slits cut into the plastic. They mature and are ready to harvest when vines turn yellow. Keep them in the ground to extend the growing season until the first frost. After that, the vines turn black. Carefully dig them up from underneath the side of the row by cutting the foliage. Cure by letting them dry out in the sun before storing. Use any damaged ones as soon as possible.

✗ **Insect Control:** Wireworms, aphids, slugs and cutworms can hurt sweet potatoes. Wireworms make small holes in potatoes that look like slug damage. If the soil is newly used, grow a line of wheat between rows to attract the wireworms. Dig up and dispose of the wheat. Cutworms feed on the base of the plant during the day and can destroy it. If plants fall over, look just beneath the soil to see if they are the cause. If so, dig up the soil around the plants and dispose of any cutworms you see. Growing ground cover will attract ground beetles that will eat the worms. To stop slugs, sink a cup of beer into the soil. The slugs crawl in and drown. For aphids, grow marigold trees to attract their predators. Also spray them off the plants with a strong water stream.

✓ **Tips:** You can harvest the potatoes in mid-summer before they reach full potential. They taste roughly the same but are a little smaller. Regularly check through the stored tubers and remove any showing signs of rot.

ooooo

❧ *SWISS CHARD* ❧

✚ **Health Power:** Chard is off the high end of the chart with its vitamin and mineral content. One cup gives 700 percent of the RDA of vitamin K, more than 100 percent of vitamin A and 50 percent of vitamin C. It is also an excellent source of magnesium, potassium, iron, fiber and more. The health potential of chard seems endless. The vitamin K, magnesium and calcium in chard give a great boost for more bone building and less bone loss. Vitamin A supports healthy vision, immune system function, lung health and protects thin membrane layers around organs and blood vessels. Minerals in chard can also help keep normal blood pressure while vitamins A, C and E do the same by preventing the build up of plaque and the blockage of blood flow in arteries. Magnesium and potassium are the main minerals that help with blood pressure and heart function by supporting muscle and nerve function. Iron is needed to deliver oxygen to tissues all over the body. Eating chard regularly also has the potential to lower high levels of cholesterol and blood sugar, mainly from its fiber content. Chard also helps the body activate crucial antioxidant molecules from the liver to help get rid of potentially dangerous metabolic wastes. Studies also suggest regular eating of vegetables like chard can slow down age-related cognitive decline. The long list of benefits shows chard is a flat out supporter of overall health.

⬆ **Vitamin and Mineral Content:**
Vitamins – K, A, C, E, B2 (Riboflavin), B6 (Pyridoxine), B1 (Thiamin), B9 (Folate), B3 (Niacin) and B5 (Pantothenic Acid)
Minerals – Magnesium, Manganese, Potassium, Iron, Copper, Calcium, Phosphorus and Zinc

⃠ **Disease Prevention:** Regularly eating chard may reduce the symptoms or the onset of osteoporosis, asthma, rheumatoid and osteoarthritis, anemia, hypertension, cardiovascular disease, diabetes, lung cancer, colon cancer and potentially many other cancers due to its antioxidants and detoxifiers, vitamins and minerals.

❦ **How to Grow:** Relatively easy to grow, Swiss chard is loaded with nutrition and seen as a delicacy in some parts of the world. You can grow two distinctly colored varieties: red and white stemmed. Although red stem is more attractive, it has no better flavor than the other. Chard needs highly fertile soil that retains moisture yet drains well. Work some organic matter into the site, like compost or planting mix, to create a nice loamy soil. The pH must be above 6.5; add lime if needed. Plant chard in mid-spring. In warmer climates, a late summer or early fall sowing works, too. Sow seeds in groups of 3 in shallow drills spacing each cluster out by 1 foot and each row by roughly 1.5 feet. Later thin out to leave the strongest seedling per cluster. Once the seedlings emerge, keep the soil moist and the bed weed free.

Harvesting can begin in mid-summer. Pull, do not cut, leaves off the plant. (Cutting makes them bleed.) It is a "cut and come again" plant. Harvest from around the outside of the plant as you need and they grow right back. They are cold hardy enough to handle light frosts, so you can harvest into the fall/winter.

✘ **Insect Control:** Slugs, caterpillars, cucumber beetles and mealy cabbage aphids may try snacking on chard. Slugs can be controlled by embedding a wide cup of beer in the soil. Slugs are attracted to it, slide in and drown. You can also remove by hand and destroy mornings and evenings. Remove caterpillars by hand, too. Watch for their eggs on the leaves and wipe them off. If infestation is uncontrollable, spray with Bt. Cucumber beetles can be removed by hand, too, but if they are too resilient, spray with rotenone. Cabbage aphids cluster on the underside of leaves. Control them by companion planting French marigolds or another smaller flowering plant. They will attract hoverflies and ladybugs that consume aphids by the score.

✓ **Tips:** Chard germinates easily. You might enjoy starting from scratch by sowing seeds directly into an outdoor planting bed. This also gives you more choice among varieties. Sow seeds in early spring, and find a recipe that works for you.

ooooo

🏵 *TARRAGON* 🏵

✚ **Health Power:** You can gain the many health benefits of tarragon by using teas, dried/fresh leaves, the essential oil and tinctures. (Tarragon mixed with isopropyl alcohol makes a good disinfectant.) Tarragon contains caffeic acid, which can stop or kill many bacteria, viruses and fungi. It makes a good cleansing disinfectant to rub on wounds or can be used as a deodorant. Components of tarragon help digestion by stimulating the secretion of digestive compounds in the saliva as well as gastric fluids (like bile and other acids) into the lower digestive tract. This stimulates faster processing of foods already in the stomach (which helps get rid of wastes and potential toxins faster) and increases appetite. Its antimicrobial action enables tarragon to kill intestinal worms. Tarragon also increases circulation, which helps distribute nutrients, oxygen, hormones and enzymes to tissues and remove toxins. Tarragon has calming properties, too. Many people use it to help relax the nerves and facilitate a good night's sleep. Despite these health benefits, use in moderation. Tarragon oil contains estragole, which is toxic at high levels. As an extra precaution, young children and pregnant women should avoid the oil. The spice is safe, as the essential oil concentrations are too small to cause harm.

↑ **Vitamin and Mineral Content:**
Vitamins – B6 (Pyridoxine), A, C and B2 (Riboflavin)
Minerals – Manganese, Iron, Calcium, Magnesium and Potassium

⊘ **Disease Prevention:** Plays a role in helping reduce the symptoms or delaying the onset of rheumatism, indigestion, anorexia, insomnia and excessive flatulence.

❦ **How to Grow:** Tarragon is a hardy perennial herb tolerant of many soil types. It comes in two varieties, French and Russian. The French has a far superior flavor for cooking purposes. Tarragon plants prefer a sheltered site with full sun and good drainage. The best way to grow is from purchased young plants. Growing French tarragon from seed is not an option, but the Russian variety sows easily. Plant them 1.5 feet apart. Water regularly as necessary to keep the soil moist. Weed also to prevent nutrient competition. Harvest the leaves throughout the season. You can store them in vinegar or dry them. If you choose vinegar, wash it off before eating, and then use the vinegar in a salad dressing. For French tarragon, put a few inches of mulch over the top to protect from direct contact with frost. They need to be lifted, divided and replanted every 3-4 years to maintain tastiness in the leaves. They should grow well enough to divide into many plants every spring. To divide them, manually lift them out and divide in half by hand or use a back-to-back garden shovel/fork. Once out, cut all the leaves down to about 2 inches from the roots and replant right away.

✖ **Insect Control:** Tarragon is generally pest free.

✓ **Tips:** For a good sleepy time tea, try it mixed with chamomile just before bedtime.

∞∞∞

❁ *THYME* ❁

✚ **Health Power:** Thyme is a healthy source of vitamin K, giving more than 60 percent of RDA in two teaspoons. It also contains iron, manganese, calcium and dietary fiber. It is an old-time remedy for chest and respiratory illness. The benefits come from the essential oils and flavonoids, which have antioxidant, antifungal and antibacterial functions. The oil thymol has antioxidant powers that help increase the good fats in cells and their membranes. It also works as an antibacterial agent against Salmonella, E. coli, Shigella and others. You can create your own surface cleaning/disinfectant spray by mixing thyme, boiling water and a little liquid soap in a spray bottle.

↑ Vitamin and Mineral Content:
Vitamins – K
Minerals – Iron, Magnesium and Calcium

⊘ Disease Prevention: Thymol oil helps fight inflammatory diseases by stopping an enzyme, elastase, from breaking down elastin, which, with collagen, affects the mechanical abilities of connective tissue, especially in the throat and lungs. Thyme also contains a collection of terpenoids, which are thought to reduce or prevent cancer tissue formation. Regularly eating thyme supports bone health and may help prevent osteoporosis and anemia.

❦ How to Grow: Thyme is more than a nice aesthetic addition to your garden. It also attracts many pollinating insects for flowers and serves as a nutritious spice. Thyme needs a sunny spot with good drainage. Ideal pH for nutrient uptake is near 7. Add lime to raise, if needed. Two popular types of thyme are used for cooking, common and lemon thyme. Sow common thyme from seed outdoors after the last frost in spring or, more commonly, buy in containers and transplant any time. They spread a lot, so plant at least a foot apart, depending on how soon you want to establish ground cover. Thyme is tolerant of poor-quality soil. A few handfuls of planting mix will ensure nice growth. Pinch the growth tips frequently to encourage shorter, denser growth. Trim back after they flower, too, and the plant will continue to produce. You can continue to pick the leaves as you want for a fresh herb to add to a variety of dishes.

✗ Insect Control: Thyme is pest free. Many insects avoid thyme, and planting it can be a great natural deterrent. Some common garden bugs, spider mites or aphids may be a problem. Spray with an insecticidal soap. You can also plant dandelions or marigolds nearby to attract ladybugs, a natural predator of aphids and mites.

✓ Tips: The leaves have more flavor dry than fresh. Dry them in a well-ventilated area before using. Thyme is a great aromatic addition to the garden. Some types can be used as a flowering ground cover. If you live in the North, you may need to protectively cover the plants with something like large evergreen branches.

∞∞∞

❧ TOMATO ❧

✚ Health Power: A great supporter of overall health. Tomatoes have a lot of vitamins C and A, plus beta-carotene and the pigment lycopene, all super antioxidants that help prevent cell damage by free radical oxygen molecules. These phytonutrients work in synergy with other vitamins and minerals in tomatoes to promote heart and bone health and protect against inflammation and a number of cancers. (The cardiovascular benefits come from helping to regulate blood pressure and reduce damage to blood vessels from oxidative stress, plaque buildup and elevated homocysteine levels.) Regularly eating tomatoes can lower cholesterol levels, promote proper fetal development and regulate blood sugar. The B vitamins help make use of the energy in food.

↑ Vitamin & Mineral Content:
Vitamins – C, A, K, B1 (Thiamin), B6 (Pyridoxine), B9 (Folate), B3 (Niacin), B2 (Riboflavin), B5 (Pantothenic Acid) and E
Minerals – Molybdenum, Potassium, Manganese, Chromium, Copper, Magnesium, Iron and Phosphorus

⊘ **Disease Prevention:** Tomatoes reduce the risk of cardiovascular disease, rheumatoid and osteoarthritis and asthma. They also help prevent cataracts and lower the risk of prostate, breast, lung, stomach, pancreatic, colon, rectal and endometrial cancers.

❧ **How to Grow:** Plant in full sun, amend the soil well with a good compost or planting mix. They prefer a pH of 6. Tomatoes grow and produce best outdoors. They can also grow in containers (minimum 15 gallons of potting soil) but not to their full potential. More soil volume is best. Start from seed indoors 6 weeks before the last frost, or buy transplants from a local nursery. Plant seedlings or transplants in space at least 2 feet square. Keep the fruit from drooping onto the ground by growing the upright varieties against canes or wire cages. Pinch out the tops after they make 3-4 groups of fruits. For bush varieties, cover the soil underneath the plants (using bark or similar) so fruits develop off the ground. They are heavy feeders and can take copious amounts of fertilizer. Keep plants moist but not sopping wet to avoid fungal diseases.

✗ **Insect Control:** Tomatoes are susceptible to tomato hornworm. Spray foliage with Bt (*Bacillus thuringiensis*) for natural control. You can also remove worms by hand early in the morning. Worms are usually on top of the foliage and are easy to remove and discard. As a general measure, you can spray with a botanical insecticide-fungicide for natural control of most insect pests and diseases, such as early blight, gray leaf spot, late blight, Septoria leaf spot, Southern blight and verticillium wilt.

✓ **Tips:** Pick or buy tomatoes fully ripe, the redder the better. Ripe tomatoes may have 4 times more beta-carotene than green, immature ones. This makes backyard tomatoes the best. You know they were not picked green and shipped to ripen weeks later.

∞∞∞

🥬 *TURNIPS* 🥬

✚ **Health Power:** Turnip roots are high in Vitamin C. With the greens, their high content of vitamins, minerals and phytonutrients are a great promoter of overall health. Turnips and turnip greens help create more bone mass by slowing osteoclastic (break down) processes and increasing osteoblastic (building) processes. Turnips and their greens are loaded with vitamins A, C and E, which reinforce immune system, maintain healthy membranes and connective tissue (for example, blood vessels and joints), protect important cells (eyes and vascular system) from free radical damage and reduce inflammation. Turnips also give dietary fiber that helps maintain healthy digestion and regulates cholesterol levels. Along with the free radical fighters, fiber promotes overall health and efficient functioning of the colon. Turnips and their greens also support heart health. The antioxidants (vitamins C, A and E) directly protect the structure and function of blood vessels and minimize the buildup of plaque on vessel walls. Vitamins B6 and folate also prevent damage to vessel walls by minimizing the potentially harmful chemical homocysteine. This vegetable also supports healthy metabolism, lung health and brain function.

↑ **Vitamin and Mineral Content (Roots and Greens):**
Vitamins – K, A, C, B9 (Folate), B6 (Pyridoxine), E, B2 (Riboflavin), B1 (Thiamin), B5 (Pantothenic Acid) and B3 (Niacin)
Minerals – Manganese, Calcium, Copper, Potassium, Magnesium, Iron and Phosphorus

⊘ **Disease Prevention:** Helps reduce symptoms or onset of osteoporosis, macular degeneration, cardiovascular disease, rheumatoid and osteoarthritis, anemia, diabetes, female liver cancer and cancers of the prostate, stomach, colon, lung, pancreas and bladder.

🌱 **How to Grow:** One of the easier root veggies to grow. You can sow turnips indoors in early winter or outdoors in mid-spring to mid-summer. Turnips prefer well-amended, fertile soil with good drainage and a pH above 6.5. If sowing indoors, you can multi-sow them by planting six seeds per tray cell or pocket made in the container. Cover seeds with a small layer of soil and/or sand. Place them in a greenhouse or under a fluorescent light in an area where the temperature is mid-60's or higher. Plant the seedlings 12 inches apart under a covering (cloche) in early spring. If sowing outdoors, create shallow drills about a foot apart and plant seeds along each drill. Cover them with a thin layer of soil and keep them well watered. After seedlings reach a couple inches tall, thin them out to 6-8 inches apart in their rows. Especially during the early stages, keep the plots weed free by hand pulling or hoeing. Mulching between the plants with some well-aged compost or other organic matter provides insulation, retains moisture, deters weeds and may give some sustenance. Harvest the first turnips when they are the size of ping pong balls. Harvest the others no larger than baseball size. For outdoor crops, they are plump and ready near mid-fall. Twist off shoots on top and store unused ones in moist sand or peat at moderate temperatures.

✗ **Insect Control:** Turnips are rather pest free. Flea beetles bother them. These little creatures eat small holes in the leaves of seedlings, which can delay harvest or even kill them. As with fleas, they leap in the air when something gets close. Use this defense against them by using a small, flat piece of wood or plastic with a sticky layer of honey or grease on it. Run the piece of wood an inch above the beetles, and watch them jump up and get stuck.

✓ **Tips:** Turnips grow best in temperatures of 50-75°F. (Any higher and the roots get woody and bitter.) Before harvesting, loosen up the soil first with a garden fork. The smaller roots are the most tender; pull them up before they get too big. Discard damaged roots, as they may spread infection to the undamaged roots in storage.

∞∞∞

🌰 *WALNUTS* 🌰

✚ **Health Power:** They lack many common vitamins and minerals, but walnuts have profound phytonutrients for your health. They are a great source of omega-3 fatty acids, an essential fat the body cannot make. Omega-3's in walnuts help protect the heart, have anti-inflammatory properties, encourage healthy brain function and help prevent many cancers. An omega-3 found in walnuts is also linked to healthy bones. Walnuts are high in fats, but these are good fats linked to lowering the risk of weight gain. They also have monounsaturated fats, which reduce the bad form of cholesterol (LDL) and the threat of clotting in arteries. Walnuts also have arginine, an essential amino acid the body cannot produce. This amino acid helps maintain smooth and elastic blood vessel walls by helping produce nitric oxide, which relaxes the smooth muscle around blood vessels. Walnuts also have many antioxidants that keep free radicals from damaging cells, especially in the cardiovascular system. Eating walnuts regularly is linked to a decrease in blood pressure. Walnuts can actually undo some of the damaging biochemical reactions caused by eating foods high in saturated fats. Cell membranes are made of fats. Introducing flexible omega-3 fatty acids increases a cell membrane's flexibility and ability to communicate and excrete wastes. This is especially important in the brain, helping us grow closer to our full cognitive potential. Walnuts give melatonin, an antioxidant that also supports healthy biorhythms. Together all these factors make walnuts a heart-smart choice.

↑ **Vitamin and Mineral Content:**
Vitamins – B6 (Pyridoxine), B9 (Folate), B1 (Thiamin), B2 (Riboflavin) and B5 (Pantothenic Acid)
Minerals – Manganese, Copper, Magnesium, Phosphorus, Zinc, Iron, and Potassium

⊘ **Disease Prevention:** A power house in preventing heart disease, atherosclerosis, high blood pressure, heart attack, stroke and gallstones. Research suggests antioxidants in walnuts, such as ellagic acid, reduce the risk of many forms of cancer.

❧ **How to Grow:** Two types of walnut trees grow, the black walnut and the Persian/English walnut. The black walnut tree grows from 50-100 feet tall. The English walnut tree grows smaller, about 40-60 feet. Both make big-spread shade trees. These trees need full sun, great drainage and a deep, highly fertile soil. Nuts are ready to harvest in the fall. Plant a seedling from a reputable nursery instead of trying to plant seeds into the ground yourself. Squirrels usually find the nut and devour it. Be sure to dig the hole deep enough for the taproot to comfortably fit in. Mulch around the trunk with a thick layer of compost or other material, but leave a space between the trunk and the mulch to keep rodents from injuring it. Water the tree thoroughly once a week, especially in dry weather when it is young. English walnuts are popularly grown for nut production, especially in California. Most cultivars are self-fertile but will give more nuts with other walnut trees nearby. Nuts are ready to harvest in the fall 3-7 years after planting the tree. You need prune only dead or diseased branches on this tree if using it for food.

✗ **Insect Control:** Some pests can infiltrate a walnut tree, but none are a large threat to a healthy tree growing in healthy soil. If leaf grubbing caterpillars become a problem, Bt (*Bacillus thurigiensis*) takes care of them. Pick up fallen sticks, husks and leaves so pests do not have a home or food over the winter.

✓ **Tips:** Check with your local nursery before buying a walnut seedling, as the tree's roots excrete the chemical juglone and may be toxic for other plants nearby. Place the walnut tree far enough from other plants that its roots cannot reach them (usually 1.5 times the height of the tree).

❧ *WATERCRESS* ❧

✚ **Health Power:** An excellent source of vitamin K and a good source of calcium, watercress helps maintain strong bones and healthy blood clotting. It also donates about half the RDA of both antioxidant vitamins A (also in the form of beta caro-tene) and C. These are key factors in protecting cells and organs from oxidative damage by free radicals. They also help support a healthy immune response, eye-sight, skin and cardiovascular system (by preventing plaque build up and main-taining elasticity in blood vessel walls). Watercress also has small amounts of vita-mins B1, B6, E and the minerals magnesium, iron, iodine and zinc. These support the thyroid gland, stimulate metabolism, synthesize red blood cells and stimulate the production of antibodies to fight infections. Watercress has the phytonutri-ents lutein and zeaxanthin, which work alongside beta-carotene and vitamin A to maintain healthy eyesight. The glucosinolates help boost and regulate the liver's production of detoxification enzymes. The phenylethyl isothiocyanates in water-cress are being studied for their potential to fight the development of cancer cells.

⬆ **Vitamin and Mineral Content:**
Vitamins – K, C and A
Minerals – Calcium, Manganese and Potassium

⊘ **Disease Prevention:** Regularly eating watercress may help reduce the risk of cardiovascular disease, heart attack, stroke, cataracts, gout, osteoporosis, lung can-cer, breast cancer and potentially many other cancers.

❦ **How to Grow:** Watercress is a great addition to soups, salads, sandwiches, dips and sauces. It grows naturally in running rivers and streams, but is also easy to cultivate in the backyard. It prefers to grow in shade with excellent water retention. Dig a trench about 1 foot deep. Layer the bottom with some aged compost/manure or planting mix. Work in some organic matter with the soil dug out and fill the trench. In early spring, sow seeds at temperature close to 55°F. If sowing indoors, use seed trays. When the seedlings get big enough, transfer them to another tray with wider spacing using a mini dibber and holding onto the leaves only. Do not touch the stems during the transfer. Plant them out in late spring to early summer spacing them out by about 4 inches. If your climate is warm enough, sow seeds outside in shallow drills. Once they grow a bit, remove the weaker ones and leave a spacing of about 4 inches. Another way is to buy a bundle of watercress, take the shoots with a couple young roots showing and plant them in the same spacing. Water generously and often. Keep the bed weed free by handpicking and/or hoe-ing. No other fertilizing is needed. Pinch the dominant shoots and remove any flowers as soon as you see them. Harvest the shoots as needed. They come back for another harvest until temperatures drop in fall.

✕ **Insect Control:** Watercress is largely pest free. If something you do not recognize begins to infest, take one of the pests to the nearest nursery and/or agricultural extension office for an ID and advice on the best treatment.

✓ **Tips:** Watercress can be grown indoors in pots with drainage holes. Place pots on an open tray of water. Refill the tray as soil soaks up water. Keep the soil damp. Prevent flowering by pruning buds immediately. Greens wither and wilt quickly. Use right after harvesting.

∞∞∞

🍉 *WATERMELON* 🍉

✚ **Health Power:** Watermelon packs a punch with important vitamins and phytonutrients. The combination of antioxidant vitamins C and A does wonders for the body. They both stop free radicals from causing damage to cells that otherwise lead to many ailments: plaque build up in arteries through the oxidation of cholesterol, increased inflammation, especially in joints, vision deterioration and cellular damage that can lead to mutations in DNA (which can become cancerous). Watermelon is also a great source of the phytonutrient lycopene, which has received much attention for its antioxidant behavior and ability to reduce the risk of many cancers. Watermelon is also a great fruit source of B vitamins, which the body uses to generate energy from sugars, carbohydrates, lipids (fats), amino acids and proteins. Another phytonutrient, citrulline (an amino acid, too) gets converted to the amino acid arginine. Higher levels of arginine are linked to relaxing blood vessels (through increased production of nitric oxide) removing the waste product ammonia and increasing cell sensitivity to the insulin molecule.

↑ **Vitamin and Mineral Content:**
Vitamins – C, A, B6 (Pyridoxine) and B1 (Thiamin)
Minerals – Potassium and Magnesium

⊘ **Disease Prevention:** Watermelon may help reduce the symptoms or prevent the onset of rheumatoid/osteoarthritis, colon cancer, asthma, heart disease, type II diabetes, erectile dysfunction, and cancers of the lung, breast, prostate, colon, rectum and endometrium.

🌱 **How to Grow:** Watermelon has the same environmental and cultivation needs as other melons (cantaloupe and honeydews) but falls in a different class. (This makes sense, since watermelon looks, tastes and feels so unlike other melons.) Watermelon cultivars have been established that can fit into a range of garden sizes. Some cultivars are even seedless. Note: Watermelon depends more than others on warm sunny weather (+75°F.) to grow. A few cultivars grow in slightly cooler climates, so check with a local nursery to see what types can grow in your area. See Melons for details on growing.

✗ **Insect Control:** Besides the pests in the Melons entry, watermelons are vulnerable to aphids and squash vine borers. Deter aphids by planting French marigolds, which attract aphid predators. Squash vine borers are white caterpillars about one inch long. See Summer-Winter Squash for how to control borers.

✓ **Tips:** Watermelon is ripe when it sounds hollow after knocking on it. Store in a cool, shady place to ensure they last as long as they can (2-3 weeks).

ооооо

❈ *WHEATGRASS* ❈

✚ **Health Power:** Wheatgrass juice or powder is a great low-calorie addition to the diet. It gives substantial vitamin C, iron and phytonutrients with little risk of adverse effects and a high potential for benefit. Within alternative medicine, wheatgrass has its strong proponents who tout its strength and versatility as a remedy. Some say wheatgrass gives them energy (by increasing metabolism), helps improve oxygen delivery to the cells (due to chlorophyll acting like hemoglobin in blood), boosts their immune system, helps improve skin conditions and wound healing (when drunk and applied topically), inhibits cancer cell development (especially liver cancer from the chlorophyll content), treats ulcerative colitis (inflammation of the colon), treats arthritis, prevents tooth decay (by holding in the mouth for 5 minutes), relieves constipation, detoxifies the blood (through high antioxidant behavior), decreases blood pressure and improves digestion. Little research has been done to support these statements. Still, give it a try and see how it makes you feel.

↑ **Vitamin and Mineral Content:**
Vitamins – C and traces
Minerals – Iron and traces

⊘ **Disease Prevention:** Drinking a shot of wheatgrass juice regularly may provide relief from or prevent the onset of rheumatoid and osteoarthritis, asthma, ulcers, heart disease, eczema, psoriasis and liver cancer. The American Cancer Society says it knows of no scientific evidence that wheatgrass can cure cancer or any disease after its onset. Wheatgrass, with its beneficial nutrients, may help alleviate symptoms and prevent the onset of many conditions.

❧ **How to Grow:** Growing wheatgrass is easy. It prefers a partly shady location, good air circulation and a temperature range of 60-75°F. This makes it an ideal candidate for indoor growing and some outdoor growing in the spring and fall. Get a growing tray and organic wheat seed from a local nursery. Soak seeds for 12 hours in a container throughout the day before planting. Rinse the seeds well and let them drain overnight. The next day, put about an inch of soil mixed with planting mix in the growing tray, dampening it by spraying it lightly as you spread the soil. Spread the wheatgrass seed on top of the soil. Water the tray with a spray bottle or a flexible spray hose from the sink. Cover the tray with an unbleached paper towel or another perforated lid (like an upside down growing tray) and spray the towel. Keep damp for 3-4 days. Generally, water once in the morning and once at night for the seed to germinate. When the seedlings reach a height of 1.5 inches, remove the paper towel or other cover and place in indirect sunlight. Temperature, humidity and air circulation will determine how frequently to water. Look underneath the tray. If the bottom is wet, do not water. A temperature of 60-75°F. is best. Harvest the wheatgrass as needed when it reaches 6-7 inches tall. Cut just above soil level and any sign of mold. Store the tray in a cool place to preserve it longer. You can juice the cuttings, dry and crush them to make powder or blend with water and strain out the foliage.

✗ **Insect Control:** Insects are not usually a problem for wheatgrass, especially if grown inside. Good air circulation and warm temperatures help prevent mold forming.

✓ **Tips:** Keep the wheatgrass seed moist to achieve good germination.

Selected References

http://www.aces.uiuc.edu/news/stories/news3066.html/

Anderson, James W. & Bryant, Carol A. Dietary Fiber: Diabetes and Obesity. *American Journal of Gastroenterology.* 1986; 81(10):898-906.

http://articles.mercola.com/sites/articles/archive/2005/10/06/how-aloe-vera-can-protect-fruits-vegetables.aspx/

Bennett, Peter. *The Purification Plan.* US: Rodale Inc., 2005.

Boutenko, Victoria. *Green for Life.* Canada: Raw Family Publishing, 2005.

Capon, Brian. *Botany for Gardeners.* Portland, OR: Timber Press, Inc., 1990.

Chen, Shirley C. et al. Phytosterol Intake and Dietary Fat Reduction are Independent and Additive in their Ability to Reduce Plasma LDL Cholesterol. *Springer Berlin / Heidelberg.* March 2009; 44(3):273-281.

http://www.ciwf.org.uk/farm_animals/default.aspx

http://www.ciwf.org.uk/your_food/default.aspx

Clarke, John D., Dashwood, Roderick H. & Emily Ho. Multi-targeted prevention of cancer by sulforaphane. *Cancer Letters.* 8 October 2008; 269(2):291-304.

Cooper, Dale A., Eldridge, Alison L., Peters, John C. Dietary Carotenoids and Lung Cancer: A Review of Recent Research. *Nutrition Reviews.* 27 April 2009; 57(5):133-145.

Cox, Jeff. *The Organic Cook's Bible: How to Select and Cook the Best Ingredients on the Market.* Hoboken, NJ: John Wiley and Sons, Inc., 2006.

Crockett, James U et al. *The Time Life Encyclopedia of Gardening: Fruits and Vegetables.* New York, New York: Time Inc., 1972.

http://www.dietaryfiberfood.com/chlorophyll.php/

http://www.dietaryfiberfood.com/h-licorice-root.php/

Dixon, Bernard. *Power Unseen: How Microbes Rule the World.* New York, NY: Macmillan Press Limited, 1996.

Don, Monty & Sarah. *From the Garden to the Table: Growing, Cooking, and Eating Your Own Food.* Guilford, CT: The Lyons Press, 2003.

http://www.elements4health.com/

http://www.everynutrient.com/

Fisher, George E. J. Micronutrients and Animal Nutrition and the Link between Application of Micronutrients to Crops and Animal Health. *Turk J Agric For.* 22 Feb 2008; 32:221-233.

Fossel, Peter V. *Organic Farming.* Minneapolis, MN: Voyager Press, 2007.

Fox, Michael W. *Beyond Evolution: The Genetically Altered Future of Plants, Animals, the Earth and Humans.* New York, NY: The Lyons Press, 1999.

Franks, Eric & Richardson, Jasmine. *Microgreens.* Layton, UT: Gibbs Smith, 2009.

http://www.freepatentsonline.com/4326523.html

Frost, Mary. *Going Back to the Basics of Human Health: Avoiding the Fads, the Trends, and the Bold-Faced Lies.* USA: Mary Frost, 2005.

http://www.fsis.usda.gov/FactSheets/Meat_&_Poultry_Labeling_Terms/index.asp/

http://www.gardenguides.com/

1000 Garden Questions and Answers. New York, NY: Workman Publishing Company, Inc., 2003.

Gates MA, Tworoger SS, Hecht JL, De Vivo I, Rosner B, Hankinson SE. A prospective study of dietary flavonoid intake and incidence of epithelial ovarian cancer. *Int J Cancer.* 30 Apr 2007; 121(10):2225-2232.

Gershuny, Grace & Smillie, Joseph. *The Soul of Soil: A Guide to Ecological Management*. Davis, CA: agAccess, 1995.

Gillman, Jeff. *The Truth About Organic Gardening*. Portland, OR: Timber Press, 2008.

Greenwood, Pippa et al., ed. *Pests and Diseases: The Complete Guide to Preventing, Identifying, and Treating Plant Problems*. New York, NY: Dorling Kindersley Publishing, Inc, 2000.

Guardia, T. Anti-inflammatory properties of plant flavonoids. Effects of rutin, quercetin and hesperidin on adjuvant arthritis in rat. *Il farmaco*. 2001; 56(9):683-.

Gupta, Umesh C., WU, Kening & Liang, Siyuan. Micronutrients in Soils, Crops, and Livestock. *Earth Science Frontiers*. September 2008; 15(5):110-125.

Hamilton, Geoff, ed. *Organic Gardening: The essential guide to growing flowers, fruit, and vegetables the natural way*. USA: DK Publishing, Inc., 2004.

http://www.herbs2000.com/herbs/herbs_guava.htm/

http://www.herbsarespecial.com.au/free-herb-information.html

Hertog, Michael G. L. et al. Flavonoid Intake and Long-term Risk of Coronary Heart Disease and Cancer in the Seven Countries Study. *Arch Intern Med*.1995; 155(4):381-386.

http://www.horseradish.org/health.html/

Kelly, Serving O. Dietary Flavonoids, Antioxidant Vitamins, and Incidence of Stroke. *Arch Intern Med*. 1996; 156(6):637-642.

Lam, Tram K. et al. Dietary quercetin, quercetin-gene interaction, metabolic gene expression in lung tissue and lung cancer risk. *Carcinogenesis*. 2010; 31(4):634-642.

Lambert, R J W. A study of the minimum inhibitory concentration and mode of action of oregano essential oil, thymol and carvacrol. *Journal of Applied Microbiology*. 2001; 91(3):453-.

Lamp'l, Joe. *The Green Gardener's Guide*. Franklin, TN: Cooling Springs Press, 2007.

Leonard, Jonathan N., ed. *The First Farmers*. USA: Time Life Inc., 1973.

http://www.livestrong.com/

Loux, Renee. *The Balanced Plate*. New York, NY: Rodale Inc., 2006.

http://lpi.oregonstate.edu/infocenter/

http://lpi.oregonstate.edu/infocenter/foods/cruciferous/

Ma, Le & Lin, Xiao-Ming. Effects of lutein and zeaxanthin on aspects of eye health. *Journal of the Science of Food and Agriculture*. 15 January 2010; 90(1):2-12.

McLeod, Judyth, ed. *Botanica's: Organic Gardening*. San Diego, CA: Laurel Glen Publishing, 2002.

http://www.mercola.com/

Merrill, Richard & Ortiz, Joe. *The Gardener's Table: A guide to Natural Vegetable Growing and Cooking*. Berkeley, CA: Ten Speed Press, 2000.

Michaels, Jillian. *Master Your Metabolism*. USA: Crown Publishing Group, 2009.

Monforte, M T, Trovato, A, Kirjavainen, S, et al. Biological effects of hesperidin, a Citrus flavonoid. (note II): hypolipidemic activity on experimental hypercholesterolemia in rat. *Il farmaco*. 2005; 50(9):595-599.

http://www.mothernature.com/

http://www.mothernature.com/Library/Ency/Index.cfm/id/1653007/

Nadeem et al. Review: Oxidant—antioxidant imbalance in asthma: scientific evidence, epidemiological data and possible therapeutic options. *Ther Adv Respir Dis*, August 2008; 2:215 - 235.

Nardi, James B. *Life in Soil: A Guide for Naturalists and Gardeners*. USA: University of Chicago Press, Ltd., 2007.

http://www.niams.nih.gov/

http://www.nih.gov/

http://www.nlm.nih.gov/medlineplus/ency/

http://www.nopalexport.com/healthbenefits.htm/

http://www.nutritiondata.com/

http://www.organicfacts.net/

P. C. H. Hollman, M. B. Katan. Dietary Flavonoids: Intake, Health Effects and Bio-availability. *Food and Chemical Toxicology*. September 1999; 37 (9-10):937-942.

http://www.peta.org/mc/factsheet_display.asp?ID=96/

Pierre, Colleen, ed. *The New Healing Foods*. USA: American Master Products/ Jerry Baker, 2005.

Pratt, Stephen & Matthews, Kathy, ed. *SuperFoods: Fourteen Foods That Will Change Your Life*. USA: Stephen G. Pratt and Kathy Matthews, Inc., 2004.

Roberts, Richard L., Green, Justin & Lewis, Brandon. Lutein and zeaxanthin in eye and skin health. *Clinics in Dermatology*. April 2009; 27(2):195-201.

Rodale's *All-New Encyclopedia of Organic Gardening*. USA: Rodale Press, Inc, 1992.

Sengupta, A. Allium vegetables in cancer prevention: an overview. *Asian Pacific J Cancer Prevention*. 2004; 5(3):237-245.

Sharma, R A. Curcumin: the story so far. *European Journal of Cancer*. 2005; 41(13):1955-.

Smith, Ed. *Theraputic Herb Manual: A guide to Safe and Effective Use of Liquid Herbal Extracts*. Williams, Oregon: Ed Smith, 2003.

http://www.southerngracefarms.com/blackberryinfo.htm/

Stahl, Wilhelm & Sies, Helmut. Lycopene: A Biologically Important Carotenoid for Humans? *Archives of Biochemistry and Biophysics*. December 1996; 336(1):1-9.

Straten, Michael V. *Organic Living*. USA: Rodale Inc., 2001.

Streppel, Martinette T. Dietary fiber intake in relation to coronary heart disease and all-cause mortality over 40 y: the Zutphen Study. *Am J Clin Nutr*. Oct. 2008; 88(4):1119-1125.

Tanaka, T. Chemoprevention of azoxymethane-induced rat colon carcinogenesis by the naturally occurring flavonoids, diosmin and hesperidin. *Carcinogenesis.* 1997; 18(5):957-.

Traka, Maria & Mithen, Richard. Glucosinolates, isothiocyanates and human health. *Springer Netherlands.* January 2009; 8(1):269-282.

Wasantwisut, E. Nutrition and Development: other micronutrients' affect on growth and cognition. *Southeast Asian J Trop Med Public Health.* 1997; 28 Suppl 2:78-82.

http://www.webmd.com/

Weickert, Martin O., & Pfeiffer, Andreas F. H. Metabolic Effects of Dietary Fiber Consumption and Prevention of Diabetes. *J. Nutr.* March 2008; 138:439-442. http://whfoods.org

Woyengo, T. A., Ramprasath, V. R. & Jones, P. J. H. Anticancer effects of phytosterols. *European Journal of Clinical Nutrition.* July 2009; 63:813-820.

Zheng, G Q. Myristicin: a potential cancer chemopreventive agent from parsley leaf oil. *Journal of Agricultural and Food Chemistry.* 1992; 40(1):107-.

Index (excludes Part 6)

NOTES